Psychosomatic Medicine

Guest Editor

JOEL E. DIMSDALE, MD

PSYCHIATRIC CLINICS OF NORTH AMERICA

www.psych.theclinics.com

September 2011 • Volume 34 • Number 3

SAUNDERS an imprint of ELSEVIER, Inc.

W.B. SAUNDERS COMPANY
A Division of Elsevier Inc.

1600 John F. Kennedy Boulevard • Suite 1800 • Philadelphia, PA 19103-2899

http://www.theclinics.com

PSYCHIATRIC CLINICS OF NORTH AMERICA Volume 34, Number 3
September 2011 ISSN 0193-953X, ISBN-13: 978-1-4557-1158-1

Editor: Sarah E. Barth

Psychiatric Clinics of North America (ISSN 0193-953X) is published quarterly by Elsevier Inc., 360 Park Avenue South, New York, NY 10010-1710. Months of issue are March, June, September, and December. Business and Editorial Offices: 1600 John F. Kennedy Blvd., Suite 1800, Philadelphia, PA 19103-2899. Periodicals postage paid at New York, NY and additional mailing offices. Subscription prices are $265.00 per year (US individuals), $473.00 per year (US institutions), $131.00 per year (US students/residents), $321.00 per year (Canadian individuals), $589.00 per year (Canadian Institutions), $399.00 per year (foreign individuals), $589.00 per year (foreign institutions), and $194.00 per year (international & Canadian students/residents). Foreign air speed delivery is included in all *Clinics'* subscription prices. All prices are subject to change without notice. **POSTMASTER:** Send address changes to *Psychiatric Clinics of North America,* Elsevier Health Sciences Division, Subscription Customer Service, 3251 Riverport Lane, Maryland Heights, MO 63043. Customer Service: 1-800-654-2452 (US). From outside the United States, call 1-314-447-8871. Fax: 1-314-447-8029. E-mail: journalscustomerservice-usa@elsevier.com (for print support) and journalsonlinesupport-usa@elsevier.com (for online support).

Reprints. For copies of 100 or more, of articles in this publication, please contact the Commercial Reprints Department, Elsevier Inc., 360 Park Avenue South, New York, New York 10010-1710. Tel.: (212) 633-3813, Fax: (212) 462-1935, E-mail: reprints@elsevier.com.

Psychiatric Clinics of North America is covered in *MEDLINE/PubMed (Index Medicus), Current Contents/Social and Behavioral Sciences, Social Science Citation Index, Embase/Excerpta Medica,* and PsycINFO.

Printed and bound by CPI Group (UK) Ltd, Croydon, CR0 4YY

Transferred to Digital Print 2011

Contributors

GUEST EDITOR

JOEL E. DIMSDALE, MD
Distinguished Professor of Psychiatry Emeritus and Research Professor, University of California, San Diego, La Jolla, California

AUTHORS

JOHN V. CAMPO, MD
Department of Psychiatry, Ohio State University and Nationwide Children's Hospital, Columbus, Ohio

DANIEL J. CLAUW, MD
Professor, Department of Anesthesiology, Chronic Pain & Fatigue Research Center, University of Michigan Medical School, Ann Arbor, Michigan

FRANCIS CREED, MD, FRCPsych, FRCP, FMed Sci
Professor of Psychological Medicine, School of Community Based Medicine, The University of Manchester, Manchester, United Kingdom

MARY LYNN DELL, MD, DMin
Associate Professor of Psychiatry, Pediatrics, and Bioethics, Case Western Reserve University School of Medicine; Director, Child and Adolescent Psychiatry Consultation Liaison Service, Rainbow Babies and Children's Hospital, Cleveland, Ohio

STUART W.G. DERBYSHIRE, PhD
Reader in Psychology, University of Birmingham, School of Psychology, Edgbaston, United Kingdom

JOEL E. DIMSDALE, MD
Distinguished Professor of Psychiatry Emeritus and Research Professor, University of California, San Diego, La Jolla, California

PER FINK, prof., MD, PhD, DMSc
The Research Clinic for Functional Disorders and Psychosomatics, Aarhus University Hospital, Aarhus, Denmark

CHARLES V. FORD, MD
Professor, Department of Psychiatry and Behavioral Neurobiology, The University of Alabama at Birmingham, Eye Foundation Hospital, Birmingham, Alabama

AFTON L. HASSETT, PsyD
Associate Research Scientist, Department of Anesthesiology, Chronic Pain & Fatigue Research Center, University of Michigan Medical School, Ann Arbor, Michigan

MICHAEL R. IRWIN, MD
Cousins Professor of Psychiatry and Biobehavioral Sciences, David Geffen School of Medicine at University of California Los Angeles (UCLA); Professor of Psychology, UCLA College of Letters and Sciences; Director, Cousins Center for Psychoneuroimmunology, Semel Institute for Neuroscience, Los Angeles, California

JAMES L. LEVENSON, MD
Professor of Psychiatry, Medicine, and Surgery; Chairman, Division of Consultation-Liaison Psychiatry; Vice Chair, Department of Psychiatry, Virginia Commonwealth University, Ricmond, Virginia

ALEXANDRA MARTIN, PhD
Associate Professor, Department of Psychosomatic Medicine and Psychotherapy, University of Erlangen-Nürnberg, University Hospital Erlangen, Erlangen, Germany

CHERYL B. MCCULLUMSMITH, MD, PhD
Director, Consult-Liaison Divison, Department of Psychiatry and Behavioral Neurobiology, The University of Alabama at Birmingham, Eye Foundation Hospital, Birmingham, Alabama

PAUL R. PURI, MD
Chief Resident, Department of Psychiatry, University of California, San Diego, California

JOHN QUERQUES, MD
Associate Director, Psychosomatic Medicine Fellowship Program, Department of Psychiatry, Massachusetts General Hospital; Assistant Professor of Psychiatry, Harvard Medical School, Boston, Massachusetts

WINFRIED RIEF, PhD
Professor, Department of Psychology, and Chair, Division of Clinical Psychology and Psychological Intervention, University of Marburg, Marburg, Germany

ANDREAS SCHRÖDER, MD, PhD
The Research Clinic for Functional Disorders and Psychosomatics, Aarhus University Hospital, Aarhus, Denmark

THEODORE A. STERN, MD
Chief, Psychiatric Consultation Service, Department of Psychiatry, Massachusetts General Hospital; Professor of Psychiatry in the field of Psychosomatic Medicine/Consultation, Harvard Medical School, Boston, Massachusetts

MARLYNN H. WEI, MD, JD
Chief Resident, Psychiatric Consultation Service, Department of Psychiatry, Massachusetts General Hospital; Administrative Chief Resident of the Massachusetts General Hospital/McLean Hospital Adult Psychiatric Residency Training Program; Clinical Fellow in Psychiatry, Harvard Medical School, Boston, Massachusetts

CHANAKA WIJERATNE, MD, FRANZCP
Consultant Psychiatrist, Academic Department for Old Age Psychiatry, Prince of Wales Hospital, Randwick; Conjoint Senior Lecturer, School of Psychiatry, University of New South Wales, Kensington, New South Wales, Australia

Contents

> Medically unexplained symptoms (MUS) provide a shaky foundation for
> the diagnosis of psychosomatic disorders. While MUS may be a key
> constituent of disorders such as conversion, such symptoms are better
> viewed as an accompanying feature rather than the basis of diagnosis.
> Medically unexplained can also be viewed as medically ignored,
> medically unexamined, or medically misunderstood. Reliability of this
> assessment is problematic. More importantly, features such as preoc-
> cupations about illness may provide a more sound basis for under-
> standing and treating psychosomatic disorders.

> There have been a number of proposals for revising the somatoform
> disorders, with some even advocating abolition of the category. Cri-
> tiques of the somatoform disorders have focused on a number of
> problems including conceptual, philosophical, empirical, and practical
> issues. Yet patients who present with multiple physical symptoms and
> excessive health concerns are common in general medical settings.
> This article documents the underuse of the somatoform diagnoses in
> clinical practice, and discusses reasons that may account for this
> relative neglect, both those applicable to the category as a whole, and
> those related to specific diagnoses.

> Somatoform disorders are common conditions, but the current diagnostic
> criteria are considered to be unreliable, based largely on medically unex-
> plained symptoms. DSM-5 is considering other possible characteristics of
> somatizers including high utilization, dissatisfaction with care, and poor
> response to reassurance. The PubMed database was searched combining
> terms such as "somatoform disorder" with "reassurance," "satisfaction,"
> and "utilization." Evidence was found to support transient but poor
> sustained response to reassurance, and for over-utilization, particularly in
> outpatient visits, though this was not specific. Future research should
> attempt to validate criteria prospectively.

The author and colleagues tested cut point scores on measures of total somatic symptoms and health anxiety of new medical out-patients, to determine whether they predicted health status and number of medical consultations. High-scoring participants had significantly more impaired health status and medical consultations. High scores were associated with dissatisfaction with the doctor's explanation of their symptoms. Whether symptoms were medically explained or not made little difference to these results; anxiety and depression were not found to have effect. The author and colleagues found support for the combination of somatic symptoms and health anxiety as proposed in DSM-V complex somatic symptom disorder.

The classification of somatoform disorders lacks clear psychological criteria that justify the classification as "mental disorder." A recent proposal for *Complex Somatic Symptom Disorder* points to the relevance of 'excessive thoughts, feelings, and behaviors related to disabling somatic symptoms and health concerns.' Reviewed evidence suggests that somatoform syndromes, excessive health concerns, and pain conditions are associated with a broad range of cognitive characteristics (eg, somatic causal symptom attributions, over-interpretation of somatic sensations/catastrophizing, the self-concept of bodily weakness), and a broad range of behavioral features (eg, avoidance of potentially symptom-provoking situations or activities, health care utilization, reassurance seeking).

Historically, how and why pain occurs has been a much-researched topic–from an early theory that a peripheral stimulus of pain passively travels "hard-wired" pathways to the brain where it is then sensed as pain, to our present knowledge that pain (especially chronic pain) is the product of a complex information processing network rather than simply signals relayed by pain fibers in nerves or pain pathways in the brain. Observations that psychiatric comorbidity is prevalent in chronic pain sufferers led many clinicians and researchers to believe that psychological stress causes chronic pain. This article explores and even challenges that concept.

The past 20 years have seen a dramatic increase in the number of functional imaging studies addressing pain. Pain experience is associated with activity in a wide range of cortical and subcortical areas and they seem to be actively involved in generating pain experience, even without a typically noxious stimulus. Several cortical and subcortical areas are associated with pain inhibition; neural imaging may reveal how the brain creates pain for some chronic pain patients. However, psychological and contextual factors are an important part of pain experience; a neural description of pain is not the same as a neural explanation.

Pain, sleep disturbance, and fatigue are common complaints in somatic disorders. This review characterizes the connections between the immune system and brain, discussing the influence of proinflammatory cytokines on somatic symptoms of pain or hyperalgesia, sleep disturbance, and fatigue. It is hypothesized that increases of peripheral inflammation markers, possibly acting in concert with stress, leads to activation of central inflammatory pathways with increased sensitization of the central nervous system to afferent signaling. These psychoneuroimmunologic pathways contribute to symptoms of pain and fatigue, and/or amplification of normal bodily sensations, which lead to distress and impairments in social, occupational, and health functioning.

Consciously simulated illnesses fall into two diagnostic categories: factitious disorders and malingering, differentiated both by motivation for behavior and by consciousness of that motivation. Factitious disorder behaviors are motivated by an unconscious need to assume the sick role, while malingering behaviors are driven consciously to achieve external secondary gains. This review discusses current controversies in diagnosis and recent research, providing further insights into the detection of simulated illnesses, and ends with a discussion of ethical and legal issues associated with factitious disorder diagnoses.

The diagnosis and treatment of mental disorders have benefited from advancements in epidemiology, genetics, pharmacology, neuroimaging and other disciplines. However, "medically unexplained" physical symptoms and somatoform disorders have defied conceptual understanding, and straightforward algorithms for clinical diagnosis and management of affected patients are lacking. The clinician must consider unique combinations of symptoms, biopsychosocial underpinnings, contexts of illness exacerbations and remissions, and the meanings of associated functional impairments to patients, families, and society. This is especially true for the young, given the additional physiological, psychological, family, educational, and environmental elements involved in pediatric somatoform disorders.

The somatoform disorders have been ignored by geriatric psychiatry because their conceptual and diagnostic difficulties are compounded in the presence of physical disease, and because of the epidemiological imperative of dementia. Given physiological and physical changes with age, older people are likely to endorse neurological and sexual somatic symptoms differently, so these symptoms seem less useful as screening items than fatigue and musculoskeletal symptoms. In older primary care samples, up to one-third of somatic symptoms cannot be attributed to a specific diagnosis even in the presence of chronic physical disease. The correlates of somatization, such as female gender, psychological disorder, and physical disease are similar to those in younger adults, but contrary to prevailing beliefs, rates of relevant somatic syndromes decline with age. Possible reasons for this decline include a tendency for older people to respond to symptoms with a normalizing rather than somatic attribution style, and to adapt better to symptoms such as chronic pain.

Similar treatment strategies have proven effective in various functional somatic syndromes such as fibromyalgia, irritable bowel syndrome, and chronic fatigue syndrome. Increasing evidence supports common etiologic factors, pathophysiologic mechanisms, and psychological features. A minority of these patients receive evidence-based treatment, mainly due to inappropriate organization of care. The authors argue for the necessity of specialized multidisciplinary psychosomatic services for bodily distress, which includes a broad range of functional somatic syndromes and somatoform disorders. The goal is for patients with bodily distress to be offered the same quality of health care as any other patient.

Teaching trainees about the practice of consultation-liaison (C-L) psychiatry involves formal didactics, bedside rounds, reviewing the literature, and the demonstration of specific skills (eg, critical thinking and self-awareness [autognosis]). Effective teaching (based on adult learning theory) about psychosomatic medicine uses problem-oriented approaches, integrates knowledge into real-life situations, and makes trainees responsible for their decisions. Discussions of differential diagnoses, work-ups, formulations (that involve biological, psychological, sociocultural, and existential perspectives) and treatment of myriad conditions seen in the general hospital create a solid foundation. Teaching C-L psychiatry is most effective with a layered approach, tailored to specific teaching forums and learning styles of trainees.

THE CLINICS ARE NOW AVAILABLE ONLINE!

Access your subscription at:
www.theclinics.com

Preface

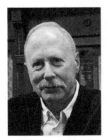

Joel E. Dimsdale, MD
Guest Editor

This issue of *Psychiatric Clinics of North America* focuses on psychosomatic medicine. The roots of psychosomatic medicine are deep and extend to topics as diverse as psychoanalysis, biological psychiatry, psychopharmacology, forensics, neuroanatomy, and medicine. In 2007, Levenson, Gitlin, and Crone edited a superb issue on psychosomatic medicine in *Psychiatric Clinics of North America*.[1] Rather than update similar topics 4 years later, this 2011 issue is intended to cover different areas so that the two issues will complement each other. The 2007 issue emphasized substantive reviews in areas such as psychiatric aspects of infertility, bariatric surgery, and pulmonary disease. The present issue principally scrutinizes cross-cutting issues in psychiatric diagnosis with reference to psychosomatic medicine. Informed by the extensive on-going discussions concerning DSM-V, the authors of this issue focus on questions such as "what are the core features of psychosomatic illness."

The issue begins with an article by Dimsdale concerning the logical problems of basing a diagnosis on the "lack of" findings or on "medically unexplained symptoms." The article raises themes echoed repeatedly throughout the issue—there are major conceptual and pragmatic problems with the cluster of somatoform diagnoses as described in DSM-IV.

Levenson further develops this theme using extensive insurance registry data from the Commonwealth of Virginia as well as the Veteran's Administration. Although psychosomatic presentations are very common, doctors do not use such diagnostic codes. In addition, psychiatric researchers have generally drifted away from studying these important clinical problems.

Puri and Dimsdale discuss the importance of focusing on patients' patterns of health care utilization and response to reassurance. The literature suggests that problems in response to reassurance form a core feature of what have been called "somatoform disorders."

Creed points out that at its heart diagnosis relies on somatic symptoms. Whereas a formal cut point in terms of number of symptoms is difficult to establish, the more somatic symptoms patients have, the worse is their quality of life. Using extensive

Psychiatr Clin N Am 34 (2011) xi–xiii
doi:10.1016/j.psc.2011.06.001
0193-953X/11/$ – see front matter © 2011 Elsevier Inc. All rights reserved.

data from international studies, this article presents important data documenting that these disorders are associated with a troubling amount of morbidity.

Martin and Rief examine the relevance of cognitive and behavioral factors in somatoform disorders. Focusing on these key features informs decisions about how to intervene, a theme that is further emphasized in the Schröder and Fink as well as the Wei, Querques, and Stern articles at the end of this issue.

Chronic pain is one of the most commonly encountered features in psychosomatic medicine. Hasset and Clauw consider the relationship between stress and chronic pain. Focusing primarily on fibromyalgia, they describe the types of studies that have been performed to shed light on this complex area.

The issue's next two articles consider a more physiological approach to understanding psychosomatic disorders. Derbyshire reviews the promise and limitations of studies that employ neural imaging as a way of understanding somatoform pain disorders. This is a burgeoning area that is capturing much attention. Irwin considers the complex interplay of inflammation in understanding somatic symptoms. Along with the neural imaging field, the characterization of inflammatory factors offers extraordinary promise in better understanding the biological substrates of psychosomatic medicine.

The next article, by McCullumsmith and Ford, visits the troubling topic of simulated illness. As pointed out by McCullumsmith and Ford and also by McDermott and Feldman[2] in the previous Psychosomatic Medicine issue, there are a host of presentations where patients simulate a disorder, sometimes for obvious material rewards and sometimes for less tangible but still meaningful rewards such as increased attention. The article also presents hard-won knowledge about how to work with these difficult patients.

The issue features two articles that consider life course in the diagnosis of somatoform disorders. As Dell and Campo point out, the presentation of symptoms

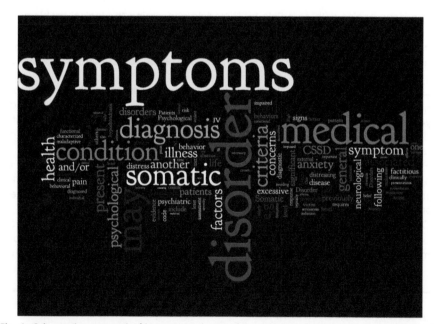

Fig. 1. Schematic portrayal of important themes for understanding proposals for change in diagnostic criteria for somatoform illness.

is different in young children, and careful involvement of the parent is vital not just for diagnosing but also for treating children with such disorders. Wijeratne considers the other end of the life course—how somatic symptoms are presented in the elderly. Because illness prevalence changes with age, symptoms such as genitourinary/gynecological symptoms are less suitable for screening purposes in studying older patients.

This issue concludes with two articles that focus not so much on the dilemmas of diagnosis but rather on treatment and education regarding these disorders. As pointed out by Schröder and Fink, there are well-established treatments for patients with somatoform disorders. They argue for specialized multidisciplinary psychosomatic services. Psychosomatic medicine is an abiding interest in consultation liaison psychiatry. The final article by Wei, Querques, and Stern describes how to educate trainees about this vital area of psychiatry that brings together so many disparate elements that shape patients' lives.

What are important developments in psychosomatic medicine? The articles in this issue and the previous issue by Levenson, Gitlin, and Crone provide some updates to that important question. **Fig. 1** uses a "wordle" diagram approach[3] to portray the scientific territory embedded in this issue. The figure clearly emphasizes the complex interweaving of symptoms, illness, health, distress, anxiety, etc that all interact in shaping the contours of psychosomatic medicine. One looks forward to seeing how this intellectual territory develops in the next 5-10 years.

Joel E. Dimsdale, MD
Department of Psychiatry
University of California, San Diego
9500 Gilman Drive, Mail Code 0804
La Jolla, CA 92093-0804, USA

E-mail address:
jdimsdale@ucsd.edu

REFERENCES

1. Levenson J, Gitlin D, Crone C. editors. Psychosomatic medicine. Psychiatr Clin North Am 2007;30(4).
2. McDermott B, Feldman M. Malingering in the medical setting. Psychiatr Clin North Am 2007;30(4):645–62.
3. www.wordle.net. Accessed May 10, 2011.

Medically Unexplained Symptoms: A Treacherous Foundation for Somatoform Disorders?

Joel E. Dimsdale, MD

KEYWORDS

• Psychiatric diagnosis • Medically unexplained • Pain

In the *DSM-IV*, medically unexplained symptoms (MUS) form the key defining feature of somatoform disorders. There are problems, however, in making MUS the "foundation" of diagnosis. I first discuss five problems that result from defining a diagnosis on the basis of the absence of a sign or symptom—in essence, a "negative" symptom. Then I suggest an alternative to MUS-based diagnoses.

PROBLEMS WITH MEDICALLY UNEXPLAINED SYMPTOMS

1. *The quality of the evaluation.* On the face of it, MUS sounds affectively neutral but the term sidesteps the quality of the medical evaluation itself. A number of factors influence the accuracy of diagnoses. Most prominently, one must consider how thorough was the physician's evaluation of the patient. How adequate was the physician's knowledge base in synthesizing the information obtained from the history and physical examination? The time pressures in primary care make it difficult to comprehensively evaluate patients and thus contribute to delays and slips in diagnosis. Similarly, physicians can wear blinders or have tunnel vision in evaluating patients.[1] Just because a patient has previously had MUS is no guarantee that the patient has yet another MUS. As a result of these factors, the reliability of the diagnosis of MUS is notoriously low.[2]

2. *The state of medical knowledge.* The considerations just posed pertain to how a diagnosis of MUS is reached. However, diagnoses are shaped by the state of medical knowledge at the time when the patient is evaluated. One "sees" what one is prepared to see or understand. If one has no tools for recognizing hepatitis C, for instance, one will not make that diagnosis until very late in the progression of the infection. New diseases are constantly arising, either totally new diseases or, more commonly, diseases that have previously not been well understood.

Department of Psychiatry, University of California, San Diego, 9500 Gilman Drive, Mail Code 0804, La Jolla, CA 92093-0804, USA
E-mail address: jdimsdale@ucsd.edu

Psychiatr Clin N Am 34 (2011) 511–513
doi:10.1016/j.psc.2011.05.003
0193-953X/11/$ – see front matter © 2011 Elsevier Inc. All rights reserved.

3. *Nonspecific symptoms as harbingers of undiagnosed illness.* Many illnesses present initially with nonspecific signs such as fatigue, long before the disease progresses to the point where laboratory and physical findings can establish a diagnosis. Thus, there is always the possibility that a patient's MUS represents an as-yet-undiagnosed disease. Interestingly, new technologies inevitably facilitate diagnosing diseases earlier in their course. Cancer screening with contemporary imaging allows the detection of smaller tumors. Advances in drug development (eg, conscious sedation) and bioinstrumentation development (eg, endoscopy) now facilitate examination of areas of the body previously "accessible" only with the use of general anesthesia. Similar advances in assay development allow simple screening with blood sampling. All of these sorts of technologies facilitate early detection and thus provide a powerful tool for understanding early nonspecific symptoms presented in conjunction with an undiagnosed disease.

   Obstructive sleep apnea provides an interesting example of revolutionary changes in perspective brought about by new ways of screening for disease. Once recognized in the severe form only, sleep apnea is now recognized to be a common disorder. Its initial presentation can frequently include nonspecific complaints of fatigue or sleepiness. How often is the undiagnosed apneic thought to have an MUS? Is it then appropriate to diagnose such a patient with a somatoform diagnosis? Is this helpful? To the extent that one believes that psychiatric intervention is good for all kinds of distress and for all chronic disease, such a diagnosis might facilitate referral and treatment. However, the question is, which is the most proximal therapy for such a patient—continuous positive airway pressure (CPAP) treatment or psychiatric referral (or both)?

4. *Mind-body dualism.* The implication of the MUS label is that we are telling the patient that "it's all in your head." Of course, that statement is quite literally true. Symptoms are processed in the brain, whether they are pain signals from a compound fracture, back spasm, or enteric distress. They are "authentic" and felt by the patient. The task of medicine is to diagnose the symptom's source and to provide appropriate treatment. Unfortunately, the implication of the "all in your head" statement is that the patient is causing or misreporting the symptom, wasting the doctor's time, or some other similarly dismissive conclusion. It is no wonder that patients are unhappy with somatoform diagnoses.[3]

5. *Heterogeneity of disease.* One needs to acknowledge that diseases are very heterogeneous. That heterogeneity may account for the variance in response to intervention. Histologically, similar tumors have different surface receptors, which affect response to chemotherapy. Particularly in chronic disease presentations such as irritable bowel syndrome or chronic fatigue syndrome, the heterogeneity of the illness makes it perilous to diagnose all such patients as having MUS and an underlying somatoform disorder.

AN ALTERNATE FORMULATION

It is true that some people are more sensitive to pain than others. That sensitivity may represent a different neural sensory amplification threshold that may be hard-wired and/or learned. One anticipates that considerable neural imaging research in these topics (see article by Stuart W.G. Derbyshire elsewhere in this issue for further exploration of this topic) will be carried out in the next 10 years. However, sensitivity to symptoms also reflects the patient's thoughts, feelings, and behaviors. The cognitive attributions of the meaning of symptoms shape the patient's help-seeking behavior (eg, headache interpreted as an aneurysm). Alternatively, the symptoms may be amplified by emotions (particularly depressive symptoms) or may be behaviorally reinforced by solicitousness from family. Grounding a psychiatric diagnosis and intervention on positive features such as thoughts, feelings, and behaviors seems more productive than basing psychiatric diagnosis and intervention on MUS—the "absence" of a medical explanation for the symptoms.

SUMMARY

Patients present with an admixture of symptoms, preconceptions, feelings, and illnesses. The task of psychiatric diagnosis is to attend to the patient's thoughts, feelings, and behaviors that are determining his/her response to symptoms, be they explained or unexplained. One hopes that future psychiatric diagnosis will focus on such features as opposed to MUS.

REFERENCES

1. Dimsdale JE. Delays and slips in medical diagnosis. Perspect Biol Med 1984;27: 213–20.
2. Rief W, Rojas G. Stability of somatoform symptoms: implications for classification. Psychosom Med 2007;69:864–9.
3. Dimsdale J, Sharma N, Sharpe M. What do physicians think of somatoform disorders? Psychosomatics 2011;52:154–9.

The Somatoform Disorders: 6 Characters in Search of an Author

James L. Levenson, MD

KEYWORDS
- Somatoform • Somatization • Conversion
- Hypochondriasis • Pain disorder

In *DSM-III, DSM-III-R,* and *DSM-IV,* there are 6 major somatoform disorders: somatization disorder, undifferentiated somatoform disorder, conversion disorder, hypochondriasis, pain disorder associated with psychological factors (code 307.80), and pain disorder associated with both psychological factors and a general medical condition (code 307.89). Their status and characterization are being re-examined as part of the development of *DSM-5.* In Luigi Pirandello's famous 1921 play *Six Characters in Search of an Author,* the performance begins as an acting company begins a rehearsal, which is disrupted by the arrival of 6 unfinished characters in search of an author to finish their story. Like Pirandello's characters, where should the somatoform disorders best appear in the diagnostic classification? What rewriting do they require?

In anticipation of the development of *DSM-5,* there have been a number of proposals for revising the somatoform disorders, with some even advocating abolition of the category, eliminating some diagnoses and reassigning others elsewhere in *DSM,* and other suggested transformations.[1–5] Critiques of the somatoform disorders have focused on a number of problems, including conceptual, philosophical, empirical, and practical issues. Yet patients who present with multiple physical symptoms and excessive health concerns that are expressed emotionally, cognitively, and behaviorally are common in general medical settings, and their frequency and the magnitude of their health care costs have been documented in an extensive evidence base over the last quarter century.[6] There is disagreement among experts regarding how to name and define the somatoform disorders, although all appear to agree on the clinical importance of the clinical phenomena.[7] However, the somatoform disorder diagnoses are greatly underused in clinical practice and in research, and the reasons why warrant careful consideration, particularly if constructive improvements are to be achieved in *DSM-5.*[4] In this essay, I demonstrate first some evidence of the underrepresentation of somatoform disorder diagnoses in clinical care and in

Department of Psychiatry, Division of Consultation–Liaison Psychiatry, Box 980268, Ricmond, VA 23298, USA
E-mail address: jlevenson@mcvh-vcu.edu

Psychiatr Clin N Am 34 (2011) 515–524
doi:10.1016/j.psc.2011.05.006
0193-953X/11/$ – see front matter © 2011 Elsevier Inc. All rights reserved.

Table 1
Frequency of use of somatoform disorders diagnoses in 28 million Wellpoint-Anthem covered lives, 2008 ($\times 100$)

Diagnosis	Frequency ($\times 100$)
Somatization disorder and undifferentiated somatoform disorder[a]	0.00199
Conversion disorder	0.00947
Hypochondriasis	0.00170
Pain disorder associated with psychological factors	0.00395
Pain disorder associated with psychological factors and a general medical condition	0.01494
Factitious disorder	0.00058
Psychological factors affecting a medical condition	0.01002

[a] Somatization disorder and undifferentiated somatoform disorder are combined because they both have the same *Diagnostic and Statistical Manual of Mental Disorders* (Fourth Edition) code, 300.81.

scholarship, and then discuss a number of reasons that may account for this relative neglect.

THE SOMATOFORM DISORDERS ARE RARELY CODED AS PRIMARY DIAGNOSES

Table 1 shows the frequencies of somatoform disorder diagnoses among 28 million enrollees in WellPoint-Anthem Blue Cross Blue Shield (WellPoint-Anthem), a major private health insurance company in the United States. This data base included all clinical encounters for the calendar year 2008 for WellPoint-Anthem enrollees in California, Colorado, Connecticut, Georgia, Indiana, Kentucky, Maine, Missouri, Nevada, New Hampshire, New York, Ohio, Virginia, and Wisconsin. For comparison, factitious disorder and psychological factors affecting a medical condition are also included. Only the first diagnosis recorded by the physician for the particular clinical service is entered, including both inpatient and ambulatory services. The diagnosis is counted only once, regardless of how many encounters there were with that diagnosis. Hence, the numbers represent what fraction of the total enrollees had any clinical services billed under that diagnosis during 1 year. The data were available for each geographic region of the United States in which WellPoint-Anthem operates, as well as by type of insurance product (eg, traditional fee-for-service, preferred provider organization, point-of-service, and health maintenance organization).

Although there was some variation by geographical region and by type of insurance product, the diagnoses were very rarely used in all regions and under all forms of insurance. Indeed, the diagnoses were so rarely used that the frequencies have been multiplied by 100 to display them with fewer zeroes after the decimal point. To put these numbers in perspective, compare them to the (albeit limited) epidemiological literature. Somatization disorder has been reported to have a lifetime prevalence of between 0.2% to 2.0% in women and less than 0.2% in men, but occurs in 1% to 5% of primary care patients (because such patients actively seek medical care, their prevalence in medical settings is higher than in the general population).[6] Yet somatization disorder and undifferentiated somatoform disorder together were recorded as a primary diagnosis in only 1 out of every 50,000 people covered by Blue Cross-Blue Shield insurance. The prevalence of hypochondriasis in the general population is thought to be 1% to 5% (American Psychiatric Association 2000),[8] and

Table 2
Proportion of Veterans Administration inpatients with each diagnosis by year (×100)

Diagnosis	Year								
	2002	2003	2004	2005	2006	2007	2008	All Years	P Value[a]
Conversion disorder	0.0447	0.0439	0.0438	0.0487	0.0519	0.0518	0.0578	0.04901	.0007
Factitious disorder	0.0222	0.0176	0.0170	0.0195	0.0188	0.0189	0.0143	0.01830	.0898
Hypochondriasis	0.0078	0.0075	0.0079	0.0082	0.0086	0.0053	0.0077	0.00756	.5916
Somatization disorder	0.0310	0.0313	0.0355	0.0277	0.0394	0.0377	0.0398	0.03465	.0058
Undifferentiated SD	0.0235	0.0243	0.0294	0.0260	0.0285	0.0322	0.0269	0.02727	.0739
Pain-psych factor[b]	0.0067	0.0052	0.0068	0.0075	0.0061	0.0083	0.0062	0.00669	.5780
Pain-psych + medical[c]	0.0098	0.0119	0.0124	0.0170	0.0160	0.0196	0.0151	0.01458	.0007
PFAMC	0.0225	0.0230	0.0246	0.0180	0.0165	0.0166	0.0124	0.01903	<.0001

Abbreviation: PFAMC, psychological factors affecting a medical condition.
[a] These *P* values are from a test for trend across years.
[b] Pain disorder associated with psychological factors.
[c] Pain disorder associated with psychological factors and a general medical condition.

such individuals also frequently seek medical attention, yet this diagnosis was primary in only 1 out of every 59,000 enrollees.

Tables 2 and **3** show the frequencies of somatoform disorder diagnoses among all veterans receiving inpatient (see **Table 2**) and outpatient (see **Table 3**) services in the Veterans Administration (VA) health care system in the United States for the years 2002 to 2008. The methodology used by the Veterans Administration is different than the one used by WellPoint-Anthem, so the numbers are not directly comparable. For outpatients, the frequency represents the number of encounters with that diagnosis as primary, divided by the total number of outpatient encounters in the VA system that year. For inpatients, the frequency represents the number of admissions with that diagnosis as primary or secondary, divided by the total number of hospital admissions that year. What is clear is that the somatoform disorders are also very infrequently used as primary diagnoses in the Veterans Administration health care system. As one would expect, the somatoform disorder diagnoses are used more often in the outpatient than inpatient setting at VA medical centers. Factitious disorder is thought to be much rarer than any of the somatoform disorders, yet it was diagnosed far more commonly in inpatient veterans than was hypochondriasis and both of the pain disorders!

These VA data also permitted testing for trends over time. There has been a small but statistically significant increase in how often inpatient veterans received diagnoses of conversion disorder, somatization disorder, and pain disorder associated with psychological factors and a general medical condition, and a decrease in psychological factors affecting a medical condition. However, there have been statistically significant decreases in almost all of the somatoform disorder diagnoses in veterans receiving outpatient care.

Table 3
Proportion of Veterans Administration outpatients with each diagnosis by year (×100)

Diagnosis	Year							All Years	P Value[a]
	2002	2003	2004	2005	2006	2007	2008		
Conversion disorder	0.0132	0.0122	0.0102	0.0110	0.0106	0.0122	0.0122	0.01162	.3942
Factitious disorder	0.0027	0.0018	0.0019	0.0024	0.0015	0.0015	0.0018	0.00191	.0003
Hypochondriasis	0.0037	0.0033	0.0030	0.0032	0.0031	0.0027	0.0026	0.00306	.0024
Somatization disorder	0.0207	0.0209	0.0192	0.0198	0.0193	0.0172	0.0172	0.01913	<.0001
Undifferentiated SD	0.0051	0.0048	0.0051	0.0056	0.0046	0.0048	0.0056	0.00508	.5995
Pain-psych factor[b]	0.0330	0.0260	0.0208	0.0355	0.0302	0.0200	0.0181	0.02608	<.0001
Pain-psych + medical[c]	0.1711	0.1639	0.1556	0.1247	0.1134	0.1196	0.1209	0.13741	<.0001
PFAMC	0.0818	0.0736	0.0621	0.0563	0.0594	0.0592	0.0698	0.06572	<.0001

Abbreviation: PFAMC, psychological factors affecting a medical condition.
[a] These P values are from a test for trend across years.
[b] Pain disorder associated with psychological factors.
[c] Pain disorder associated with psychological factors and a general medical condition.

One limitation of both of these data sets is that they only include the primary diagnosis recorded for the clinical encounter by the physician. It is possible that the physician recognized the presence of a somatoform disorder but did not record it, or recorded it as a secondary diagnosis. Furthermore, there is no way to determine whether these diagnoses were correctly made. Nevertheless, there is a large difference between the order of magnitude of how often such patients present for medical care and how often somatoform disorder diagnoses are recorded in the medical record. The VA data permit looking for time trends, and overall, these diagnoses declined in use over recent years in ambulatory settings, which is where most patients with somatoform disorders present for diagnosis and care.

THE SOMATOFORM DISORDER DIAGNOSES ARE UNDERSTUDIED

The somatoform disorders are underrepresented in the medical literature as well. **Fig. 1** shows how many entries there were in Medline for the years 2000 to 2010 with titles containing the terms *somatization disorder, undifferentiated somatoform disorder, conversion disorder,* and *hypochondriasis.* All entries have been included, regardless of article type. These 4 diagnoses combined appeared in the title of 21 entries in 2000 and 35 in 2010. Although the number of entries for conversion disorder has risen over the past decade, the others remain essentially unchanged, with almost no entries for undifferentiated somatoform disorder. Conversion disorder was most frequent, with a total of 145 titles during this period. Comparison to the corresponding numbers for trichotillomania (405), Tourette's syndrome (366), and pathological gambling (378) for the same period (2000–2010) further illustrates the neglect the somatoform disorders have suffered in the medical literature.

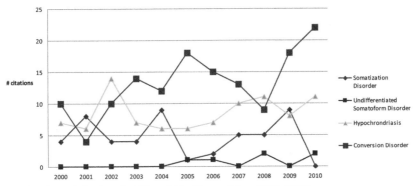

Fig. 1. Number of citations in titles of Medline entries, 2000–2010.

Psychological factors affecting a medical condition and the pain disorders were not included in **Fig. 1** for the following reasons: *Psychological factors affecting a medical condition* has appeared only once (2007) in a title in all Medline years. *Psychological factors affecting a physical condition* (PFAPC), the name for this diagnosis in *DSM-III*, appeared in the title of only 5 entries, all between 1989 to1993, and all of these were authored by members of the *DSM-IV* PFAPC Work Group. A count of titles containing *pain disorder* is complicated by observing that many of the entries refer to painful conditions that are not considered to be mental disorders. It is noteworthy that about half of the entries even in 2009 and 2010 that do relate to pain disorder as a mental disorder, refer to it in their titles as *somatoform pain disorder,* which was the *DSM-III* term replaced in *DSM-IV* in 1980. These articles are mainly by non-US authors, reflecting the continued use of that name as *persistent somatoform pain disorder* in *International Classification of Diseases, Tenth Revision.*

GENERAL REASONS WHY SOMATOFORM DISORDER DIAGNOSES ARE NOT USED MORE OFTEN

So why are somatoform disorder diagnoses not used more frequently? One reason is a problem with the names themselves, starting with the category name, *somatoform.* This term appeared in a small number of articles prior to *DSM-III*, with the first Medline listing as a text word in a German article in 1966,[9] but somatoform was first used to refer to a set of disorders during the development of *DSM-III*.[10] All words start out as artificial constructions, but they naturally evolve, survive, and thrive if they are useful and clear for communication. Many clinicians find the term *somatoform* confusing, and it is even more obtuse to patients. The confusion was increased by *DSM-IV* assigning the same coding number (300.81) to somatization disorder and undifferentiated somatoform disorder. Even psychiatrists mix up "somatoform disorder" with "somatization disorder," both in clinical usage and in publications, referring to somatoform disorder as if it was a specific diagnosis.[11,12] Another common error resulting from the intrinsic confusion of the terms is the substitution of somatoform for somatization in undifferentiated somatoform disorder (eg, undifferentiated somatization disorder).[13] Even the report of the recommendations of the expert members of the Conceptual Issues in Somatoform and Similar Disorders work group contains that mistake.[1]

Another reason for underdiagnosis of somatoform disorders is related to cross-cultural issues. Neologisms do not translate well if at all, and jargon does not travel well cross culturally. Although cultural factors can influence how patients perceive, report, and seek care for physical symptoms, somatoform disorders do occur in similar patterns in different cultures.[14,15] Therefore, it is important that diagnostic names be understandable conceptually and linguistically when translated from English into other languages. In cross-cultural psychiatry, one recognized principle is that the simpler and less abstract a construct is, the more cross culturally applicable and translatable it will be. It is especially problematic to translate abstractions like somatoform that are not in common use. Indeed, undifferentiated somatoform disorder was a particularly bad choice as a diagnostic term, as it is completely unintelligible after translation into Chinese (Sing Lee, personal communication, 2010). Some would assert it was already unintelligible in English.

REASONS WHY SPECIFIC SOMATOFORM DISORDER DIAGNOSES ARE NOT USED MORE OFTEN
Somatization Disorder

Somatization disorder has been problematic for clinicians when applying its diagnostic criteria, with its long symptom counts that were hard enough to remember even without the changes that occurred between *DSM-III*, *DSM-III-R* (Third Edition, Revised*)*, and *DSM-IV*. *DSM-III* required at least 13 symptoms from a list of a possible 35 symptoms. *DSM-IV* reduced the number to 8, but imposed a pattern requirement of 4 pain symptoms, 2 gastrointestinal symptoms, 1 neurological symptom and 1 sexual symptom, thereby rendering the criteria very unwieldy even for experts, let alone time-pressured primary care physicians. The required counts (and pattern) seemed arbitrary, and it is now clear that somatization exists along a spectrum, rather than the categorical approach taken in *DSM*.

There is an extensive evidence base demonstrating that there is a continuous relationship between the number of somatic symptoms and psychiatric comorbidity, functional impairment, psychosocial risk factors, and health care use. There is no clear symptom count threshold to justify using it as a specific cut point, and simply counting the number of bodily symptoms seems a strange way to make a psychiatric diagnosis.[1] Because of the large number of somatic symptoms required for somatization disorder, most "somatizers," that is, patients in medical settings with problematic somatic symptoms and illness behavior, did not meet criteria for the diagnosis. In the pursuit of *DSM* criteria for somatization disorder with optimal construct validity and reliability, too much generalizability was sacrificed.

Undifferentiated Somatoform Disorder

This diagnosis was created in recognition that somatization disorder would only capture a small minority of somatizing patients, which was true, but the diagnosis has never caught on. "Undifferentiated" seems more appropriate to histology than psychiatry. As noted above, undifferentiated somatoform disorder does not translate into other languages well. It is difficult to remember the difference between undifferentiated somatoform disorder and somatoform disorder, not otherwise specified, and if one can, it seems to be a distinction without a meaningful difference.

Conversion Disorder

The term *conversion disorder* has limitations as well that have reduced its usage. It implies a particular etiological hypothesis, specifically a psychoanalytic concept of somatic representation of repressed unconscious affect, impulses, memories, or conflicts. Although it may be correct in some instances, the conversion hypothesis is unproven, and there are other plausible theories.[16] The name is not well accepted by patients and many clinicians and researchers do not use it; only 34% of neurologists use it when describing patients with a psychogenic movement disorder.[17] In the research literature, the terms *psychogenic, functional, non-epileptic, medically unexplained,* and *dissociative* are more widely used.[16] Although neurologists often refer to conversion symptoms as "psychogenic," they are reluctant to use either term as an explanation to patients.[17]

Hypochondriasis

Hypochondriasis is derived from the plural form of the Greek word *hypochóndrios,* referring to the upper abdomen, reflecting the ancient belief that the upper abdominal viscera were the seat of melancholy and other emotional disturbances. It took on its modern meaning in the 19th century, although the concept was considerably older, already widely recognized at the time of Moliere's 1673 play *Le Malade Imaginaire* (*The Imaginary Invalid*). Like *hysteria,* another term originating in ancient Greek medicine from the attribution of psychological illness to abdominal/pelvic organs, hypochondriasis is not a patient-friendly term. Physicians rarely use this diagnosis in talking with patients because it is perceived by patients as a dismissal of their symptoms, that physicians believe they are imagining or making them up. It is difficult enough to reassure the patient with excessive health anxiety and to explain how illness can arise without an underlying medical disease, even without this stigmatizing term.

Pain Disorders

The *DSM-IV* pain disorders diagnoses assume that some pains are just associated with psychological factors, some with medical diseases or injuries, and some with both. But this assumes one can clinically make such distinctions with reliability and validity, a proposition with little evidence. For example, a study of chronic pain patients, found "no significant difference between pain disorder associated with both psychological factors and a general medical condition (code 307.89) and pain disorder associated with psychological factors (code 307.80) with regard to the pain duration, intensity, and type and the level of disability and educational level."[18] Boland[19] observed that with each *DSM* edition, the concept of pain disorder was broadened and gradually moved away from the original idea of "psychogenic pain." Although this appears to have increased use of the diagnosis clinically, it did not solve the problems of reliability and validity. The current *DSM* pain disorder diagnoses are stuck in mind-body dualism. Indeed, psychological factors influence *all* forms of pain. Furthermore, most patients with chronic pain attribute their pain to a combination of factors, including somatic, psychological, and environmental influences.[20] Finally, it is unclear why pain (vs other somatic symptoms like fatigue, weakness, dizziness, etc) warrants separate diagnoses in *DSM*. Patients presenting with unexplained pain are very similar to patients with other unexplained somatic symptoms.[21]

Conceptual Problems

The boundaries between categories within the somatoform disorders are unclear. Although the goal of diagnostic classification is to "carve nature at its joints," this is difficult to do throughout much of psychiatry, and especially so for the somatoform disorders. Physicians are unlikely to use diagnoses that they cannot keep straight in their minds. Even in our own literature, there is a common practice of lumping the somatoform disorders together.[22]

Conceptually, somatoform disorders were fundamentally defined by symptoms that lack medical explanation.[23] However, in patients presenting with somatic symptoms, the exclusion of a medical explanation does not per se allow one to infer that the symptoms are psychologically explained. Our ability to reliably exclude medical causation is far from perfect. Diagnosing by exclusion fosters dichotomous thinking—that is, deciding whether a symptom is either psychogenic or caused by a medical disease—which overlooks the possibility that it may be both, which is very often the case. Finding a medical explanation for a symptom does not exclude coexisting influences of psychological factors, for instance, the significant effects of depression on symptoms of diabetes mellitus.[24] To diagnose a psychiatric disorder, there should be some affirmative evidence of psychological dysfunction.

In placing the emphasis on ruling out a medical explanation for symptoms, the DSM approach to somatization disorder and undifferentiated somatoform disorder fostered excessive diagnostic testing by nonpsychiatric physicians, who (1) did not want to miss a significant medical disorder, and (2) were more comfortable looking for diseases they understood than addressing psychiatric ones they did not. With "medically unexplained symptoms" as a central concept, it is not surprising that many physicians confused somatoform disorders with factitious disorder and malingering.

UNDERUSE OF THE SOMATOFORM DIAGNOSES BY NONPSYCHIATRIC PHYSICIANS

Nonpsychiatric physicians have become more knowledgeable about psychiatric illnesses and more often recognize and treat them than 25 years ago. One important factor in that evolution has been the marketing of psychiatric medications directly to primary care and other physicians by the pharmaceutical industry, which included extensive support for continuing medical education. These marketing and educational initiatives were focused on mental disorders likely to be encountered in general medical settings for which medications could be prescribed, that is, mood and anxiety disorders, attention-deficit disorder, and insomnia.

Although there is evidence that some patients with somatoform disorders benefit from psychotropic medication,[6] this was apparently not judged to be a fruitful market by the pharmaceutical industry. Hence, primary care physicians were trained to screen for symptoms of depression and anxiety and became more comfortable doing so. Education and direct-to-consumer advertising reduced the stigma associated with those disorders. In contrast, nonpsychiatric physicians (and many psychiatrists, it must be acknowledged) are less comfortable making diagnoses of the somatoform disorders, as they know little about how to diagnose them, and even if diagnosed, are uncertain how to treat them. It is much easier to "explain" mood and anxiety disorders as "a chemical imbalance," "a deficiency of a neurotransmitter," than it is to explain the concepts of somatization and conversion.

Primary physicians are also afraid that patients will be upset, even insulted by a somatoform diagnosis that seems to convey that the physician thinks nothing is really wrong with them. Not knowing how to effectively explain a somatoform diagnosis, physicians may indeed communicate "it's all in your head," with resulting harm to the doctor-patient relationship. There have been no public campaigns to destigmatize the somatoform disorders.

Finally, nonpsychiatric physicians tend to practice in a linear reflexive deductive manner from diagnosis to treatment, for instance, infection to antibiotic, hypertension to antihypertensive, depression to antidepressant. There is no parallel simple reflexive intervention for somatoform disorders, further disincentivizing diagnosis. Why make a diagnosis if there is no medicine to prescribe for it (sic)?

SUMMARY

The somatoform disorder diagnoses are used very uncommonly by physicians, both in recording a diagnosis in the chart, and in discussion with patients. This is not because the phenomena they try to capture are rare; on the contrary, they are very common. The somatoform disorders have also been the subject of much less research than their frequency and impact on quality of life and health care utilization warrant, and they have been left out of almost all community-based psychiatric epidemiology studies.

If such underuse and inattention are to be remedied, there is a need for diagnoses that are (1) user friendly for nonpsychiatric clinicians, (2) nonstigmatizing and acceptable to patients, (3) not grounded in mind-body dualism, (4) based on the presence of abnormal phenomena, not just the absence of an apparent medical cause, and (5) measurably reliable and valid. Significant changes in how we classify, name, and define criteria for the previously named somatoform disorders under the new rubric *somatic symptom disorders* have been proposed[4,16] that are hoped to increase the utility of diagnoses in clinical care and research. It is important to note, however, that such changes cannot eliminate stigmatization of patients and deficiencies in treatment. Simply changing terms and criteria will not change how clinicians think or practice, let alone systems of care.[25] The term *somatoform* is not stigmatizing— it is how somatizing patients are treated by their health care providers. A purely medical approach to evaluation and treatment in such patients leads to serial negative tests, ineffective interventions, and mutual doctor-patient frustration. The reinforcement of somatic attribution sometimes originates more from physicians intently pursuing their investigations for organic disease, rather than the patient.

REFERENCES

1. Kroenke K, Sharpe M, Sykes R. Revising the classification of somatoform disorders: key questions and preliminary recommendations. Psychosomatics 2007;48:277–85.
2. Mayou R, Kirmayer LJ, Simon G, et al. Somatoform disorders: time for a new approach in DSM-V. Am J Psychiatry 2005;162:847–55.
3. Fink P, Schroder A. One single diagnosis, bodily distress syndrome, succeeded to capture 10 diagnostic categories of functional somatic syndromes and somatoform disorders. J Psychosom Res 2010;68:415–26.
4. Dimsdale J, Creed F. DSM-V Workgroup on Somatic Symptom Disorders: the proposed diagnosis of somatic symptom disorders in DSM-V to replace somatoform disorders in DSM-IV–a preliminary report. J Psychosom Res 2009;66:473–6.
5. Fava GA, Fabbri S, Sirri L, et al. Psychological factors affecting medical condition: a new proposal for DSM-V. Psychosomatics 2007;48:103–11.
6. Abbey SE, Wulsin L, Levenson JL. Somatization and somatoform disorders. In: Levenson JL, editor. American psychiatric publishing textbook of psychosomatic medicine. Washington, DC: Psychiatric Publishing; 2011.
7. Hiller W, Rief W. Why DSM-III was right to introduce the concept of somatoform disorders. Psychosomatics 2005;46:105–8.
8. American Psychiatric Association. Diagnostic and statistical manual of mental disorders. Fourth edition, text revision. Washington, DC: American Psychiatric Association; 2000. p. 505.
9. Leonhard K. [Prevention of neuroses]. Psychiatr Neurol Med Psychol Beih 1966;4–5: 222–31 [in German].
10. Hyler SE, Spitzer RL. Hysteria split asunder. Am J Psychiatry 1978;135:1500–4.

11. Mouradian MS, Rodgers J, Kashmere J, et al. Can rt-PA be administered to the wrong patient? Two patients with somatoform disorder. Can J Neurol Sci 2004;31:99–101.
12. Bankier B, Aigner M, Bach M. Alexithymia in DSM-IV disorder: comparative evaluation of somatoform disorder, panic disorder, obsessive-compulsive disorder, and depression. Psychosomatics 2001;42:235–40.
13. Grabe HJ, Meyer C, Hapke U, et al. Specific somatoform disorder in the general population. Psychosomatics 2003;44:304–11.
14. Gureje O, Simon GE, Ustun TB, et al. Somatization in cross-cultural perspective: a World Health Organization study in primary care. Am J Psychiatry 1997;154:989–95.
15. Gureje O, Ustun TB, Simon GE. The syndrome of hypochondriasis: a cross-national study in primary care. Psychol Med 1997;27:1001–10.
16. Stone J, LaFrance WC, Brown R, et al. Conversion disorder: current problems and potential solutions for DSM-5. J Psychosom Res, in press.
17. Espay AJ, Goldenhar LM, Voon V, et al. Opinions and clinical practices related to diagnosing and managing patients with psychogenic movement disorders: an international survey of movement disorder society members. Mov Disord 2009; 24:1366–74.
18. Aigner M, Bach M. Clinical utility of DSM-IV pain disorder. Compr Psychiatry 1999; 40:353–7.
19. Boland RJ. How could the validity of the DSM-IV pain disorder be improved in reference to the concept that it is supposed to identify? Curr Pain Headache Rep 2002;6:23–9.
20. Hiller W, Heuser J, Fichter MM. The DSM-IV nosology of chronic pain: a comparison of pain disorder and multiple somatization syndrome. Eur J Pain 2000;4:45–55.
21. Birket-Smith M, Mortensen EL. Pain in somatoform disorders: is somatoform pain disorder a valid diagnosis? Acta Psychiatr Scand 2002;106:103–8.
22. Arnold IA, de Waal MW, Eekhof JA, et al. Somatoform disorder in primary care: course and the need for cognitive-behavioral treatment. Psychosomatics 2006; 47:498–503.
23. Hiller W, Cebulla M, Korn HJ, et al. Causal symptom attributions in somatoform disorder and chronic pain. J Psychosom Res 2010;68:9–19.
24. Ludman EJ, Katon W, Russo J, et al. Depression and diabetes symptom burden. Gen Hosp Psychiatry 2004;26:430–6.
25. Levenson JL. A rose by any other name is still a rose. Journal of Psychosomatic Research 2006;60:325–6.

Health Care Utilization and Poor Reassurance: Potential Predictors of Somatoform Disorders

Paul R. Puri, MD[a],*, Joel E. Dimsdale, MD[b]

KEYWORDS

- Somatoform disorder • DSM • Utilization • Satisfaction
- Reassurance

INTRODUCTION

Somatoform disorders have been one of the most troublesome diagnostic categories in the DSM. Many objections have been raised to the current conceptualization of the spectrum, from its lack of empirical foundation[1] to its heterogeneity and promotion of mind-body dualism.[2] Re-examining the distinctive qualities of somatoform disorders may yield a more validated approach to the spectrum.

Current thinking involves a redrawing of the diagnostic criteria for somatoform disorders. This redrawing, with particular emphasis on Complex Somatic Symptom Disorder (CSSD), emphasizes three attributes: somatic symptoms, excess concern with symptoms and illness, and abnormal health care utilization.[3] The reconceptualization of DSM-V shifts focus away from defining somatoform disorders primarily on the basis of Medically Unexplained Symptoms (MUS). Attempting to diagnose somatization by the presence or absence of MUS, or an absolute number of symptoms, is prone to error, as symptom recall is unreliable and there is no clean cut point in terms of number of symptoms. Syndromes based simply on medically unexplained symptoms have been shown to have poor reliability at long-term follow-up, with only 22% of those meeting criteria at baseline still meeting criteria at 5 years.[4] With outpatients with a somatoform disorder using up to twice the medical resources compared with outpatients without a somatoform disorder,[5,6] there is a tremendous need for well validated diagnostic criteria, and an opportunity to examine psychobehavioral aspects of somatoform disorders.

The authors thank Wayne Bardwell, PhD, Murray Stein, MD, and Scott Matthews, MD for helpful comments and criticisms.

[a] Department of Psychiatry, University of California, San Diego, CA, USA

[b] Department of Psychiatry, University of California, San Diego, 9500 Gilman Drive, Mail Code 0804, La Jolla, CA 92093-0804, USA

* Corresponding author. UCSD Box #9116A, 9500 Gilman Drive, La Jolla, CA 92093, USA

E-mail address: ppuri@ucsd.edu

Psychiatr Clin N Am 34 (2011) 525–544
doi:10.1016/j.psc.2011.05.011
0193-953X/11/$ – see front matter © 2011 Elsevier Inc. All rights reserved.

Clinical experience has suggested that somatoform patients have excessive concern, which does not seem to respond well to traditional interventions such as reassurance. Potentially inherent in this poor response is an underlying dissatisfaction with care received. Dissatisfaction and ongoing concern with symptoms would logically lead to pursuit of alternative care, "doctor shopping," or other ways of over-utilizing the health care system. The prevalence of somatoform disorders has long been thought to be high among over-utilizers or frequent attenders.[7] The evidence to support each criterion (over-utilization, poor response to reassurance, and poor satisfaction with care) as a distinctive aspect of somatization, however, should be evaluated critically. While these criteria are supported by clinical observation and are mentioned in earlier versions of the DSM, they have not been included in the current CSSD criteria. This paper is an exploratory evaluation of the literature and evidence to support these three patterns in somatoform patients, to examine if adequate evidence exists to incorporate them into future diagnostic criteria.

METHODS

The PubMed database was queried combining search terms "Somatoform," "Somatoform disorders," or "Hypochondriasis" for subject population. These results were then narrowed in subsequent independent searches by adding terms "Utilization," "Patient Satisfaction," and "Reassurance," searched in any field. The term "Somatoform" was used to include underlying relevant research conditions in the search such as multisomatoform disorder, which might be excluded if limited to MeSH term "Somatoform disorders." Hypochondriasis was added due to the finding in the literature of hypochondriasis as a trait that might be independent of the full disorder and not be found in a search for "Somatoform disorders." No limitation was made on years of publication, in order to maximize the inclusion of relevant literature that might antedate current DSM discussions. Other articles were obtained through inspection of bibliographies of relevant articles and authors. Individual abstracts or full articles were inspected to determine relevance to intended inquiry. Exclusion criteria included lack of new empiric data, such as review articles or editorials, or if the study failed to address the clinical question, such as studying clinician satisfaction rather than patient satisfaction. Rating of response to reassurance (positive or negative) was based on the stated positive or negative findings within each paper. Patient satisfaction findings in studies were coded by reviewer as clearly satisfied, clearly dissatisfied, or mixed. Utilization findings were broken down into forms of utilization, and then examined for any findings supportive of higher utilization in patients with somatoform conditions.

RESULTS

Search results are summarized in **Table 1**. A large number of citations were found on each search topic, but when search terms were combined, the resultant number of citations was markedly smaller. For example, while over 11,000 articles were found on somatoform related topics, when limited to English and combined with the keyword of reassurance, only 56 results were found. Total study results from each search are illustrated in **Table 1**. Papers varied in design, approach, and subjects. We will discuss separately observations on reassurance, dissatisfaction, and utilization. Several promising areas were noted which warrant further study for examination of utilization patterns.

Reassurance

A Pubmed search on somatizers and reassurance identified 59 relevant papers. Limiting results to English reduced the total to 56 studies. Thirty-four of these studies

Search Terms	Somatoform Search [Somatoform OR Somatoform Disorders OR Hypochondriasis]	Reassurance	Patient Satisfaction	Utilization [subheading]
Table 1 Pubmed independent searches				
Total Results	11836	2821	62207	108153
Limited to English	8605	2696	56651	98586
Somatoform search AND Reassurance	56			
Somatoform search AND Patient Satisfaction	116			
Somatoform search AND Utilization	240			

were excluded due to lack of relevant or new data. Twenty-two studies remained, the results of which are summarized in **Table 2**.

There was a strong trend in the studies suggesting a trait problem with sustained reassurance in somatoform patients, with 12 of the 22 studies reporting clear findings of poor response to reassurance. Reassurance seeking behavior was also noted in several studies. Four studies reported temporary relief of health anxiety from reassurance, but also that anxiety recurs and the temporary relief further drives reassurance seeking behavior. For instance, **Fig. 1** illustrates a subject's rating of anxiety before reassurance, immediately after with improvement, and subsequent rise in anxiety back to baseline. Few studies showed evidence of long-term benefit from reassurance. One editorial questioned the idea of poor reassurance response in somatizers, pointing out that reassurance has a broad range of quality, and that poor response to reassurance is a product of low quality reassurance from the provider.[8] An older editorial by Sapira[9] discussed a similar approach of "Reassurance Therapy," namely that certain criteria must be met for reassurance to be effective. These include getting a detailed description of the symptom, eliciting the emotional meaning of the symptom, examining the patient, making a diagnosis, and explaining the pathophysiology of the symptom.

A sub-group analysis found a number of studies examining populations with distinct somatoform disorders. It was interesting to note that 3 studies examined conversion disorder patients, and these were the only studies that did demonstrate improvement with reassurance. Of the 7 studies found examining patients with hypochondriasis, six had poor response to reassurance, and one had temporary response followed by increased drive to complete a checking behavior. There were no studies found that supported a clear effectiveness from reassurance in reducing health anxiety longitudinally in non-conversion disorder patients. Some data did support decreased utilization after reassurance,[10] though there were also conflicting data showing worsening from reassurance.[11]

Satisfaction

The Pubmed search on somatizers and satisfaction produced 137 papers, which were reduced to 115 papers once limited to English. Abstracts and papers were individually inspected, and 73 papers were excluded which did not appear to examine somatoform disorders, hypochondriasis, or satisfaction with health care. Many

Table 2
Summary of studies found examining response to reassurance

Study	Subjects	Responsive to Reassurance	Other Findings
Verschuur et al, 2008[53]	General population after natural disaster, with high health anxiety	Mixed	After a physical exam, subjects were reassured early on, but anxiety recurred by 12 weeks
Abramowitz and Moore, 2007[54]	Hypochondriacs performing safety behaviors (like reassurance seeking)	Mixed	Following a safety behavior, pt's had a large spike in desire to complete
Aggarwal et al, 2006[55]	Pt's with syndromes classified as somatizers (IBS, chronic fatigue, etc)	Mixed	Conditions all had high health anxiety and reassurance seeking behavior.
Salmon et al, 2005[51]	Primary care patients with MUS	Mixed	Pt's wanted more emotional support, but not more explanation or reassurance
Reid et al, 2001[56]	Primary care patients with MUS	Mixed	>80% of GP's feel that GP's should manage MUS pt's, and are using reassurance largely.
Pilowsky, 1993[57]	Pain clinic patients, psychiatric inpt's	Mixed	Testing Illness Behavior Questionnaire to test response to reassurance. Useful in these populations.
Salkovskis and Warwick, 1986[52]	Hypochondriacal pt's. Case examples to support theory.	Mixed	Presents idea of immediate effective reassurance, followed by return of anxiety, perpetuating pursuit of more reassurance.
Hausteiner et al, 2009[58]	MUS pt's referred for allergy workup	No	Also higher disease conviction
Morgan et al, 2008[59]	General population after a public health scare, with high health anxiety	No	Those with high health anxiety didn't respond well to reassurance
Fontenelle et al, 2006[60]	Body Dysmorphic Disorder pt's	No	Longitudinally had reassurance seeking behaviors, but didn't assess response to reassurance
Wearden et al, 2006[61]	Hypochondriacs	No	Association between hypochondriasis, reassurance seeking, and negative affectivity
Rief et al, 2006[62]	MUS pt's, compared to healthy and depressed controls	No	Heard audio report about a condition rejecting medical explanations, but pt's recalled the report improperly as stating likely the cause was medical

(continued on next page)

Table 2
(continued)

Study	Subjects	Responsive to Reassurance	Other Findings
Dowrick et al, 2004[11]	Primary care patients with MUS	No	Reassurance and normalization without explanation was not helpful, even making pt's worse.
Noyes et al, 2003[14]	Hypochondriacal pt's in primary care	No	Hypochondriasis modestly associated with poor physician-pt relationship, poor reassurance and satisfaction
Speckens et al, 2000[48]	Primary care patients with MUS	No	Using the Reassurance Questionnaire, showed poor reassurance, but this was not associated to utilization
Gulhati and Minty, 1998[63]	Mothers of children with MUS	No	Even mothers of these children responded poorly to reassurance
Barsky et al, 1993[64]	Hypochondriacal pt's in primary care	No	Hypochondriacs believe health involves being absolutely symptom free.
Logsdail et al, 1991[65]	Hypochondriacs with illness phobia of having AIDS. Case series	No	Had either temporary or poor response to reassurance, but would continue to seek it.
Warwick and Marks, 1988[66]	Pt's with hypochondriasis or illness phobia. No controls.	No	Subjects had sought reassurance repeatedly from providers, prior to treatment (exposure).
Al-Sharbati et al, 2001[67]	Conversion disorder case study	Yes	Reassurance part of therapy, effective
Hop et al, 1997[68]	Conversion disorder case series	Yes	Reassurance was helpful in a number of cases
Ophir et al, 1990[69]	Other Conversion Disorder	Yes	Responsive to reassurance.

excluded articles mentioned the term "satisfaction" superficially or examined life satisfaction rather than patient satisfaction. Results overall were quite mixed on satisfaction in somatizers, with a trend towards finding general satisfaction with care rather than dissatisfaction. The remaining studies are summarized in **Table 3**. Twenty studies were found that had strong findings of satisfaction with medical care, and twelve studies were found with clearly low satisfaction with care.

A majority of studies noted specific patient characteristics or characteristics of their medical care that predicted satisfaction. For instance, one study noted poorer satisfaction in patients or parents of patients with a mixture of somatization and a comorbid medical condition,[12] and another study found that presence of a chronic psychiatric disorder predicted low satisfaction with care.[13] One study found that

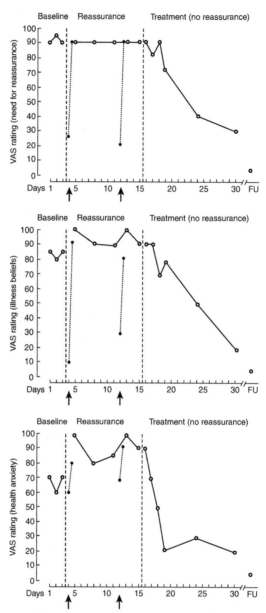

Fig. 1. Displays a case of hypochondriasis and self-rated anxiety before and after reassurance. Anxiety was reduced immediately, with a quick increase in anxiety soon thereafter and a tapering over time (*Adapted from* Salkovskis PM, Warwick HM. Morbid preoccupations, health anxiety and reassurance: a cognitive-behavioural approach to hypochondriasis. Behav Res Ther 1986;24:597–602; with permission.).

hypochondriasis was modestly associated with poor satisfaction in primary care patients,[14] while another study found no effect on satisfaction of surgery patients.[15] Hypochondriacs in another study made equal numbers of positive statements about their doctors as did controls, but made more negative statements than controls.[16]

Table 3			
Summary of studies found examining satisfaction with care			
Study	Sample Population	Satisfied with Care	Findings
Muller et al, 2008[17]	Multisomatoform pt's	Mixed	+ Depression or anxiety led to worse satisfaction
Hayden et al, 2005[15]	Hypochondriacal pt's getting a surgery	Mixed	At baseline pt's presumed would be dissatisfied. Got different surgery and had better satisfaction.
Persing et al, 2000[16]	Primary care pt's	Mixed	Hypochondriacal pt's made more negative statements about physicians
Jackson et al, 1999[70]	Military and Civilian Primary Care Pt's	Mixed	Satisfaction in somatizers not specifically mentioned. Unmet expectations in general decreased satisfaction.
Salmon et al, 1999[49]	Somatizing primary care pt's	Mixed	Pt's satisfied with tangible physical explanations, and explanations that made them feel empowered.
Downes-Grainger, 1998[71]	Somatizers in a surgery clinic	Mixed	Pt's feeling more understood and satisfied with the explanation of illness was associated with decreased psychiatric symptoms, but not decreased somatic
Riaz et al, 1998[23]	Pt's with PNES	Mixed	Following diagnosis of their seizures as psychogenic, pt.'s were more dissatisfied with the dx, but still more satisfied than not with treatment
Jones et al, 1989[72]	Internal Medicine inpt's	Mixed	Physicians believed illness was influenced by psychological factors if illness was less medically severe, and patients less satisfied with care
Johnson et al, 1989[20]	Pt's post-gynecologic surgery, getting PCA	Mixed	Self-perceived external locus of control associated with lower satisfaction with care
Kasteler et al, 1976[73]	Doctor Shoppers	Mixed	Lack of confidence in a specific doctor associated with shopping
Rosendal et al, 2007[74]	Somatizing primary care pt's	No	Only 30% highly satisfied. No data given on how many actively dissatisfied.
Lawoko and Soares, 2006[12]	Parents of children with heart disease	No	Somatizing patients had 0.83 odds ratio of being satisfied.
Frostholm et al, 2005[75]	Somatizing primary care pt's	No	Not knowing what was wrong, or having more symptoms predicted dissatisfaction
Hasler et al, 2004[13]	Psychiatric pt's	No	Somatizers had lower satisfaction than other disorders (like affective)
Noyes et al, 2003[14]	Hypochondriacal pt's in primary care	No	Modest correlation with poor satisfaction

(continued on next page)

Table 3
(continued)

Study	Sample Population	Satisfied with Care	Findings
Guo et al, 2002[42]	Self-referred pt's	No	Less satisfied with prior providers in particular
Garcia-Campayo and Sanz-Carillo 2000[76]	Pt's seeking alternative medicine	No	Somatoform pt's were less satisfied, but didn't have more hypochondriasis than others
Sumathipala et al, 2000[77]	Pt's with MUS	No	Baseline low satisfaction with care.
Godden, 1999[78]	BDD by proxy	No	Mother of pt viewed her as disfigured, sought further care and a lawsuit over perceived disfigurement.
Butler and Rollnick, 1996[79]	Case study of somatizer	No	Presumed problem with communication style.
Sato et al, 1995[80]	Doctor Shoppers	No	Low satisfaction with prior illness explanation, but seeking relief of symptoms.
Barsky et al, 1991[19]	Hypochondriacal pt's in primary care	No	Small sample size and response rate. More anxious and depressed than controls.
van Bokhoven et al, 2009[81]	Somatizing primary care pt's	Yes	Ordering tests did not improve satisfaction
Wieske et al, 2008[82]	Self-referred vs tertiary referral pt's	Yes	Only 9% of pt's intended to seek a second opinion
Jackson and Kroenke, 2008[4]	Multisomatoform pt's	Yes	At 5 years, only 21% still met criteria for diagnosis.
Tignol et al, 2007[83]	Pt's seeking cosmetic surgery	Yes	No difference in surgery in patients with vs without Body Dysmorphic Disorder
Zojaji et al, 2007[84]	Pt's seeking rhinoplasty	Yes	55.1% satisfaction rate. Lowest satisfaction in those with obsessive and psychasthenic personality traits.
Dirkzwager and Verhaak, 2007[85]	MUS pt's, controls, other high utilizers	Yes	Somatizers were quite positive about their care, though lower than controls. Only 10% of somatizers actively dissatisfied.
Jackson and Passamonti, 2005[86]	MUS pt's followed from onset	Yes	Pt's satisfied with resolution of symptoms. Lack of illness worry good prognostic factor. Most pt's with MUS did not have a mental illness
Eytan et al, 2004[87]	Pt's on a medical/psychiatric unit	Yes	High satisfaction overall. Those with personality disorders had lower but not low satisfaction with care.
Veale et al, 2003[88]	Pt's seeking rhinoplasty	Yes	No difference in satisfaction in BDD vs non-BDD pt's.
Klapow et al, 2001[89]	Somatizing primary care pt's	Yes	All patients reported satisfaction in the "good" range

(continued on next page)

Study	Sample Population	Satisfied with Care	Findings
Hartz et al, 2000[90]	MUS pt's in primary care	Yes	Satisfaction with care ranged from 54–79% based on aspect of satisfaction.
Lidbeck, 1997[91]	Somatizers	Yes	75% were very satisfied with a CBT/Relaxation training program.
Kroenke et al, 1997[18]	Multisomatoform pt's	Yes	Whole primary care sample had 76% highly satisfied. MSD once adjusted for psychiatric comorbidity was not a factor in satisfaction.
Wyshak and Barsky, 1995[37]	Hypochondriacal pt's in primary care	Yes	Three quarters of patients were very satisfied with care. Over half said care just about perfect. Higher depression predictive of worse satisfaction.
Camara, 1991[92]	Outpt's in a C/L clinic	Yes	Subjects had high satisfaction. No breakdown of subjects by diagnosis.
Schweickhardt et al, 2005[21]	Somatizing pt's	Yes	3 groups of somatizers. One with high emotional and physical stress, one with high emotional, and one with low both. High stress groups improved with tx, but low stress group worsened in depression after tx, though stayed satisfied.
Morriss et al, 1999[22]	MUS pt's in primary care	Yes	GP's were trained to treat somatizers. Pt's had high satisfaction at baseline, no better after the intervention.
Phillips et al, 1996[93]	Ob/Gyn pt's seen on a Psychiatry C/L service	Yes	83% of pt's found the C/L consultation quite helpful or very helpful. No breakdown of satisfaction by diagnosis.
van der Feltz-Cornelis et al, 1996[94]	Primary care somatizers, seen by a C/L psychiatrist	Yes	Over 91% of patients were satisfied with care.
Smith et al, 1986[95]	Primary care pt's with somatization d/o	Yes	Adding psychiatric consultation to primary care reduces costs in somatizers, without reducing satisfaction

Table 3
(continued)

Abbreviations: BDD, body dysmorphic disorder; PCA, patient controlled analgesia; PNES, psychogenic non-epileptic seizures.

Overall, no particular type of somatoform disorder patient was more or less likely to be satisfied with their medical care.

Presence of another psychiatric disorder, particularly anxiety or depression, may modify this relationship. One study looking at multisomatoform disorder found that presence of depression or anxiety was associated with more dissatisfaction with care,[17] though another study found that once anxiety and depression were controlled for, this effect disappeared.[18] This observation is in line with a study that showed hypochondriacs were more depressed, anxious, and dissatisfied with care.[19] Some factors associated with dissatisfaction with care were poor communication, perception of uncertainty about condition (not knowing what was wrong), presence of more symptoms, and external perceived locus of control.[20]

Thus, convergence of findings is not established despite the clinical impression of poor satisfaction in somatizers. A study by Schweickhardt and colleagues[21] may help explain this discrepancy. Primary care physicians underwent a training course in treating somatizers. They found three groups in the somatizing population: those with high emotional and physical distress; those with high emotional distress, minimal physical distress, and low satisfaction; and those with physical distress, low anxiety, and low satisfaction with physical functioning. In the course of treatment, those with anxiety had decreased anxiety and increased satisfaction with emotional functioning. Those with physical distress and low satisfaction during treatment began to attribute the cause of their problems to emotional rather than physical factors, and had an increase in stress and anxiety. Interestingly their satisfaction with care and self-reported therapeutic success increased, as did their feeling of being understood. In other words the groups with only physical distress (the deniers of psychological distress) became more anxious and aware of emotional distress as they were treated, but also became more satisfied with care. This complex effect may mask true benefits of treatment.

Adding to this complexity, educating somatizers about how psychosocial problems can lead to physical symptoms led to lower satisfaction with care in one study, though they still were very satisfied.[22] Riaz and colleagues[23] studied non-epileptiform seizure patients. Following diagnosis, their feelings about care were neutral or negative. At one year follow-up, however, satisfaction was more positive.

These diverse studies indicate that a simple relationship between somatization and satisfaction is not supported by the literature, but that a more textured analysis is needed to understand the mixed levels of satisfaction in somatizers.

Utilization

Utilization studies were quite heterogeneous, in terms of measurement of utilization and in subject populations of somatoform and other medical or psychiatric conditions. Two hundred twenty-two papers were found from search criteria described above. Eighty-five studies were excluded for lack of empirical data or lack of utilization measures. Some studies were excluded that measured pathways to referral for psychiatric evaluation as a form of utilization. Analysis found that 96 studies examined somatoform patients. Outpatient visit frequency was the most consistently elevated form of utilization found, with all studies examining this variable showing high utilization in somatizers. Other studies examined high utilization in nonsomatizers, suggesting high utilization may be sensitive but not specific to somatizers. Selection bias was also suspected, however, because many studies intentionally studied high utilizers as their sample population.

Other types of higher utilization were inconsistent in somatizers, possibly indicating subgroups of somatizers. Mental health visits in particular did not appear to be higher for somatizers compared to controls (normals or patients with other psychiatric conditions). Utilization measures and positive findings in somatoform patients are summarized in **Fig. 2**. Because there are so many criteria for high utilization, we provide further detail below on the findings based on measures of utilization, to illustrate the complexity of defining abnormal utilization.

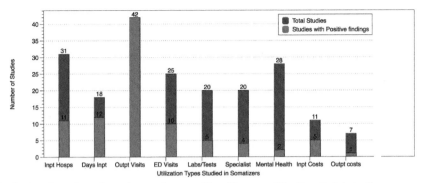

Fig. 2. Number of studies using each type of health care utilization. Total studies compared to studies showing higher utilization in somatizers (positive findings).

Utilization Breakdown

The definition of a frequent attender or high utilizer varies greatly throughout the medical literature. While some studies simply focus on selecting the top utilizers by percent (range 3–15%),[24,25] there are over a hundred different definitions of frequent attenders in various studies.[26] For example, one study examined total health expenditures in a set period (1 or 2 years), where a high utilizer had greater than two standard deviations higher expenditures than that of the average person in that society.[27] This of course begins the dilemma of delineating what is abnormal, which typically does not take into account variables such as comorbidities. Defining abnormal utilization must begin with defining how to measure general utilization, and then examining the impact of various definitions of abnormal utilization, particularly in somatoform disorders.

Time

The first step in measuring utilization involves identifying its components. Intuitively, utilization involves use of clinician time and health care resources. Clinician time can be difficult to measure, as self-reporting of time spent lacks standardization, and is difficult to track on a larger scale or accurate basis. Other factors are routinely tracked within the medical system. Utilization reviews by health care administrators have alternate methods of assessing and predicting severity of illness, such as by classifying patients into Diagnosis-Related Groups (DRG). Administrators performing utilization review examine specific types of patients by diagnosis in order to predict resource use and utilization, using factors such as principal diagnosis, complications, procedure, age, sex, and discharge status.[28] This aids administrators to predict utilization in typical illnesses, but has somewhat less utility for somatoform disorders, as they can be heterogeneous in complaints and not fall into a clear DRG. Each criterion used has benefits and drawbacks in being applied to somatoform patients.

Costs

Many studies have indicated significantly higher costs in those who are recognized as somatizing, even if only meeting criteria for a DSM-IV-TR Somatoform NOS diagnosis.[4] In a primary care study, patients with psychiatric conditions had significantly more primary visits than those without, and patients with undifferentiated somatoform disorder had approximately 30% more visits than patients with other psychiatric conditions.[10]

Measures of higher overall costs do not identify specific aspects of utilization that are particular for somatizers, however. Individuals with high overall costs may have recently had an organ transplant, but may be utilizing their resources at an appropriate level. Therefore overall costs can be both arbitrary and nonspecific. Analyses controlling for comorbidities and disease severity would be a more fruitful examination of costs. Most studies break down utilization and health care costs based on acuity of care, and by location.

Inpatient

Inpatient admissions are commonly measured by number of admissions, number of hospital days annually, and days per admission.[29–31] This may aid in identifying indicators such as short hospital stays, but no studies were found that examined the pattern of inpatient stays in somatizers. Further breakdown of inpatient expenses could include the number and cost of extensive medical tests.

High inpatient utilizers may fit a special subpopulation, such as patients with somatic symptoms manifesting in ways that require invasive procedures or repeated medical evaluation. No data were found on how representative they are of general somatizing high utilizers.

Outpatient

The most studied form of utilization in somatizers was outpatient utilization. There exists some evidence that somatizers may visit multiple outpatient locations (emergency rooms, primary care doctors), with a trend in the literature towards different sites based on gender and culture.[32–34] Studies of outpatient utilization include number of outpatient visits (over a defined time period ranging from 6 months to 2 years)[35–37] and total medication costs.[31,33] Cutoffs for the number of visits per year qualifying as high utilization varies between authors, from 7–12.[34] Some may argue that this does not account for comorbidities, but a study examining utilization in the chronically medically ill found that while disease/symptom severity and complications do affect utilization, disease duration and comorbidities do not.[38]

Specialist referrals

One area of utilization that may be easier to distinguish, and potentially even more characteristic of somatizers, is the use of referral to specialists or subspecialists. This is a large area of cost and one which is believed to have a relatively low yield in terms of treatment changes or formal diagnoses for patients with medically unexplained symptoms (somatizers).[39] Their use of specialists has been found to be elevated, even when controlling for medical comorbidities.[5,40] Somatizers often have symptoms from multiple organ systems, which likely leads to referrals to a variety of specialists and subspecialists. No research was found that distinguished a cutoff, however, on number of referrals or number of subspecialists seen.

Self-referrers

An additional subcategory of high utilization is that of self-referral. This has multiple possible forms. It has long been believed that those with somatoform disorders can "doctor-shop," seeking second and third opinions from other physicians. DSM-III identified this as a characteristic seen in several somatoform disorders, though did not identify this as a diagnostic criterion.[41] A further way to potentially distinguish somatizers with over-utilization would be to measure not only total number of visits, but percent of visits initiated by the patient, as opposed to those initiated by another physician.[8] This clearly also relates to use of specialists, when available, via self-referral.

In countries with a socialized health care model, self-referrers are defined as those who change doctors without a referral, especially during a single illness episode, and is considered a possible indicator of abnormal illness behavior and somatization.[42] Again, a consistent cutoff for an acceptable amount of self-referral was not found.

Emergency

The number of emergency room visits has also been evaluated as a measure of utilization. Studies vary in their definition of high utilization of ED services, ranging from 4–7 or more ED visits in a year.[43] Cultural issues should not be discounted, as access to care differs greatly across cultures. Many studies were performed in the UK, where primary care is a standardized first point of contact; thus, the population seeking emergency care may differ greatly from that in the US.

A gender difference in emergency room utilizers may also exist between cultures. In a UK study looking at users of emergency services, there was a predominance of men, regardless of level of utilization.[43] The high utilizers had multiple problems, but not more diagnoses of actual somatoform disorders. This somewhat conflicts with the common belief that high-utilizing somatizers are predominantly women. In the US, women are more likely to be high utilizers of primary care.[36,44]

The emergency department can also be distinguished from outpatient care by its high level of acuity. Somatizers and high utilizers may use the emergency department for inappropriate issues on multiple occasions. Objective criteria for emergency room use includes the Canadian Triage and Acuity Scale (CTAS) and the Hospital Urgencies Appropriateness Protocol (PAUH). The CTAS, for example, classifies emergency care in levels, based on acuity (waiting time allowed before being examined by the physician, risk of death, vital signs, pain level, possibility of complications, and origin of the injury).[33] Those with lower scores would be classified into a lower level of acuity, which when combined with frequency of visits may represent a specific type of high utilizer or inappropriate utilizer. Use of emergency services simply because of convenience of location indicates that at least a subpopulation of low acuity high utilizers may just have a low threshold for physician visits, which has been found elsewhere as a factor in higher utilizers seeking treatment.[45] Neither the CTAS nor the PAUH have been studied in somatizers specifically, though both appear to be useful methods of identifying patients with low acuity. It would be helpful if future trials examined these variables in relation to somatizers.

Overall, emergency room utilization does not seem to distinguish somatizers from non-somatizers, due to a variety of reasons. Other patient groups overuse emergency services, based on factors such as convenience and location, as well as health care access. If future studies focused on the number of symptoms for presentation and repeat presentations for identical conditions, then patterns may emerge in somatizers.

Diagnostic testing

The cost of medical testing (laboratory tests, imaging) is frequently considered a marker of utilization. A commonly noted belief is that somatizers have more medical testing that is not productive of a diagnosis. The studies found were mixed. Many studies mentioned diagnostic testing in their measures. One study noted negative workups, but no difference in costs in hospitalized somatizers versus hospitalized non-somatizers.[46] Reid and colleagues[39] found that within a group of high utilizers, primary care somatizers had more brain CTs, exercise ECG, endoscopy, and abdominal ultrasounds performed, and that these were often requested by the patients. This contrasted with results of a study by Thomassen and colleagues,[47] which showed patients with somatoform disorders had less testing than patients with other mental illnesses, and no more than patients with other medical conditions. Furthermore, Jyväsjärvi and colleagues[34] examined somatizing and non-somatizing frequent attenders, and found no difference in the number of labs or tests ordered. This may be due to specialists ordering a standard workup regardless of complaints. The somatizers may not have warranted the workup but still received an identical one to those with a medical illness. As with many of the studies, the lack of consistent findings is more likely due to the lack of studies rather than actual negative studies. A majority of studies that examined medical workup did not examine how to distinguish somatizers, but instead focused on the benefit of an intervention to reduce utilization in high utilizers.

DISCUSSION

Somatoform disorders are disabling for patients, and challenging and time consuming for medical providers. In the absence of well validated diagnostic criteria, the conditions are not only difficult to diagnose, but difficult to treat. DSM-V may redefine the diagnostic criteria, moving away from medically unexplained symptoms as the core construct. Our review of the literature suggests that somatizers have poor sustained response to reassurance, and higher utilization patterns, especially in outpatient care. In addition, somatizers appear to have increased numbers of nonproductive medical workups. On the other hand, there are less data to suggest that somatizers are consistently more dissatisfied with care than non-somatoform patients, or that more tests/procedures are ordered for them.

Limitations exist within our review. Studies included were only in English. There are repeated suggestions in the literature that cultural influences need to be evaluated; including different medical systems, different acceptability of having physical or mental illness, as well as different gender roles. A formal meta-analysis was not completed because study designs and patient populations were far too heterogeneous. Abnormal illness behavior, while including the criteria explored here, should be recognized to include other psychobehavioral facets that may be worthy of evaluation, such as illness preoccupation.

The issue of comorbidities also requires further investigation. Presence of medical comorbidities is generally expected to result in greater utilization of medical resources. However, not all medical conditions increase the need for health care use. The distinction could be made between conditions that cause morbidity and those that don't; disease severity, symptom severity, and complications increased utilization, but disease duration and comorbidities did not. Depression and psychological distress were the strongest predictors of hospitalizations and physician visits, even though chronic psychiatric patients were excluded.[38] This is an under-explored issue, that becomes important when considering predictive models in patients with somatoform disorders. However, it also suggests another conundrum: does the chronic medical illness worsen the psychological distress, or does the baseline psychiatric illness result in worse preoccupation with their physical symptoms?

Studies are needed that prospectively attempt to identify somatizers using criteria of high utilization or poor response to reassurance. Examination of self-referrers appears to have potential but is an understudied area as well. Furthermore, studying poor responders to reassurance and examining for subcategories of patients could be productive. It would be useful to examine an outpatient population and identify those with high utilization patterns in any of the mentioned aspects of utilization. Subjects identified, as well as normal utilizers, could be tested for health anxiety and response to reassurance immediately and longitudinally, as well as other psychiatric comorbidities.

One relatively large study based in the UK did attempt to evaluate distinctive styles of utilization and developed an extensive algorithm to predict somatizers, but found only moderate predictive ability.[40] This may be due to cultural and gender differences in utilization, which warrant further investigation. A UK-based study, where there is a nationalized health care system, may not generalize to the US, since many in the US do not have access to a primary care provider.

Another attempt to predict somatizers examined medical records using an independent examiner, as the gold standard, to identify somatizing patients. Statistical analysis yielded a model of predicting somatization weighted by various criteria. These criteria included gender (females were far more common), number of visits (cutoff of minimum 6 visits in a year), and percent of visits with "somatization potential" (based on complaints in the musculoskeletal, nervous, GI system, or "ill-defined complaints"). Varying the coefficient weights of different variables in the equation led to different sensitivities and specificities,[44] but these weightings pertain only to the specific study population and may not be generalizable. Similar equations could be created for various populations using other factors such as reassurance seeking.

Increasing use of standardized instruments would advance the field. There are well validated measures such as the Whitely Index (WI), Illness Attitude Scales (IAS), and Somatosensory Amplification Scale (SSAS). Each studies independent but overlapping domains. In comparison, the Reassurance Questionnaire (RQ) is one of the few to specifically examine response to reassurance.[48] There is a logical difficulty in studying alternative diagnostic criteria for somatoform disorders, since in the current nomenclature MUS is a central construct, but most people find it highly questionable and unreliable. Inclusion of studies in a review such as this one must be based on some criteria, and so many of the articles found inevitably rely on the use of MUS to define their study population. This creates an ongoing dilemma of determining the generalizability and validity of any conclusions drawn from the literature. If new criteria are established for what used to be called somatoform disorders, it is possible that the conclusions from this review may need to be modified.

SUMMARY

Redefining somatoform disorders challenges assumptions. While the goal is to escape the use of medically unexplained symptoms as diagnostic criteria, validation of any other criteria inevitably returns to MUS as selection criteria in referring to the current research literature. This tautology is just one of many challenges inherent in critically examining research on somatoform disorders.

Utilization is measured in many domains, and in none of those domains is there an agreed-upon cutoff for what qualifies as over-utilization. Furthermore many areas of utilization include significant experimental error ("noise,") (ie, other over-utilizers who are not somatizers) and this must be controlled for in the analysis. Nonetheless, somatizers do appear to utilize more heavily than non-somatizers, and this relationship may become more pronounced as the defining criteria for somatoform disorders are revised. Some areas of utilization deserve special attention, including self-referral, both to primary care for an ongoing illness episode, as well as to specialists. If a condition is not deemed necessary by the primary care physician for scheduled follow-up or referral, that in itself could be suggestive of somatization when the patient pursues further care. Other possible indices of utilization include emergency room visits for illness episodes that are not deemed of a severity to require emergency care, but on a repeated basis for the same condition.

Finally, research could be directed towards evaluating somatizing sub-groups. Somatizers as a whole are likely heterogeneous, and some seek explanation of their symptoms,[11,49] some alleviation,[50] and others emotional support.[51] Their patterns of utilization could vary based on what they seek.

REFERENCES

1. Rief W, Hiller W. Toward empirically based criteria for the classification of somatoform disorders. J Psychosom Res 1999;46:507–18.
2. Noyes R Jr, Stuart SP, Watson DB. A reconceptualization of the somatoform disorders. Psychosomatics 2008;49:14–22.
3. Dimsdale J, Creed F; DSM-V Workgroup on Somatic Symptom Disorders. The proposed diagnosis of somatic symptom disorders in DSM-V to replace somatoform disorders in DSM-IV–a preliminary report. J Psychosom Res 2009;66:473–6.
4. Jackson JL, Kroenke K. Prevalence, impact, and prognosis of multisomatoform disorder in primary care: a 5-year follow-up study. Psychosom Med 2008;70:430–4.
5. Barsky AJ, Orav EJ, Bates DW. Somatization increases medical utilization and costs independent of psychiatric and medical comorbidity. Arch Gen Psychiatry 2005;62:903–10.
6. Barsky AJ, Ettner SL, Horsky J, et al. Resource utilization of patients with hypochondriacal health anxiety and somatization. Med Care 2001;39:705–15.
7. Schrire S. Frequent attenders–a review. Fam Pract 1986;3:272–5.
8. Starcević V. Reassurance and treatment of hypochondriasis. Gen Hosp Psychiatry 1991;13:122–7.
9. Sapira JD. Reassurance therapy. What to say to symptomatic patients with benign diseases. Ann Intern Med 1972;77:603–4.
10. Harding KJ, Skritskaya N, Doherty E, et al. Advances in understanding illness anxiety. Curr Psychiatry Rep 2008;10:311–7.
11. Dowrick CF, Ring A, Humphris GM, et al. Normalisation of unexplained symptoms by general practitioners: a functional typology. Br J Gen Pract 2004;54:165–70.
12. Lawoko S, Soares JJF. Psychosocial morbidity among parents of children with congenital heart disease: a prospective longitudinal study. Heart Lung 2006;35:301–14.
13. Hasler G, Moergeli H, Bachmann R, et al. Patient satisfaction with outpatient psychiatric treatment: the role of diagnosis, pharmacotherapy, and perceived therapeutic change. Can J Psychiatry 2004;49:315–21.
14. Noyes R Jr, Stuart SP, Langbehn DR, et al. Test of an interpersonal model of hypochondriasis. Psychosom Med 2003;65:292–300.
15. Hayden JD, Myers JC, Jamieson GG. Illness behavior and laparoscopic antireflux surgery: tailoring the wrap to suit the patient. Dis Esophagus 2005;18:378–82.
16. Persing JS, Stuart SP, Noyes R Jr, et al. Hypochondriasis: the patient's perspective. Int J Psychiatry Med 2000;30:329–42.
17. Muller JE, Wentzel I, Nel DG, et al. Depression and anxiety in multisomatoform disorder: prevalence and clinical predictors in primary care. S Afr Med J 2008;98:473–6.
18. Kroenke K, Spitzer RL, deGruy FV 3rd, et al. Multisomatoform disorder. An alternative to undifferentiated somatoform disorder for the somatizing patient in primary care. Arch Gen Psychiatry 1997;54:352–8.
19. Barsky AJ, Wyshak G, Latham KS, et al. Hypochondriacal patients, their physicians, and their medical care. J Gen Intern Med 1991;6:413–9.
20. Johnson LR, Magnani B, Chan V, et al. Modifiers of patient-controlled analgesia efficacy. I. Locus of control. Pain 1989;39:17–22.

21. Schweickhardt A, Larisch A, Fritzsche K. Differentiation of somatizing patients in primary care: why the effects of treatment are always moderate. J Nerv Ment Dis 2005;193:813–9.
22. Morriss RK, Gask L, Ronalds C, et al. Clinical and patient satisfaction outcomes of a new treatment for somatized mental disorder taught to general practitioners. Br J Gen Pract 1999;49:263–7.
23. Riaz H, Comish S, Lawton L, et al. Non-epileptic attack disorder and clinical outcome: a pilot study. Seizure 1998;7:365–8.
24. Smits FTM, Wittkampf KA, Schene AH, et al. Interventions on frequent attenders in primary care. A systematic literature review. Scand J Prim Health Care 2008;26: 111–6.
25. Smits FTM, Mohrs JJ, Beem EE, et al. Defining frequent attendance in general practice. BMC Fam Pract 2008;9:21.
26. Hulka BS, Wheat JR. Patterns of utilization. The patient perspective. Med Care 1985;23:438–60.
27. Hiller W, Fichter MM. High utilizers of medical care: a crucial subgroup among somatizing patients. J Psychosom Res 2004;56:437–43.
28. Aronow DB. Severity-of-illness measurement: applications in quality assurance and utilizationreview. Med Care Rev 1988;45:339–66.
29. Zhang M, Booth BM, Smith GR. Services utilization before and after the prospective payment system by patients with somatization disorder. J Behav Health Serv Res 1998;25:76–82.
30. Diefenbach GJ, Robison JT, Tolin DF, et al. Late-life anxiety disorders among Puerto Rican primary care patients: impact on well-being, functioning, and service utilization. J Anxiety Disord 2004;18:841–58.
31. Labott SM, Preisman RC, Popovich J, et al. Health care utilization of somatizing patients in a pulmonary subspecialty clinic. Psychosomatics 1995;36:122–8.
32. Carret MLV, Fassa ACG, Domingues MR. Inappropriate use of emergency services: a systematic review of prevalence and associated factors. Cad Saude Publica 2009; 25:7–28.
33. Frayne SM, Yu W, Yano EM, et al. Gender and use of care: planning for tomorrow's Veterans Health Administration. J Womens Health (Larchmt) 2007;16:1188–99.
34. Jyväsjärvi S, Joukamaa M, Väisänen E, et al. Alexithymia, hypochondriacal beliefs, and psychological distress among frequent attenders in primary health care. Compr Psychiatry 1999;40:292–8.
35. Martin RC, Gilliam FG, Kilgore M, et al. Improved health care resource utilization following video-EEG-confirmed diagnosis of nonepileptic psychogenic seizures. Seizure 1998;7:385–90.
36. de Waal MWM, Arnold IA, Eekhof JAH, et al. Follow-up study on health care use of patients with somatoform, anxiety and depressive disorders in primary care. BMC Fam Pract 2008;9:5.
37. Wyshak G, Barsky A. Satisfaction with and effectiveness of medical care in relation to anxiety and depression. Patient and physician ratings compared. Gen Hosp Psychiatry 1995;17:108–14.
38. de Boer AG, Wijker W, de Haes HC. Predictors of health care utilization in the chronically ill: a review of the literature. Health Policy 1997;42:101–15.
39. Reid S, Wessely S, Crayford T, et al. Frequent attenders with medically unexplained symptoms: service use and costs in secondary care. Br J Psychiatry 2002;180:248–53.
40. Barsky AJ, Orav EJ, Bates DW. Distinctive patterns of medical care utilization in patients who somatize. Med Care 2006;44:803–11.

41. American Psychiatric Association. Diagnostic and Statistical Manual of Mental Disorders. 3rd edition. Author; 1980.

42. Guo Y, Kuroki T, Yamashiro S, et al. Illness behaviour and patient satisfaction as correlates of self-referral in Japan. Fam Pract 2002;19:326–32.

43. Williams ER, Guthrie E, Mackway-Jones K, et al. Psychiatric status, somatisation, and health care utilization of frequent attenders at the emergency department: a comparison with routine attenders. J Psychosom Res 2001;50:161–7.

44. Smith RC, Gardiner JC, Armatti S, et al. Screening for high utilizing somatizing patients using a prediction rule derived from the management information system of an HMO: a preliminary study. Med Care 2001;39:968–78.

45. Mewes R, Rief W, Brähler E, et al. Lower decision threshold for doctor visits as a predictor of health care use in somatoform disorders and in the general population. Gen Hosp Psychiatry 2008;30:349–55.

46. deGruy F, Crider J, Hashimi DK, et al. Somatization disorder in a university hospital. J Fam Pract 1987;25:579–84.

47. Thomassen R, van Hemert AM, Huyse FJ, van der Mast RC, Hengeveld MW. Somatoform disorders in consultation-liaison psychiatry: a comparison with other mental disorders. Gen Hosp Psychiatry 2003;25:8–13.

48. Speckens AEM, Spinhoven P, Van Hemert AM, Bolk JH. The Reassurance Questionnaire (RQ): psychometric properties of a self-report questionnaire to assess reassurability. Psychol Med 2000;30:841–7.

49. Salmon P, Peters S, Stanley I. Patients' perceptions of medical explanations for somatisation disorders: qualitative analysis. BMJ 1999;318(7180):372–6.

50. Barsky AJ, Cleary PD, Sarnie MK, Klerman GL. The course of transient hypochondriasis. Am J Psychiatry 1993;150:484–8.

51. Salmon P, Ring A, Dowrick CF, et al. What do general practice patients want when they present medically unexplained symptoms, and why do their doctors feel pressurized? J Psychosom Res 2005;59:255–60.

52. Salkovskis PM, Warwick HM. Morbid preoccupations, health anxiety and reassurance: a cognitive-behavioural approach to hypochondriasis. Behav Res Ther 1986; 24:597–602.

53. Verschuur MJ, Spinhoven P, Rosendaal FR. Offering a medical examination following disaster exposure does not result in long-lasting reassurance about health complaints. Gen Hosp Psychiatry 2008;30:200–7.

54. Abramowitz JS, Moore EL. An experimental analysis of hypochondriasis. Behav Res Ther 2007;45:413–24.

55. Aggarwal VR, McBeth J, Zakrzewska JM, et al. The epidemiology of chronic syndromes that are frequently unexplained: do they have common associated factors? Int J Epidemiol 2006;35:468–76.

56. Reid S, Whooley D, Crayford T, et al. Medically unexplained symptoms–GPs' attitudes towards their cause and management. Fam Pract 2001;18:519–23.

57. Pilowsky I. Dimensions of illness behaviour as measured by the Illness Behaviour Questionnaire: a replication study. J Psychosom Res 1993;37:53–62.

58. Hausteiner C, Bornschein S, Bubel E, et al. Psychobehavioral predictors of somatoform disorders in patients with suspected allergies. Psychosom Med 2009;71:1004–11.

59. Morgan OW, Page L, Forrester S, et al. Polonium-210 poisoning in London: hypochondriasis and public health. Prehosp Disaster Med 2008;23:96–7.

60. Fontenelle LF, Telles LL, Nazar BP, et al. A sociodemographic, phenomenological, and long-term follow-up study of patients with body dysmorphic disorder in Brazil. Int J Psychiatry Med 2006;36:243–59.

61. Wearden A, Perryman K, Ward V. Adult attachment, reassurance seeking and hypochondriacal concerns in college students. J Health Psychol 2006;11:877–86.
62. Rief W, Heitmüller AM, Reisberg K, et al. Why reassurance fails in patients with unexplained symptoms–an experimental investigation of remembered probabilities. PLoS Med 2006;3:e269.
63. Gulhati A, Minty B. Parental health attitudes, illnesses and supports and the referral of children to medical specialists. Child Care Health Dev 1998;24:295–313.
64. Barsky AJ, Coeytaux RR, Sarnie MK, et al. Hypochondriacal patients' beliefs about good health. Am J Psychiatry 1993;150:1085–9.
65. Logsdail S, Lovell K, Warwick H, et al. Behavioural treatment of AIDS-focused illness phobia. Br J Psychiatry 1991;159:422–5.
66. Warwick HM, Marks IM. Behavioural treatment of illness phobia and hypochondriasis. A pilot study of 17 cases. Br J Psychiatry 1988;152:239–41.
67. Al-Sharbati MM, Viernes N, Al-Hussaini A, et al. A case of bilateral ptosis with unsteady gait: suggestibility and culture in conversion disorder. Int J Psychiatry Med 2001;31:225–32.
68. Hop JW, Frijns CJ, van Gijn J. Psychogenic pseudoptosis. J Neurol 1997;244:623–4.
69. Ophir D, Katz Y, Tavori I, et al. Functional upper airway obstruction in adolescents. Arch Otolaryngol Head Neck Surg 1990;116:1208–9.
70. Jackson JL, O'Malley PG, Kroenke K. A psychometric comparison of military and civilian medical practices. Mil Med 1999;164:112–5.
71. Downes-Grainger E, Morriss R, Gask L, et al. Clinical factors associated with short-term changes in outcome of patients with somatized mental disorder in primary care. Psychol Med 1998;28:703–11.
72. Jones LR, Mabe PA, Riley WT. Physician interpretation of illness behavior. Int J Psychiatry Med 1989;19:237–48.
73. Kasteler J, Kane RL, Olsen DM, et al. Issues underlying prevalence of "doctor-shopping" behavior. J Health Soc Behav 1976;17:329–39.
74. Rosendal M, Olesen F, Fink P, et al. A randomized controlled trial of brief training in the assessment and treatment of somatization in primary care: effects on patient outcome. Gen Hosp Psychiatry 2007;29:364–73.
75. Frostholm L, Fink P, Oernboel E, et al. The uncertain consultation and patient satisfaction: the impact of patients' illness perceptions and a randomized controlled trial on the training of physicians' communication skills. Psychosom Med 2005;67:897–905.
76. García-Campayo J, Sanz-Carrillo C. The use of alternative medicines by somatoform disorder patients in Spain. Br J Gen Pract 2000;50:487–8.
77. Sumathipala A, Hewege S, Hanwella R. Randomized controlled trial of cognitive behaviour therapy for repeated consultations for medically unexplained complaints: a feasibility study in Sri Lanka. Psychol Med 2000;30:747–57.
78. Godden D. Body dysmorphic disorder by proxy. Br J Oral Maxillofac Surg 1999;37:331.
79. Butler C, Rollnick S. Missing the meaning and provoking resistance; a case of myalgic encephalomyelitis. Fam Pract 1996;13:106–9.
80. Sato T, Takeichi M, Shirahama M, et al. Doctor-shopping patients and users of alternative medicine among Japanese primary care patients. Gen Hosp Psychiatry 1995;17(2):115–25.
81. van Bokhoven MA, Koch H, van der Weijden T, et al. Influence of watchful waiting on satisfaction and anxiety among patients seeking care for unexplained complaints. Ann Fam Med 2009;7:112–20.

82. Wieske L, Wijers D, Richard E, et al. Second opinions and tertiary referrals in neurology: a prospective observational study. J Neurol 2008;255:1743–9.

83. Tignol J, Biraben-Gotzamanis L, Martin-Guehl C, et al. Body dysmorphic disorder and cosmetic surgery: evolution of 24 subjects with a minimal defect in appearance 5 years after their request for cosmetic surgery. Eur Psychiatry 2007;22:520–4.

84. Zojaji R, Javanbakht M, Ghanadan A, et al. High prevalence of personality abnormalities in patients seeking rhinoplasty. Otolaryngol Head Neck Surg 2007;137(1):83–7.

85. Dirkzwager AJ, Verhaak PF. Patients with persistent medically unexplained symptoms in general practice: characteristics and quality of care. BMC Fam Pract 2007;8:33.

86. Jackson JL, Passamonti M. The outcomes among patients presenting in primary care with a physical symptom at 5 years. J Gen Intern Med 2005;20(11):1032–7.

87. Eytan A, Bovet L, Gex-Fabry M, et al. Patients' satisfaction with hospitalization in a mixed psychiatric and somatic care unit. Eur Psychiatry 2004;19:499–501.

88. Veale D, De Haro L, Lambrou C. Cosmetic rhinoplasty in body dysmorphic disorder. Br J Plast Surg 2003;56:546–51.

89. Klapow JC, Schmidt SM, Taylor LA, et al. Symptom management in older primary care patients: feasibility of an experimental, written self-disclosure protocol. Ann Intern Med 2001;134:905–11.

90. Hartz AJ, Noyes R, Bentler SE, et al. Unexplained symptoms in primary care: perspectives of doctors and patients. Gen Hosp Psychiatry 2000;22:144–52.

91. Lidbeck J. Group therapy for somatization disorders in general practice: effectiveness of a short cognitive-behavioural treatment model. Acta Psychiatr Scand 1997;96:14–24.

92. Camara EG. A psychiatry outpatient consultation-liaison clinic. Experience at the Cleveland Clinic Foundation. Psychosomatics 1991;32:304–8.

93. Phillips N, Dennerstein L, Farish S. Psychological morbidity in obstetric-gynaecology patients: testing the need for expanded psychiatry services in obstetric-gynaecology facilities. Aust N Z J Psychiatry 1996;30:74–81.

94. van der Feltz-Cornelis CM, Wijkel D, Verhaak PF. Psychiatric consultation for somatizing patients in the family practice setting: a feasibility study. Int J Psychiatry Med 1996;26:223–39.

95. Smith GR Jr, Monson RA, Ray DC. Psychiatric consultation in somatization disorder. A randomized controlled study. N Engl J Med 1986;314:1407–13.

The Relationship Between Somatic Symptoms, Health Anxiety, and Outcome in Medical Out-Patients

Francis Creed, MD, FRCPsych, FRCP, FMed Sci

KEYWORDS

- Somatization • Medically unexplained symptoms
- Health anxiety • Health care utilization • Outcome

INTRODUCTION

Somatic symptom disorders, also known as "somatoform" disorders, are common, distressing to patients, families, and physicians but surprisingly understudied. The definitions of these disorders include impairment and/or treatment seeking, but the relationship between the symptoms and cognitive characteristics of these disorders and later outcome has not been assessed adequately in prospective studies. In particular, it is not clear whether somatic symptoms, the hallmark of somatization, and health anxiety (hypochondriasis) have similar relationships with health status, medical treatment seeking, and satisfaction with care. These relationships are important in clinical practice in order to decide which disorders will resolve spontaneously and which will require psychological treatment. They are relevant also to the examination of the somatoform disorders in preparation for DSM-V.[1]

One of the aims of the current revision of the DSM is to incorporate a dimensional approach to diagnosis in addition to the categorical one.[2] This is useful for research and many of the findings in the field of psychosomatics indicate that the relevant variables, such as number of somatic symptoms, physiological measures, and outcomes are distributed as continuous variables.[3-9] The clinical utility of the dimensional approach is a little less clear, however, as cut points on relevant scales have not been reliably established.

It is well recognized that blood pressure is distributed in the population as a continuous variable but there have also been established cut point values, above which complications are more likely. Similar cut points have not been established adequately in the field of somatic symptoms and health anxiety, although these are

The author has no conflicts of interest to disclose.

School of Community Based Medicine, The University of Manchester, Jean McFarlane Building, Oxford Road, Manchester M13 9PL, UK

E-mail address: francis.creed@manchester.ac.uk

Psychiatr Clin N Am 34 (2011) 545–564
doi:10.1016/j.psc.2011.05.001
0193-953X/11/$ – see front matter © 2011 Elsevier Inc. All rights reserved.

central to the somatic symptom disorders.[1] This paper aims to assess whether it is possible to establish cut points on the dimensions of total somatic symptom count and health anxiety that are meaningfully related to outcome. The data come from a study which has been published previously[10–12] but all the analyses in this paper are original. The current study also includes a broader range of outcomes than most previous similar studies; we have studied health status, frequency of medical consultations, and satisfaction.

Although somatic symptoms and health worries are ubiquitous, it is necessary to identify a threshold above which these phenomena are associated with impairment and frequent medical help-seeking. In primary care a threshold for the number of somatic symptoms which corresponds to a provisional diagnosis of "somatization" has been ascertained. Using the PHQ-15, Kroenke identified the top third and the top 10% of scorers to assess the relationship between a high number of bothersome somatic symptoms (PHQ-15) and impaired health status, time off sick, and frequent medical consultations.[13] Scores of 5, 10, and 15 on PHQ-15 were said to correspond with a low, medium, and high somatic symptom severity. The data showed nicely that number of somatic symptoms and outcome are closely correlated and both appear to be continuously distributed. Barsky used a cut point on the PHQ-15 questionnaire to provide a 'provisional diagnosis of somatoform disorder' (approximately 20% of primary care patients) when demonstrating the association between total somatic symptom count with high health care costs and impaired function, after adjustment for confounders.[14,15]

There are 2 important aspects of these studies that are relevant to this paper. First, the PHQ-15 is a self-administered questionnaire and measures all somatic symptoms; there is no attempt to identify "medically unexplained symptoms," so the questionnaire yields a total somatic symptom score. This is important as the definition of somatoform disorders in previous versions of DSM has relied solely on 'medically unexplained' symptoms and less is known about the predictive power of total somatic symptom count.

Second, most previous assessments of the association between a high total somatic symptom count and impaired health status have used cross-sectional analyses preventing any conclusions about causality. Furthermore, the analyses of association with health care use have employed retrospective, not prospective, measures of health care, although we need to know the predictive value of somatic symptoms and health anxiety. The 2 studies that have used a prospective design have shown that, after adjusting for confounders: (a) somatic symptoms predicted subsequent impairment and (b) a combined measure of somatic symptoms and hypochondriacal cognitions predicted health care use.[15,16] The latter study did not identify the relative contribution of somatic symptoms and health anxiety to subsequent outcome; these are probably overlapping concepts.[16–18]

The study described here used prospective measures of health care use and health status. This is in line with the notion that treatment seeking and impairment should not be regarded as diagnostic criteria for somatoform disorders but they should be regarded as outcome measures.[19]

Although the dimensional approach is appropriate to establish relationships between variables in research, establishing appropriate thresholds is required to identify patients for treatment and to establish the prevalence of a disorder in a given population. There have been problems with determining prevalence because the threshold for diagnosing DSM-IV somatization disorder was too high for primary care or population-based studies.[20] A variety of alternative measures has led to a very wide variation in the prevalence of somatoform disorders in primary care.[21] Similarly, the use of a cut point on measures of health anxiety has led to widely differing estimates of the prevalence of hypochondriasis.[18,20,22–24] The data from a clinic study, such as the one described here, cannot establish prevalence of a disorder, which requires a population-based study, but can contribute to our understanding of which clinic patients have clinically significant multiple somatic symptoms and health anxiety.

The present study concerned new patients at secondary and tertiary gastroenterology, cardiology, and neurology clinics where patients with persistent 'medically unexplained' symptoms are common as well as patients with serious organic disease. The first aim of this study was to assess whether cut points could be established on measures of total somatic symptom count and health anxiety measures that predicted subsequent outcome. The prospective design meant that we used number of somatic symptoms and health anxiety at first clinic visit as predictors of outcomes; the latter were health status 6 months later and number of medical consultations during the 6 months following first clinic visit. In a subsample we obtained measures of satisfaction 2 weeks after first clinic visit.[12] We also compared whether there were differences between patients whose presenting symptoms could be attributed to well recognized physical diseases and those with 'medically unexplained' symptoms.

Our previous study indicated somewhat different relationships between somatic symptoms and health anxiety with outcome. That association was linear for somatic symptoms and outcome. However, for health anxiety, it was only the highest scores (top 10%) that were associated with poor outcome.[10] We used cut points derived from that study in the present one, but we performed more detailed analyses that adjusted for relevant baseline scores of the outcome measures in addition to other confounders. Our previous study suggested that the relationship between somatic symptoms, health anxiety, and outcome was similar for symptoms explained and not explained by organic disease. We checked this further in the present study as this is implicit in the proposed DSM-V complex somatic symptom disorder.[1]

Our analyses aimed to answer the following questions: (1) Is the correlation between number of somatic symptoms and outcomes similar to that between health anxiety and outcomes and, in addition, are these similar for patients with explained and unexplained symptoms? (2) Do the patients who score above the cut points on the somatic symptom and health anxiety scores have worse outcomes, and is this regardless of whether the symptoms were explained? (3) Do the patients who had *both* high number of somatic symptoms and marked health anxiety have the worst outcomes of all? (4) Are somatic symptoms score and health anxiety score independent predictors of outcome when adjustment is made for confounders, including anxiety and depression?

METHOD

The sample comprised consenting new patients attending the neurology, gastroenterology, and cardiology out-patient departments of 2 large hospitals in the UK.[10,11] These clinics receive referrals from primary care and other out-patient clinics, ie, secondary and tertiary referrals. We approached all new patients at these clinics if they were: aged 18–75 years, physically and mentally able to complete questionnaires in English, and clearly symptomatic; we excluded asymptomatic patients (eg, those with hypertension or heart murmur detected at routine screening) as our questionnaires referred to current symptoms.

Six months after the index appointment, patients were mailed a more limited set of questionnaires to measure outcomes. A subsample completed satisfaction questionnaires 2 weeks after the initial clinic visit.[12] This substudy was performed only in the neurology and cardiology clinics.

Also at about 6 months, 2 clinicians, who were blind to the questionnaire data, independently reviewed the case notes and classified patients' presenting complaints as either 'medically unexplained symptoms' or 'symptoms explained by demonstrable abnormality' (indicating recognized pathologic or pathophysiologic abnormality) according to the stated doctor's opinion in the notes and the results of investigations.[25]

At first clinic visit participants completed the following self-administered questionnaires. A short socio-demographic questionnaire collected data including age, sex, marital status, socio-economic status (low SES was defined as >22 on Goldthorpe and Hope classification[26]), employment status, ethnicity, and presenting symptom(s).

The Hospital Anxiety and Depression Scale (HADS) is a measure of anxiety and depression (7 questions for each) that is suitable for medical patients as it avoids physical items (eg, weight loss, pain) that might be caused by physical illness and is a valid and reliable tool in clinical populations.[27,28]

The Illness Perception Questionnaire (IPQ) assesses individuals' beliefs about their illness. The 'Somatic symptom' scale lists 12 bodily symptoms (henceforth referred to as somatic symptom score), which the respondent might currently experience and attribute to their current illness. These are: pain, nausea, breathlessness, weight loss, fatigue, stiff joints, sore eyes, headaches, upset stomach, sleep difficulties, dizziness, and loss of strength. Each is rated on a 4-point scale indicating how often they experience them. The total somatic symptom score used in this study is the number of symptoms that were marked as present "all the time" or "frequently."[29]

The Health Anxiety Questionnaire (HAQ) focuses specifically on concerns about health, with questions covering health worry and preoccupation, fear of illness and death, reassurance-seeking behavior, and interference with life/activities.[30] It was developed for medical groups and is based on the cognitive-behavioral model of health anxiety. It is intended to reflect a range of severity of health anxiety. Cluster analysis led to 4 subscores: health worry and preoccupation, fear of illness and death, reassurance seeking behavior, and interference with life.[30] High scores indicate greater anxiety about health.

Outcomes

The 36-item Short-Form health survey 36 (SF-36) is a widely used generic measure of health status.[31] It can be scored as 2 summary scores representing physical and mental components of health status: each score ranges from 50 to 0, with low scores indicating poor health.[32] In this study we report the physical and mental component summary scores. The questionnaire also asked whether the patient felt their symptoms(s) had improved or not. We report results here comparing those whose symptoms had improved at follow-up compared to those whose symptoms were the same or worse.

Number of medical consultations over the 6 months subsequent to first clinic visit was derived from the GP and hospital records. Since all patients were treated under the National Health Service, we had access to all primary and secondary care records for each patient and we included the total number of medical consultations for the 12 months prior to and 6 months after the date of the index clinic visit (visits to the GP, hospital out-patients, and Accident and Emergency Department).

Satisfaction with initial clinic visits was assessed by questionnaire 2 weeks after the appointment.[12] We quote here data for the communication and explanation subscales. The first recorded the patients' *satisfaction* with the doctor's manner, willingness to answer questions, and the extent to which s/he tried to understand the patient's concerns and worries. The *explanation* subscale measured satisfaction with the doctor's explanation of the cause of symptoms, planned further investigations and future appointments. Each item on the questionnaire is rated from 1 = completely satisfied to 4 = very dissatisfied, so a high score represents dissatisfaction.[12]

Statistical Analyses

All data were entered and analysed on SPSS, version 16.0. Descriptive data are presented as mean and standard deviation (SD), or standard error of mean (SEM) for ANCOVA analyses, for normally distributed data, and as median and inter-quartile range (IQR) for other data. The analyses employed the following variables as predictors of outcome: (a) total somatic symptom score, (b) Health Anxiety Questionnaire (HAQ) score (as total score and as subscales 'fear of illness and death,' 'health worry and preoccupation,' 'reassurance seeking behavior,' 'interference with life').

The following were used as outcome measures: (a) number of medical consultations during subsequent 6 months (log transformed for multivariate analyses), (b) scores at follow-up for SF-36 physical and mental component scores, (c) scores on the satisfaction scales for explanation by the doctor and doctor-patient communication,[12] (d) symptomatic improvement versus same or worse.

The first analysis compared the association between our predictors and outcomes using Spearman correlation coefficient. This analysis was repeated for patients with medically explained or unexplained symptoms separately.

The second analysis examined whether using cut points on the somatic symptom and health anxiety scales produced groups that differed in outcome. We used cut points derived from our previous study (somatic symptom score of 9 or more, HAQ score of 30 or more),[10] and ANCOVA to adjust for baseline variable of the relevant outcome measure. We used log transformed number of medical consultations for this analysis.

The third analysis assessed whether patients who had *both* high number of somatic symptoms and marked health anxiety had worse outcomes. The sample was divided into 4 groups: high somatic symptom score only, high health anxiety score only, both scores high, neither score high. In order to obtain reasonable numbers for analysis, we used the cut point of 9 or above to define "high" somatic symptoms, and 24 or above on the HAQ to define high health anxiety. The continuous outcome variables were compared across these 4 groups and statistical significance of difference was adjusted, using ANCOVA adjusting for age, sex, and medically unexplained versus explained symptoms in addition to relevant baseline value. Chi-square test was used for categorical measures.

In order to assess whether somatic symptoms and health anxiety were independent predictors of outcome after adjustment for confounders, we used multiple linear regression with each of the outcome variables in turn as the dependent variable (log transformed number of medical consultations, physical and mental component follow-up scores, satisfaction scores). The independent variables were age, sex, marital status (divorced, married or widowed vs remainder), low socio-economic status versus remainder, medically explained or unexplained symptoms, SF-36 physical function score (as measure of physical disability), 4 subscales of HAQ, number of somatic symptoms, Hospital Anxiety and Depression total score, Model 1 included SF-36 scale for physical function (to adjust for physical disability) as well as demographic features, somatic symptoms, and health anxiety. In model 2 total HADS (anxiety and depression) score was entered also as these are known to be associated with somatoform disorders.

The project had approval from Central Manchester Ethical Committee (Reference No. CM/96/169) and all participants signed consent after full explanation.

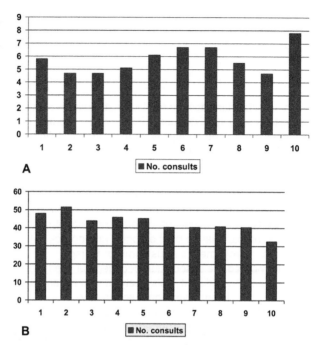

Fig. 1. The number of consultations (*A*) for 6 months after index clinic visits and (*B*) follow-up SF-36 mental component score by HAQ total score divided into deciles. *1* = decile with lowest HAQ score and *10* = decile with highest HAQ score.

The consent included completion of questionnaires on 2 occasions and examination of case notes to identify frequency of medical consultations and nature of presenting symptoms.

RESULTS

Of the 383 patients approached at their first clinic visit, 292 (76.2%) joined the study. The mean age of the sample was 47.2 (SD = 13.6) years; 55% were female, 58% married or cohabiting, and 21% separated, widowed or divorced. Forty-six percent were of lower socio-economic status and 91.9% were white Caucasians. Of the 292 participants 113 (38.7%) had medically unexplained symptoms.

Association Between Health Anxiety, Number of Consultations and Health Status

Fig. 1A shows the relationship between Health Anxiety Questionnaire score, displayed as deciles, and the mean number of medical consultations over subsequent 6 months. **Fig. 1**B is similar but shows data for the SF-36 mental component score at follow-up. For the 10% with highest HAQ score (top decile) the median (interquartile range) number of medical consultations was 8 (4–9) compared with 5 (2–7) for the remainder [P = .003 Mann Whitney] and the mean SF-36 mental component scores were 32.6 (SD = 13.5) and 44.1 (11.2) respectively [P = .001]. For other deciles, HAQ was not clearly associated with increases in consultations or adverse effects on quality of life.

Anxiety and Depression Scores in Patients with Medically Explained and Unexplained Symptoms

Patients with medically unexplained symptoms had higher anxiety and depression scores than those with explained symptoms (17.4 [SD = 8.9] vs 13.2 [7.1], $P<.001$). There was no difference between the groups on somatic symptom score (7.7 [3.0] vs 7.8 [2.9]). Patients with medically unexplained symptoms had a higher HAQ score (17.4 [1.2] vs 14.7 [9.6], $P = .030$), but this difference disappeared after adjustment for anxiety and depression (15.5 [SEM = 0.8] vs 15.8 [0.6], $P = .77$).

Outcome Measures

Medical consultation data were collected from the records of 275 (94%) of the 292 participants. The median number of visits to the GP and hospital (out-patients and accident and emergency) over the 6 months following initial clinic visit was 5 (range: 1–28) of which 3 (range 1–17) were to primary care.

The SF36 physical and mental component summary scores at follow-up were available for 200 participants (68.5%); the mean scores (SD) were 39.7 (12.5) and 43.4 (11.6) respectively. These scores indicate considerable impairment—comparable with chronic pain conditions such as back pain, arthritis, heart disease, and severe irritable bowel syndrome.[33–37] A quarter (51/200, 25.5%) scored less than 30 on the physical component scale (2 SD below population norm) and 24.5% (49/200) scored less the 35 on the mental component scale (1.5 SD below norm). Forty-three percent (82/191) of participants reported that their symptoms had improved at follow-up.

Patient Satisfaction

The mean score for satisfaction with the doctors' explanation of the symptoms was 13.4 (SD = 3.9). This represents reasonable satisfaction.[12] For example, participants who reported complete satisfaction on the questionnaire item regarding "what your doctor told you about what was wrong with you?" had a mean total satisfaction score for explanation of 11.5 whereas those who very dissatisfied on this item scored 21.8. Twenty-one of 145 (14.5%) scored 1 SD or more above the mean, indicating dissatisfaction.

The mean score for satisfaction with doctor-patient communication was: 19.3 (SD = 7.4). This corresponds with only fair satisfaction as, for example, on the item concerning the doctor's understanding of the patient's concerns, those completely satisfied scored 5.0 compared to 37.8 for those very dissatisfied. Twenty-two out of 145 participants (15.2%) scored 1 SD above the mean.

Do Somatic Symptoms and Anxieties Predict Outcomes?

Table 1 provides an overview of the relationship between predictors and outcomes using continuous scores and correlation coefficient. Baseline total somatic symptoms score was significantly associated with all outcomes except symptom improvement and satisfaction with doctor-patient communication. Similarly, HAQ interference with life (indicating bodily symptoms that prevent enjoyment, working, and concentration) predicted all outcomes except satisfaction with doctor-patient communication.

The HAQ subscale 'reassurance seeking behavior' did not predict outcome. Both 'fear of illness and death' and 'health worries and preoccupation' scores predicted mental component score at follow-up and the latter predicted dissatisfaction with the doctor's explanation of symptoms.

When these correlation coefficients were repeated separately for patients with medically explained and unexplained symptoms, the correlation coefficients were very similar

Table 1
Significant correlations (Spearman correlation coefficient) between predictors and outcomes

Predictors	Health Anxiety Questionnaire			
	Somatic Symptom Count	Fear of Illness and Death	Health Worries and Preoccupation	Interference with Life
Outcomes				
Number of medical consultations subsequent 6 months	r = 0.32 P<.001	—	—	r = 0.28 P<.001
SF PCS follow-up score	r = −0.54 P<.001	—	—	r = −0.49 P<.001
MCS follow-up score	r = −0.37 P<.001	r = −0.22 P<.002	r = −0.33 P<.001	r = −0.43 P<.001
Satisfaction score - mean (SD): Explanation Communication	r = 0.36 P<.001 —	— —	r = 0.26 P = .001 —	r = 0.38 P<.001 —

Abbreviations: MCS, Mental component score; PCS, Physical component score.
The negative sign indicates that the correlation is negative, ie, higher somatic symptom score or greater health anxiety are associated with reduced (impaired) health status (SF scores). The remaining correlations indicate that higher somatic symptom score or greater health anxiety are associated with greater number of medical consultations and greater dissatisfaction.

in the 2 groups but group sizes were, of course, smaller. For patients with medically explained symptoms the association (Spearman r) between total somatic symptom score, SF physical and mental summary scores, and number of consultations were −0.49, −0.51, and 0.35 (all P<.001). Corresponding data for medically unexplained symptoms were comparable: −0.49 (P<.001), −0.27 (P = .020), and −0.33 (P = .001).

For patients with medically explained symptoms the association (Spearman r) between HAQ interference with life score and number of consultations was: 0.18 (P = .016) whereas for patients with medically unexplained symptoms the association was stronger: 0.42 (P<.001). Only the latter correlation coefficient (medically unexplained symptoms) remained significant after adjustment for anxiety and depression.

Similarly, for patients with medically explained symptoms the association between HAQ health worry and preoccupation score with mental component score and satisfaction with doctor's explanation were −0.24 (P = .006) and 0.22 (P = .0029) respectively. On the other hand for patients with medically unexplained symptoms the correlations were: −0.42 (P< .001) and 0.40 (P = .002). All of the 4 correlation coefficients mentioned in this paragraph became nonsignificant after adjustment for anxiety and depression.

CUT POINT SCORES AND PREDICTION OF OUTCOME

A cut point score of 9 on the somatic symptom scale identified 24.7% of the sample. This group had significantly more medical consultations during the subsequent 6 months than the remainder and had significantly lower (more impaired) scores on both physical and mental summary scores at follow-up even after adjustment for relevant baseline values (Table 2, top half).

Ten percent of the sample scored 30 or more on the Health Anxiety Questionnaire and these participants also had significantly higher consultation rate and greater impairment after adjustment for relevant baseline values (Table 2, bottom half).

Table 2
Outcome measures by group, based on cut point scores (Somatic symptom score of 9 or more in top half of table and health anxiety score of 30 or more in bottom half of the table). SF-36 follow-up scores are adjusted for relevant baseline value and number of consultations is adjusted for number of consultations in previous 12 months

	IPQ Somatic Symptom Score 9+	IPQ Somatic Symptom Score <9	P Value[a]
Median number of medical consultations (IQR)	6 (4–9) (N = 65)	4 (2–6) (N = 210)	.018[a,b]
SF PCS follow-up score: mean (SEM)	37.3 (1.27) (N = 52)	40.5 (0.7) (N = 146)	.038[a]
SF MCS follow-up score: mean (SEM)	40.0 (1.4) (N = 52)	44.6 (0.8) (N = 146)	.006[a]
Satisfaction score: mean (SD):	(N = 55)	(N = 90)	
Explanation	15.0 (3.5)	12.6 (3.6)	P = .001
Communication	20.8 (7.8)	18.3 (7.0)	P = .49
7 or more consultations during follow-up 6 months	33/65 (50.8%)	61/211 (28.9%)	χ^2 = 10.57, P = .001
Symptom(s) Improved at follow-up	15/50 (30.0%)	67/141 (47.5%)	χ^2 = 4.62, P = .032
	HAQ Total 30+	**HAQ Total <30**	
Median number of medical consultations (IQR)	8 (4–9 (N = 26)	5 (2–7) (N = 247)	.027[a,b]
SF PCS follow-up score	39.6 (0.6) (N = 13)	43.2 (2.3) (N = 184)	.14[a]
MCS follow-up score	37.3 (2.7) (N = 13)	43.7 (0.7) (N = 184)	.026[a]
Satisfaction score, mean (SD):	(N = 17)	(N = 126)	
Explanation	15.5 (3.9)	13.2 (3.7)	P = .021
Communication	21.4 (8.1)	18.9 (7.3)	P = .20
7 or more consultations during follow-up 6 months	17/26 (65.4%)	75/247 (30.4%)	χ^2 = 12.9, P<.001
Symptom(s) Improved at follow-up	4/15 (26.7%)	77/174 (44.3%)	χ^2 = 1.74, P = .19

Abbreviations: MCS, mental component score; PCS, physical component score; SEM, standard error of mean.
[a] Adjusted for relevant baseline value of outcome measure.
[b] Assessed using log transformed number of consultations.

Those participants with scores above cut point on somatic symptom and health anxiety scales had higher scores (greater dissatisfaction) with the explanation provided by the doctor for their symptoms and subsequent management (see **Table 2**); there was no difference for satisfaction with doctor-patient communication.

The proportion of participants with 7 or more consultations during the 6-month follow-up period was significantly greater for those with scores above cut point on somatic symptoms than the remainder; there was 2-fold difference in this proportion for the health anxiety groups (**Table 2**, penultimate row).

Symptom improvement was significantly less likely only for the participants with a high somatic symptom score.

Examining these relationships separately for patients with symptoms explained or unexplained yielded small groups. The associations between high somatic symptom score and medical consultations, and the physical and mental component score were significant only for patients with medically explained symptoms. The association between high health anxiety score and 7 or more consultations was found only in those with medically unexplained symptoms.

Combining the Groups with Somatic Symptom and Health Anxiety Scores above Cut Points

The sample was divided into 4 groups: below cut point score on both scales (group A), above cut point on health anxiety only (group B), above cut point on somatic symptoms scale only (group C) and above cut point on both scales (group D).

A high consultation rate and impairment on the physical summary score were associated with a high somatic symptom count, whether or not it was accompanied by high health anxiety (Groups C and D: top 2 rows of **Table 3A**). These differences did not reach statistical significance after adjustment for baseline values in addition to other confounders, but numbers in the groups were small.

Impairment on the mental component score was apparent in all 3 groups with high scores on either scale (groups B–D) but greatest in the group with high scores on both scales (group D) (**Table 3A**, third row).

Only in group D were the satisfaction scores (adjusted only for age, sex, and medically (un) explained symptoms) clearly raised, indicating dissatisfaction with both the doctor's explanation of the symptoms and doctor-patient communication (**Table 3A**, fourth row). These differences were significant in spite of the small numbers.

In the unadjusted analyses (**Table 3B**) it can be seen that symptomatic improvement was rare in patients who scored above cut point for both somatic symptoms and health anxiety (Group D: **Table 3B**, top row). The majority of group D had a follow-up mental component score 1.5 SD below population norm, indicating significantly greater impairment than the other groups. Half had 7 or more consultations over the subsequent 6 months. Nearly half of group D expressed clear dissatisfaction with the doctor's explanation compared to less than 13% of groups A–C (**Table 3B**, fifth row). There was no significant difference in satisfaction with doctor-patient communication.

There was no significant difference in the proportion of patients with medically unexplained symptoms across groups A–D and the results reported above were similar for patients with medically explained or unexplained symptoms. For example, the proportion of participants in groups B–D who reported that their symptoms had improved was 13/44 (29.5%) for those with medically explained symptoms and 8/28 (28.6%) for those with medically unexplained symptoms. The corresponding proportions for group A were 52.7% and 43.5% respectively.

Group D was associated with low socio economic status and showed a trend towards greater proportion with divorced, separated, or widowed status but there was no difference on the other socio-demographic characteristics.

Predicting Quality of Life, Number of Consultations, and Satisfaction Using Multivariate Analysis to Adjust for Relevant Confounders

The results of the multiple regression analyses are shown in **Tables 4–7**. These results are shown for model 1, which included SF-36 scale for physical function (to adjust for physical disability) as well as demographic features, somatic symptom, health anxiety. In model 2 total HADS (anxiety plus depression) score was also entered, as they are known to be associated with somatoform disorders. The

Table 3

A. Comparison of 4 groups according to high health anxiety, high somatic symptom count or both. Means (standard error of means) shown for outcome scores (number of consultations, physical, and mental component scores and satisfaction) adjusted for age, sex, medically explained or unexplained symptoms and relevant baseline value

	Group A Neither High Health Anxiety or High Somatic Symptom Count	Group B High Health Anxiety Only	Group C High Somatic Symptom Count Only	Group D Both High Health Anxiety & High Somatic Symptom Count	Adjusted P Value
Median (IQR) number of medical consultations over subsequent 6 months	4 (2–6)\nn = 176	4 (2–8)\nn = 31	7 (4–8)\nn = 47	7 (4–9)\nn = 18	P = .073[a]
Mean SF36 Physical Component Score mean (SEM)	40.6 (0.76)\n(n = 126)	42.4 (1.9)\n(n = 19)	36.9 (1.4)\n(n = 40)	37.9 (2.4)\n(n = 12)	P = .060
Mean SF36 Mental Component Score mean (SEM)	44.9 (0.9)\n(n = 126)	42.4 (2.2)\n(n = 19)	40.7 (1.5)\n(n = 40)	36.7 (2.9)\n(n = 12)	P = .016
Satisfaction score[b]—mean (SEM):	(n = 74)	(n = 14)	(n = 40)	(n = 15)	
Explanation	12.5 (0.4)	12.6 (0.9)	14.2 (0.5)	17.2 (0.9)	P<.001
Communication	17.8 (0.8)	19.8 (1.9)	20.1 (1.1)	23.5 (1.8)	P = .029

[a] Assessed using log transformed number of consultations and P adjusted for number of consultations in 12 months prior to index clinic visit.
[b] P adjusted for age, sex and medically explained vs unexplained symptoms only.

Table 3

B. Comparison of 4 groups according to high health anxiety, high somatic symptom count, or both. Categorical measures of outcome and socio-demographic characteristics of the groups. Percentages for categorical variables with chi-square and P value

	Group A Neither High Health Anxiety or High Somatic Symptom Count	Group B High Health Anxiety Only	Group C High Somatic Symptom Count Only	Group D Both High Health Anxiety & High Somatic Symptom Count	Unadjusted P Values
Symptom(s) Improved at follow-up	59/120 (49.2%)	7/19 (36.8%)	13/39 (33.3%)	2/11 (18.2%)	$\chi^2 = 6.41$, $P = .093$
SF-36 Physical score 30 or less	21/123 (17.1%)	6/20 (30%)	18/40 (45.0%)	5/11 (45.5%)	$\chi^2 = 15.0$, $P = .002$
SF-36 mental score 35 or less	21/126 (16.7%)	6/20 (30%)	14/41 (34.1%)	8/11 (72.7%)	$\chi^2 = 20.26$, $P < .001$
7 or more consultations during follow-up 6 months	47/177 (27%)	12/31 (38.7%)	24/47 (51.1%)	9/18 (50%)	$\chi^2 = 12.88$, $P = .005$
Marked dissatisfaction (score in top 15%) Explanation	9/74 (12.2%)	1/14 (7.5%)	3/40 (7.5%)	7/15 (46.7%)	$\chi^2 = 15.46$, $P = .001$
Number (%) women	104/186 (55.9%)	15/33 (45.5%)	32/52 (61.5%)	11/21 (52.4%)	$\chi^2 = 2.21$, $P = .53$
Medically unexplained symptoms	71/186 (33.1%)	15/33 (45.5%)	17/52 (32.7%)	10/21 (47.6%)	$\chi^2 = 2.15$, $P = .54$
Separated, widowed or divorced	37/183 (20.2%)	4/30 (13.3%)	10/52 (19.2%)	13/21 (42.9%)	$\chi^2 = 7.28$, $P = .063$
Low socio-economic status	63/165 (38.1%)	14/25 (56%)	29/50 (58%)	13/19 (68.4%)	$\chi^2 = 11.81$, $P = .008$
White Caucasian	170/186 (91.4%)	25/33 (75.8%)	47/52 (90.4%)	18/21 (85.7%)	$\chi^2 = 7.36$, $P = .061$

Table 4
Multiple linear regression to predict follow-up SF-36 physical component score

	Model 1 with Somatic Symptom Score			Model 2 Including Anxiety and Depression		
	B	SE	Sig	B	SE	Sig
Age	−0.127	0.053	0.018	−0.12	0.053	0.028
SF-36 physical function score	0.20	0.027	<0.001	0.20	0.027	<0.001
HAQ interference with life	−0.753	0.31	0.016	−0.89	0.32	0.006
IPQ somatic symptom score	−1.28	0.26	<0.001	−1.42	0.27	<0.001
HADS total score				0.158	0.11	0.16

Not included in final model: Sex, medically (un)explained symptoms, divorced, separated or widowed status, SES, HAQ health worry and preoccupation subscale score.

outcomes measures were used in turn as the dependent variable (physical and mental component scores, number of medical consultations, and satisfaction scores).

In each table the variables that were significant independent predictors of the relevant outcome are shown plus the regression coefficient for HADS total score (anxiety plus depression), which is included in every table. The variables that were not significant in either model are listed below each table.

Table 4 shows that the significant independent predictors of SF36 physical component score were age, baseline SF Physical function score (physical impairment), HAQ interference with life scale and total somatic symptoms score. HADS anxiety and depression score and the other variables listed below **Table 4** were not included in the final model.

Table 5 shows that only age and total HADS anxiety and depression score were predictors of SF36 mental component scale. HAQ health worry and preoccupation, HAQ interference with life scale, and total somatic symptoms score were significant predictors in model 1, but their predictive effect on mental component score was mediated by anxiety and depression.

Table 6 shows that female sex and number of somatic symptoms were predictors of a high number of medical consultations. **Table 7** shows that age, sex, and somatic

Table 5
Multiple linear regression to predict follow-up SF-36 mental component score

	Model 1 with Somatic Symptom Score			Model 2 Including Anxiety and Depression		
	B	SE	Sig	B	SE	Sig
Age	−0.21	0.064	0.001	−0.17	0.058	0.005
HAQ health worry and preoccupation 10 +	−4.23	2.07	0.043			
HAQ interference with life	−0.96	0.37	0.011	−0.31	0.35	0.38
IPQ somatic symptom score	−0.97	0.31	0.002	−0.31	0.30	0.30
HADS total				−0.75	0.12	<0.001

Not included in final model: Sex, medically (un)explained symptoms, divorced, separated or widowed status, SES, baseline SF-36 physical function score.

Table 6
Multiple linear regression to predict number of consultations

	Model 1 with Somatic Symptom Score			Model 2 Including Anxiety and Depression		
	B	SE	Sig	B	SE	Sig
Sex	−0.107	0.033	0.001	−0.108	0.033	0.001
HAQ interference with life	0.014	0.008	0.077	0.14	0.08	0.090
IPQ somatic symptom score	0.02	0.06	0.002	0.020	0.007	0.004
HADS total score				<0.001	0.003	0.99

Not included in final model: Age, medically (un)explained symptoms, divorced, separated or widowed status, SES, baseline SF-36 physical function score, HAQ health worry and preoccupation score.

symptoms score predicted satisfaction on the explanation scale; HAQ health worry and preoccupation score predicted satisfaction until HADS score was added to the model. These variables had a Variance Inflation Factor under 3 suggesting that collinearity was not a problem.

In summary, these analyses (see **Tables 4–7**) show that number of somatic symptoms is an independent predictor of all 4 outcomes (physical and mental component scores, number of medical consultations, and (dis)satisfaction with doctor's explanation). HAQ interference with life subscale score is an independent predictor of physical component score and the HAQ health worry and preoccupation score predicts (dis)satisfaction until HADS total score is added to the model. Anxiety and depression (HADS total score) is an independent predictor of mental component score only.

DISCUSSION

In relation to our first aim, we have shown that, among patients attending medical out-patient clinics, identification of those who score above cut point points for total somatic symptoms count and for health anxiety produces clinically meaningful groups with worse outcomes than the remainder. These findings are robust in the

Table 7
Multiple linear regression to predict satisfaction with doctor's explanation

	Model 1 with Somatic Symptom Score			Model 2 Including Anxiety and Depression		
	B	SE	Sig	B	SE	Sig
Age	0.067	0.024	0.007	0.061	0.024	0.014
Sex	−0.187	0.593	0.002	−1.195	0.59	0.001
HAQ health worry and preoccupation 10 +	2.025	0.75	0.008	1.465	0.814	0.074
IPQ somatic symptom score	0.36	0.123	0.004	0.281	0.131	0.034
HAD total score				0.083	0.049	0.093

Not included in final model: Medically (un)explained symptoms, divorced, separated or widowed status, SES, baseline SF-36 physical function score, HAQ interference with life.

sense that many of the associations between the predictors and poor outcomes remained significant after controlling for the baseline value of the relevant outcome measure (see **Table 2**) as well as adjusting for a number of other confounders (see **Tables 4–7**). It is interesting that a high somatic symptom score is clearly associated with poor outcome in all 4 of our outcome measures whereas HADS anxiety and depression score was a predictor for only 1 outcome, the mental component score.

Our data suggest that the relationships between total somatic symptom count, health status, and consultation rate were similar for patients whose symptoms were medically explained or not explained. This suggests that the relationship between predictors and outcome is similar whatever the aetiology of the symptoms. The relationship between high health anxiety and poor outcome appears somewhat stronger in those with "medically unexplained" symptoms than the remainder, though this appears to be the result of the higher anxiety and depression scores in this group. In the multivariate analyses where we included medically explained or unexplained symptoms as a variable, this did not appear as an independent predictor.

Before discussing the results further it is necessary to recognize the limitations of this study. The results are based on secondary analyses of an existing dataset, which was not collected for this purpose. In particular, the numbers of participants was rather small in those groups that are defined by a very high health anxiety score and in the analyses of satisfaction data, which were limited to patients attending two of the clinics. The limited numbers restricts the statistical power of the study. Therefore we must be aware of the possibility of Type II errors but the statistical associations we have found, even after adjustment for confounders, are interesting.

The population we studied seems typical of patients attending secondary or tertiary referral specialist medical clinics and is quite severely impaired.[38] This means that the results cannot be extrapolated to other populations, especially primary care and population based samples. In addition, we did not use standardized research interviews so it was impossible to identify people with DSM-IV somatoform disorders. We lacked also detailed information on the number and type of medical diagnoses, which is a potential confounder. The response rate was just adequate.

On the other hand, the study has a number of strengths. It is rare to have such a wide range of outcome measures in a single prospective study. This allowed us to examine health status, health care use and satisfaction, which are the relevant outcomes in this group, although it did lead us to perform a large number of analyses. Since these analyses concerned separate dimensions of outcome, it was not necessary to use a Bonferroni correction but entering closely related variables into multiple regression could have led to a problem of collinearity, though this did not appear to be the case. We used recognized measures of somatic symptoms and health anxiety, though these have not been used widely in this context so we cannot compare our results directly with those of previous studies.[13–15] Number of medical consultations was derived from medical notes rather than participants' memory. The data set was reasonably complete for those participants who joined the study.

Our results extend the very limited prospective data showing that number of somatic symptoms, with or without health anxiety, are predictors of high health care use and impaired health status.[15,16,39] Most previous work examining this relationship has concerned people with medically unexplained symptoms only but we have shown that the relationship between number of somatic symptoms and poor outcomes holds also in people with serious physical illness. This has been shown in several previous prospective studies, which did not adjust for confounders,[40–44] and 1 recent cross-sectional study of people with cancer and pain or depression that did make these adjustments.[45]

We cannot decide from these data whether the cut point scores that we chose were optimal. This would require a much larger sample in which different thresholds could be compared. Our cut point on the somatic symptoms scale identified just under 25% of the sample. This is a larger proportion than the 14–20% used in some previous studies but since our sample came from secondary and tertiary clinics, rather than primary care, one would expect a higher proportion to have a troublesome number of somatic symptoms. In fact, reporting 9 different somatic symptoms which are present most or all of the time is a high symptom burden.[40,41,43,45,46] Our cut point score on the health anxiety scale was much higher (identifying only the top 10%) because we found that only at this high level of health anxiety was there an association with impaired outcome in our previous study (see **Fig. 1**).

The measures of somatic symptoms and health anxiety are not truly independent of each other because the HAQ interference with life scale actually asks whether bodily symptoms impaired the respondent's ability to enjoy themselves, concentrate, and work. This is a measure of burdensomeness of somatic symptoms. It is interesting that both number of somatic symptoms and their burdensomeness were independently associated with outcome in the first model of the regression analyses.

We had expected that anxiety and depression would be included as an independent predictor of all outcomes but this turned out to be true only for mental component score; it was not a predictor of physical score, number of medical consultations, or satisfaction (see **Tables 4, 6,** and **7**). Our data do not support the notion that multiple somatic symptoms is primarily a manifestation of depression and anxiety.[47]

Compared to participants with scores below cut points on both scales, those participants who scored 9 or more on the total somatic symptoms count and/or 30 or more on the HAQ had approximately 3 times the chance of marked impairment and marked dissatisfaction and nearly twice the chance of having frequent medical consultations. This suggests that these scores would have clinical utility as in clinical practice the clinician requires a readily applied measure that will indicate which patients are likely to have a poor outcome and, therefore, might benefit from additional, psychological treatment. In this context it is not necessary to make adjustments for severity of physical illness or presence of anxiety or depression; the clinician simply needs to identify the patients who are at risk of poor outcome and might benefit from further treatment. A consultation rate of 7 during 6 months equates to 14 consultations per year, which is similar to the 12–14 visits in the previous year reported by the "high somatization" patients of previous studies.[13,14]

The results of this study have implications for the proposed DSM-V diagnosis of complex somatic symptoms disorder. In view of its clear association with poor outcomes, it is appropriate that numerous bothersome somatic symptoms should be a key feature of this disorder. It appears appropriate also to include all somatic symptoms, not just those that have been rated as "medically unexplained."

There is some support for the addition of health anxiety as another key feature of the complex somatic symptoms diagnosis, partly because of the considerable overlap between numerous somatic symptoms and high health anxiety and partly because these 2 measures were independent predictors of several outcomes in our multiple regression analyses. Furthermore, our participants who had both numerous somatic symptoms and high health anxiety were much more likely to express dissatisfaction with the doctor-patient communication and the doctor's explanation of the symptoms and their planned treatment. This would correspond to the 'difficult' doctor-patient relationship that has been associated with patients who have this kind of disorder. It does seem appropriate to have a high threshold for inclusion of health anxiety in the diagnosis; 2 out of 3 features of health anxiety are required in complex somatic symptoms disorder (http://www.dsm5.org/ProposedRevisions/Pages/proposedrevision.aspx?rid=368).

There has been very little previous work assessing outcome in people who have both numerous somatic symptoms and a high health anxiety score, but our data in this respect must be regarded as preliminary because of small numbers (group D in **Table 3**). This analysis must be repeated in larger samples. In a population-based sample of over 700, however, it was shown that both somatic symptoms score and health anxiety contributed as independent predictors to a high consultation rate in primary care over the subsequent year after adjustment for confounders, including physical and psychiatric illness.[48] Like ours, that study found that subsequent consultation rate was more closely associated with number of somatic symptoms than health anxiety. That study found that for every 10 unit increase in health anxiety score, an individual was likely to consult 1.5 times more frequently but for every 5-unit increase on the Somatic Symptom Scale, patients consulted almost 3 times as often. Thus the same relationships between predictors and outcome that we found appear to hold in primary care though the optimal cut point scores on scales of somatic symptoms and health anxiety might be lower in that setting.

SUMMARY

Our findings suggest that cut point scores on scales of somatic symptoms and health anxiety have clinical utility as they predict outcome. Our data also suggest that the relationship between these predictors and outcomes hold for both medically explained and unexplained symptoms. We did not find evidence that general anxiety and depression were responsible for these predictor-outcome relationships. Further work is needed to test the optimal cut point scores in primary and secondary health care settings and in population-based samples. There is some support for the combination of somatic symptoms and health anxiety as proposed in DSM-V complex somatic symptoms disorder.

ACKNOWLEDGMENTS

This work was funded by the Central Manchester NHS Trust R&D Directorate and the Functional Gastrointestinal Disorders Working Group.

REFERENCES

1. Dimsdale J, Creed FH, DSM-V Workgroup on Somatic Symptom Disorders. The proposed diagnosis of somatic symptom disorders in DSM-V to replace somatoform disorders in DSM-IV–a preliminary report. J Psychosom Res 2009;66:473–6.
2. Regier DA. Dimensional approaches to psychiatric classification: refining the research agenda for DSM-V: an introduction [review]. Int J Methods Psychiatr Res 2007;16 (Suppl 1):S1–5.
3. Farmer AD, Aziz Q, Tack J, et al. The future of neuroscientific research in functional gastrointestinal disorders: integration towards multidimensional (visceral) pain endophenotypes? J Psychosom Res 2010;68:475–81.
4. Luppino FS, van Reedt Dortland AK, Wardenaar KJ, et al. Symptom dimensions of depression and anxiety and the metabolic syndrome. Psychosom Med 2011;73: 257–64.
5. Kroenke K, Spitzer RL, Williams JB, et al. The Patient Health Questionnaire Somatic, Anxiety, and Depressive Symptom Scales: a systematic review. Gen Hospital Psychiatry 2010;32:345–59.

6. Hansen HS, Rosendal M, Oernboel E, et al. Are medically unexplained symptoms and functional disorders predictive for the illness course? A two-year follow-up on patients' health and health care utilisation. J Psychosom Res 2011;71(1):38–44.

7. Voigt K, Nagel A, Meyer B, et al. Towards positive diagnostic criteria: a systematic review of somatoform disorder diagnoses and suggestions for future classification. J Psychosom Res 2010;68:403–14.

8. Wijeratne C, Hickie I, Davenport T. Is there an independent somatic symptom dimension in older people? J Psychosom Res 2006;61:197–204.

9. Mattila AK, Saarni SI, Alanen E, et al. Health-related quality-of-life profiles in nonalexithymic and alexithymic subjects from general population. J Psychosom Res 2010; 68:279–83.

10. Jackson J, Fiddler M, Kapur N, et al. Number of bodily symptoms predicts outcome more accurately than health anxiety in patients attending neurology, cardiology, and gastroenterology clinics. J Psychosom Res 2006;60:357–63.

11. Fiddler M, Jackson J, Kapur N, et al. Childhood adversity and frequent medical consultations. Gen Hosp Psychiatry 2004;26:367–77.

12. Jackson J, Kincey J, Fiddler M, et al. Differences between out-patients with physical disease and those with medically unexplained symptoms with respect to patient satisfaction, emotional distress and illness perception. Br J Health Psychol 2004;9:433–46.

13. Kroenke K, Spitzer RL, Williams JB. The PHQ-15: validity of a new measure for evaluating the severity of somatic symptoms. Psychosom Med 2002;64:258–66.

14. Barsky AJ, Orav EJ, Bates DW. Somatization increases medical utilization and costs independent of psychiatric and medical comorbidity. Arch Gen Psychiatry 2005;62: 903–10.

15. Harris AM, Orav EJ, Bates DW, et al. Somatization increases disability independent of comorbidity. J Gen Intern Med 2009;24:155–61.

16. Barsky AJ, Ettner SL, Horsky J, et al. Resource utilization of patients with hypochondriacal health anxiety and somatization. Med Care 2001;39:705–15.

17. Kirmayer LJ, Robbins JM. Three forms of somatization in primary care: prevalence, co-occurrence, and sociodemographic characteristics. J Nerv Ment Dis 1991;179:647–55.

18. Peveler R, Kilkenny L, Kinmonth AL. Medically unexplained physical symptoms in primary care: a comparison of self-report screening questionnaires and clinical opinion. J Psychosom Res 1997;42:245–52.

19. Sartorius N. Disability and mental illness are different entities and should be assessed separately. World Psychiatry 2009;8:86.

20. Creed F, Barsky A. A systematic review of somatisation and hypochondriasis. J Psychosom Res 2004;56:391–408.

21. Lynch DJ, McGrady A, Nagel R, et al. Somatization in family practice: comparing 5 methods of classification. Prim Care Companion J Clin Psychiatry 1999;1:85–9.

22. Noyes R Jr, Hartz AJ, Doebbeling CC, et al. Illness fears in the general population. Psychosom Med 2000;62:318–25.

23. Rief W, Hessel A, Braehler E. Somatization symptoms and hypochondriacal features in the general population. Psychosom Med 2001;63:595–602.

24. Looper KJ, Kirmayer LJ. Hypochondriacal concerns in a community population. Psychol Med 2001;31:577–84.

25. Reid S, Crayford T, Richards S, et al. Recognition of medically unexplained symptoms–do doctors agree? J Psychosom Res 1999;47:483–5.

26. Goldthorpe J, Hope K. The social grading of occupations: a new approach and scale. Oxford: Oxford University Press; 1974.

27. Zigmond AS, Snaith RP. The hospital anxiety and depression scale. Acta Psychiatr Scand 1983;67:361–70.

28. Bjelland I, Dahl AA, Haug TT, et al. The validity of the Hospital Anxiety and Depression Scale. An updated literature review. J Psychosom Res 2002;52:69–77.
29. Weinman J, Petrie K, Moss-Morriss R, et al. The illness perception questionnaire: a new method for assessing the cognitive representation of illness. Psychol Health 1996;11:114–29.
30. Lucock MP, Morley S. The health anxiety questionnaire. Br J Health Psychol 1996:1; 137–50.
31. Ware JE Jr, Sherbourne CD. The MOS 36-item short-form health survey (SF-36). I. Conceptual framework and item selection. Med Care 1992;30:473–83.
32. Ware JE, Kosinski M, Keller SD. SF-36 physical and mental health summary scales: a user's manual. Boston: The Health Institute; 1994.
33. Rosenzweig S, Greeson JM, Reibel DK, et al. Mindfulness-based stress reduction for chronic pain conditions: variation in treatment outcomes and role of home meditation practice. J Psychosomatic Research 2010;68:29–36.
34. Dickens CM, McGowan L, Percival C, et al. Contribution of depression and anxiety to impaired health-related quality of life following first myocardial infarction. Br J Psychiatry 2006;189:367–72.
35. Creed F, Fernandes L, Guthrie E, et al. The cost-effectiveness of psychotherapy and paroxetine for severe irritable bowel syndrome [see comment]. Gastroenterology 2003;124:303–17.
36. Myint PK, Luben RN, Surtees PG, et al. Relation between self-reported physical functional health and chronic disease mortality in men and women in the European Prospective Investigation into Cancer (EPIC-Norfolk): a prospective population study. Ann Epidemiol 2006;16:492–500.
37. Wolfe F, Hassett AL, Katz RS, et al. Do we need core sets of fibromyalgia domains? the assessment of fibromyalgia (and other rheumatic disorders) in clinical practice. J Rheumatol 2011;38(6):1104–12.
38. Creed FH, Barsky A, Leiknes KA. Epidemiology: prevalence, causes and consequences. In: Creed F, Henningsen P, Fink P, editors. Medically unexplained symptoms, somatisation and bodily distress: developing better clinical services. Cambridge: Cambridge University Press; 2011. p. 1–42.
39. Sha MC, Callahan CM, Counsell SR, et al. Physical symptoms as a predictor of health care use and mortality among older adults. Am J Med 2005;118:301–6.
40. Dickens C, McGowan L, Percival C, et al. Negative illness perceptions are associated with new-onset depression following myocardial infarction. Gen Hosp Psychiatry 2008;30:414–20.
41. Stafford L, Berk M, Jackson HJ. Are illness perceptions about coronary artery disease predictive of depression and quality of life outcomes? J Psychosom Res 2009;66: 211.
42. Juergens MC, Seekatz B, Moosdorf RG, et al. Illness beliefs before cardiac surgery predict disability, quality of life, and depression 3 months later. J Psychosom Res 2010;68:553–60.
43. Bijsterbosch J, Scharloo M, Visser AW, et al. Illness perceptions in patients with osteoarthritis: change over time and association with disability. Arthritis Rheum 2009;61:1054–61.
44. Scharloo M, Baatenburg de Jong RJ, Langeveld TP, et al. Quality of life and illness perceptions in patients with recently diagnosed head and neck cancer. Head Neck 2005;27:857–63.
45. Kroenke K, Zhong X, Theobald D, et al. Somatic symptoms in patients with cancer experiencing pain or depression: prevalence, disability, and health care use. Arch Intern Med 2010;170:1686–94.

46. Katon W, Lin EH, Kroenke K. The association of depression and anxiety with medical symptom burden in patients with chronic medical illness. Gen Hosp Psychiatry 2007;29:147–55.
47. Mayou R, Kirmayer LJ, Simon G, et al. Somatoform disorders: time for a new approach in DSM-V [see comment]. Am J Psychiatry 2005;162:847–55.
48. Kapur N, Hunt I, Lunt M, et al. Psychosocial and illness related predictors of consultation rates in primary care–a cohort study. Psychol Med 2004;34:719–28.

Relevance of Cognitive and Behavioral Factors in Medically Unexplained Syndromes and Somatoform Disorders

Alexandra Martin, PhD[a],*, Winfried Rief, PhD[b]

KEYWORDS

- Illness worry • Pain • Somatic symptoms
- Causal attribution • Catastrophizing • Fear-avoidance

INTRODUCTION

Many physical complaints cannot be accounted for by any known specific pathophysiology or known disease; 25–80% of all symptoms presented in the primary care setting are considered to be of unclear origin.[1] Even in the general population unspecific somatic symptoms are experienced very often.[2] Though the majority of these symptoms are transient phenomena that do not require further treatment, in some people these bodily complaints persist over years, resulting in severe distress and disability. Reviewing the existing longitudinal studies, evidence suggests that especially the presence of multiple symptoms (rather than single symptoms) of unclear origin is associated with chronic course and higher degrees of functional disability at follow-up.[3,4] Moreover, it has been postulated that the presence of cognitive and behavioral features in patients with somatic symptoms is associated with higher disability, symptom persistence, and increased health care needs.[5] In this paper, we will summarize psychological features that are considered to be of relevance in the context of somatoform disorders, and that could be candidates for classification criteria for patients with complex syndromes.

[a] Department of Psychosomatic Medicine and Psychotherapy, University of Erlangen-Nürnberg, University Hospital Erlangen, Schwabachanlage 6, D-91054 Erlangen, Germany
[b] Department of Psychology, Division of Clinical Psychology and Psychological Intervention, University of Marburg, Gutenbergstraße 18, D-35037 Marburg, Germany
* Corresponding author.
E-mail address: Alexandra.martin@uk-erlangen.de

Psychiatr Clin N Am 34 (2011) 565–578
doi:10.1016/j.psc.2011.05.007
0193-953X/11/$ – see front matter © 2011 Elsevier Inc. All rights reserved.

Current and Future Classification of Somatoform Disorders

Although rarely used as a diagnosis in the US, medically unexplained somatic symptoms are supposed to be classified as somatoform disorder (SFD), if the symptoms have resulted in significant distress or psychosocial impairment. The main characteristic of Somatoform Disorders, according to the Diagnostic and Statistic Manual of Mental Disorders DSM IV,[6] is the existence of physical symptoms that cannot be fully explained by a known general medical condition or the direct effects of a substance. If a related general medical condition exists, the physical complaints or resulting social or occupational impairment need to exceed what would be expected from physical findings.

The Somatic Symptom Disorders Work Group of the APA is developing an improved classification proposal for DSM-5. Their first suggestion is to rename the category to 'Somatic Symptom Disorders' including not only the (former) somatoform disorders, but also subsuming 'psychological factors affecting medical condition,' and 'factitious disorders,' because all of them involve presentations of physical symptoms and/or concerns about medical illness. The Work Group further suggests classifying somatization disorder, hypochondriasis, undifferentiated somatoform disorder, and pain disorder under one common diagnosis called *complex somatic symptom disorder* (CSSD), based on the consideration that these disorders share many features like somatic symptoms and cognitive distortions (**Box 1**).

CSSD is drafted as a disorder characterized by chronic distressing or disabling somatic symptoms and also an excessive or maladaptive response to these symptoms (see **Box 1**). Compared to DSM-IV, it is a major change to omit the previous core criterion of somatoform disorders (lack of explicability of somatic symptoms) because of its implicit mind-body dualism and the unreliability of the decision to consider symptoms as "medically unexplained" (see **Box 1**, criterion A).

Box 1
Complex Somatic Symptom Disorder (CSSD)

Complex Somatic Symptom Disorder (APA, www.dsm5.org; Updated January 14, 2011).

To meet criteria for CSSD, criteria A, B, and C are all necessary.

A. **Somatic symptoms:** One or more somatic symptoms that are distressing and/or result in significant disruption of daily life.

B. **Excessive thoughts, feelings, and behaviors related to these somatic symptoms or associated health concerns:** At least two of the following are required to meet this criterion:

   1. High level of health-related anxiety

   2. Disproportionate and persistent concerns about the medical seriousness of one's symptoms

   3. Excessive time and energy devoted to these symptoms or health concerns

C. **Chronicity:** Although any one symptom may not be continuously present, the state of being symptomatic is chronic (at least 6 months).

For patients who fulfill the CSSD criteria, the following optional specifiers may be applied to a diagnosis of CSSD where one of them dominates the clinical presentation:

   1. Predominant somatic complaints (previously somatization disorder)

   2. Predominant health anxiety (previously hypochondriasis)

   3. Predominant pain (previously pain disorder)

CSSD focuses attention on the excessive or maladaptive response to the symptoms which is expressed in 'excessive thoughts, feelings, and behaviors related to these somatic symptoms or associated health concerns,' namely 'high level of health-related anxiety,' 'disproportionate and persistent concerns about the medical seriousness of one's symptoms,' and 'excessive time and energy devoted to these symptoms or health concerns' (see DSM-5 proposal, criterion B). The CSSD proposal acknowledges the importance of defining positive classification criteria, namely psychological factors, to improve the current classification of somatoform disorders.

The aim of this review is to provide an overview of the evidence regarding possible cognitive and behavioral candidate criteria, and to discuss the empirical validity to include or omit some of these features.

COGNITIVE FACTORS
Causal Symptom Attributions

Many authors consider the inflexible attribution of somatic symptoms to potential biomedical causes as a central characteristic of patients with somatoform disorders. Indeed, there is accumulating evidence that subjects with medically unexplained symptoms or somatoform disorders have the tendency to attribute their bodily symptoms predominantly to somatic causes as compared to psychosocial aspects[7-11] (see overview in **Table 1**). However, the majority of the studies also show that patients with somatoform symptoms do not hold simplistic, monocausal assumptions, but consider multiple causes as relevant to their symptoms—and many affected people consider additional psychological factors to be causative of their symptoms. Correlates of the report of psychosocial symptom causation are comorbid depression and anxiety in subjects with unexplained symptoms.[8-12]

Some studies have not found evidence for a stronger tendency to somatic causal attributions in patients suffering from 'medically unexplained symptoms' compared to patients with somatic symptoms of known pathophysiology.[13,14] This implies that causal attribution style may not be a sufficient classification criterion for somatoform disorders, as it lacks specificity in comparisons with other somatic conditions.[13] In relation to the CSSD proposal, however, the distinction between 'explained' and 'unexplained' pathophysiology is of less relevance. To qualify as a diagnostic criterion it would be important to show the possible impact of the subjective causal attribution on clinical course or outcome. Some findings from cross-sectional as well as from prospective studies suggest that patient's somatic attributions are a crucial factor associated with disability and chronic course of the condition:

Patients with somatoform disorders reporting predominantly biomedical causes felt more incapacitated by their bodily symptoms than did patients with psychosocial causal attributions, and their comorbid depressive symptoms were unchanged at 6-month follow-up.[8]

In addition, biomedical and vulnerability causal attributions in primary care patients with somatoform symptoms seem to be associated with various aspects of illness behavior, such as the subjective need for medical examinations, increased expression of symptoms, increased illness consequences, and bodily scanning,[11] and increased health care use (see review in Rief and Broadbent[15]).

Additional evidence for the role of causal explanations results from investigations in related syndromes, such as irritable bowel syndrome (IBS), chronic fatigue syndrome (CFS), and pain: Somatic attributions were associated with reduced physical quality of life and symptom severity in IBS,[16] and with symptom severity over time in a prospective study with patients suffering from CFS.[17] Preliminary data also

Table 1
Causal symptom attribution in patients with somatoform disorders (SFD) or with medically unexplained symptoms (MUS)

Authors	Setting	Sample	Control Group(s)	Assessment of Causal Attributions: Recall Method (instrument)	SFD/MUS Report Mainly Somatic Attributions	SFD/MUS Report Psychosocial/Mixed Attributions to a Significant Degree	Major Results
Duddu et al, 2003[7]	Psychiatry outpatients	SFD	DEP, Normal Controls	prompted (Q)	+		Disorder-specificity of attribution styles: SFD had highest somatic, depressed patients higher psychological and normal controls have highest normalizing attribution score. Experience of recent symptoms, diagnosis of SFD and lack of normalizing attributions were predictors of higher somatosensory amplification degrees.
Groben & Hausteiner, 2011[13]	Allergy clinic	SFD	NoSFD	spontaneous (I); prompted (Q)	(+); –	+; +	Lack of specificity: Patients with SFD presenting for an allergy diagnostic work-up were no more likely than non-somatoform control patients to report somatic explanations for their symptoms.
Henningsen et al, 2005[8]	Tertiary care, psychosomatic medicine and orthopedic	SFD	DEP/ANG	prompted (I)	+	+ (associated with DEP/ANG)	Pure SFD patients explained symptoms mainly with organic causal attributions, patients with pure depression/ anxiety mainly with psychosocial causes, and in diagnostic overlap group (SFD and DEP/ANG) they chose mixed causal attributions.

			PAIN				
Hiller et al, 2010[12]	Tertiary care, psychosomatic and pain clinics	SFD		prompted (I)		+ (associated with DEP)	Patients with predominantly organic perceived causes felt more incapacitated by their bodily symptoms than patients with psychosocial causal attributions. Patients with psychosocial perceived causes were less depressed at 6 months follow-up. On average, SFD patients chose 2.57 different attributions for each symptom. SFD patients attributed most of their symptoms to mental/emotional problems (46.9%) and somatic disease (41.1%). SFD and chronic pain showed distinguishable attribution patterns. Depression correlated positively with psychological/ stress attributions and negatively with somatic attributions.
Martin et al, 2007[9]	Tertiary care, psychosomatic hospital, inpatient	SFD	–	spontaneous (I)	+	+ (associated with DEP)	SFD patients reported significantly more somatic than psychological attributions; however psychological attributions were common too. The number of somatoform symptoms was positively associated and depression severity negatively associated with a tendency to report somatic attributions. Treatment gains were not worse in SFD patients with a predominantly somatic attribution style.

Table 1
(continued)

Authors	Setting	Sample	Control Group(s)	Assessment of Causal Attributions: Recall Method (instrument)	SFD/MUS Report Mainly Somatic Attributions	SFD/MUS Report Psychosocial/Mixed Attributions to a Significant Degree	Major Results
Nimnuan et al, 2001[10]	Tertiary care, general hospital, specialties, outpatient	MUS	noMUS	prompted (Q)	+	+	MUS patients were more likely to attribute their illness to physical causes as opposed to lifestyle factors. But many patients consider lifestyle and psychological attributions to be causally relevant, too. Physical attribution was associated with an increased risk of having MUS, but not psychological attributions.
Rief et al, 2004[11]	Primary care	SFD	noSFD	prompted (Q)	+	+ (associated with DEP/ANG)	SFD had increased scores on vulnerability and organic illness beliefs, though most patients reported multiple illness attributions. Comorbidity with depression and anxiety was associated with more psychological attributions. Organic and vulnerability causal attributions were associated with illness behavior (need for medical diagnostic examinations, increased expression of symptoms, increased illness consequences, bodily scanning)

		MUS	noMUS	prompted (Q)	−	+	
Taylor et al, 2000[14]	Primary care						MUS- patients were *no more likely* to report physical attribution than patients with explained symptoms. Instead, nearly half of MUS patients acknowledged emotional factors as causative while only one quarter of patients with explained symptoms did so. Regression analyses revealed that presentation with unexplained symptoms is predicted by abnormal attachment style, high GHQ psychopathology, and a tendency to make non-physical attribution of symptoms

Abbreviations: Sample: ANG, anxiety disorder; DEP, depression; MUS, medically unexplained symptoms; PAIN, chronic pain disorder; SFD, somatoform disorder.
Assessment instrument: I, interview; Q, questionnaire.
Assessment method: prompted, prompted/cued recall; spontaneous, free recall.

indicate a higher risk of developing a chronic pain disorder after acute herpes zoster infection in those subjects with greater physical disease conviction at the beginning.[18]

These findings indicate the prognostic significance of assessing patient's causal attribution as a complementary feature of clinical evaluation in subjects suffering from unspecific somatic symptoms. Yet the vast majority of studies have been conducted in clinical settings and a selection bias cannot be ruled out. Therefore we conducted a study based on a general population sample rather than a help-seeking sample.[5] Results confirmed the utility of ten psychological variables to identify subjects with somatic symptoms who needed medical help and/or were seriously disabled, and a "bias for somatic illness attributions" was one of them.

Together, these findings support the relevance of subjective causal symptom attribution on course, health care seeking, and outcome of symptoms in subjects suffering from somatic symptoms that cannot fully be explained by a known medical condition. The generalizability is still limited by the small number of prospective studies, and only little is known about the differential impact of illness related cognitions in groups with established diseases as compared to somatoform disorders. It seems possible that not only beliefs about the origin of the symptoms, but other illness beliefs—namely assumptions about 'low symptom controllability,' 'expectation of chronicity,' 'perceived consequences' of the health problem, and emotional representations—affect health related quality of life and also predict long-term outcome.[19,20]

Catastrophizing Cognitive Style and Cognitions

Catastrophizing is considered as the tendency to over-interpret the likelihood and/or intensity of potential negative consequences of symptoms. Patients with a catastrophizing cognitive style anticipate, ruminate, magnify, and feel helpless about terrible outcomes. This concept is negatively associated with the ability to tolerate pain and other symptoms. Pain catastrophizing has consistently been associated with pain disability in pain patients, as well as in the general population (see reviews[21,22]). Prospective studies have demonstrated that initial pain catastrophizing is related to higher pain intensity in a variety of situations, eg, during a subsequent painful procedure, after surgery, and in the long-term adjustment to lower-limb amputation.[21,22] The psychological variable pain catastrophizing is closely related to brain activity after experimental pain.[23] Sullivan and colleagues[24] provided experimental support that initial levels of pain catastrophizing were related to subsequent activity intolerance. Thus, there is robust empirical evidence for the relevance of the cognitive process of catastrophizing for immediate and long-term related outcomes in pain conditions. Therefore catastrophizing can be considered to be a useful classification feature for CSSD.

Many patients with medically unexplained symptoms have a tendency to over-interpret physical sensations.[25] Such patients believe that being healthy is defined by the total absence of any physical sensations, or they show other signs of an over-exclusive cognitive concept of health.[26] Barsky and colleagues[27] compared patients with hypochondriasis to a non-hypochondriasis group; they found that hypochondriacs believed good health to be relatively symptom-free, and vice versa every somatic symptom indicates a sickness. Together with the fact that some physical symptoms are normal and up to 80% of the general population report at least some somatic complaints for the last 7 days,[2] an over-exclusive concept of health provides the basis for misinterpreting somatic sensations as signs of serious medical conditions, and searching treatment for these complaints.

Further cognitive aspects have been discussed in the context of somatoform disorders. Patients with somatoform complaints show a stronger *self-concept of bodily weakness*, which appears to be specific compared to patients with other mental disorders.[25] However, this self-concept may also be a consequence of severe disability due to symptoms rather than a distinct factor in somatoform disorders, and one study showed that it might not be common across the different manifestations of somatoform disorders.[28] Special interactional patterns have been also reported to characterize patients with somatoform symptoms, with distrust being more prominent compared to healthy controls. This can offer a link to increased rates of personality disorders in somatoform disorders.[29] However, these additional cognitive styles need further evaluation, especially about their specificity for somatoform disorders.

BEHAVIORAL CHARACTERISTICS

The current proposals for the classification of CSSD or somatoform disorders do not place much emphasis on behavioral aspects, even though behavioral features have been frequently investigated in somatoform and pain conditions. Therefore we will also address the role of behavioral variables in this context.

Illness behavior, described initially by Mechanic,[30] focuses on how patients react to symptoms or cope with their illness. The individual illness behavior is considered as a learned behavior; in this sense, illness behavior is not just a reflection of the biomedical illness processes, but strongly depends on learning and environmental influences. Illness behavior covers features such as health care use, taking medication, being disabled at work or social activities, avoidance of physical activity, and expression of symptoms to significant others. Pilowsky[31,32] summarized behavioral aspects that might contribute to the maintenance of the disorder with—a newly introduced term— "abnormal illness behavior." The expression "abnormal" is supposed to describe that the illness behavior goes far beyond what would be expected by the biomedical condition. In the following, we address the empirical evidence for single features of illness behavior, such as health care utilization, avoidance behavior, and disability at activities in patients with somatoform disorders.

Health Care Utilization

There is considerable evidence that patients with somatoform symptoms or illness worry have increased rates of medical utilization (see review[33]). Higher medical utilization is reflected in more primary care visits, more specialty visits, more emergency department visits, more hospital admissions, and overall higher inpatient and outpatient costs. Health care utilization is higher in somatizing patients compared to other patient groups, a fact that underlines the specificity of these criteria.[34] The majority of studies were based on patients from treatment facilities, and it is questionable whether this biases the results. More recently, a number of studies have been conducted in general population samples confirming the finding of increased health care utilization and costs in subjects reporting medically unexplained symptoms[35–37] or illness worry.[38,39] The report of Martin and Jacobi[38] suggests an almost 2-fold number of health care visits to GP offices in subjects reporting persistent illness worry (but not fulfilling full criteria of hypochondriasis) compared with subjects without illness worry. A large prospective study showed that the degree of somatization at baseline predicted an increase of inpatient (+39.9%) and outpatient (+11.9%) costs at 5-year follow-up.[35]

However, the specificity of the association of somatoform disorders with treatment costs has been questioned by other studies, highlighting that other mental disorders are also associated with increased health care utilization.[37] Depression and anxiety co-occur with somatoform syndromes, and both syndromes are also associated with increased health care costs. Few studies determined the effect of somatoform disorders on medical care utilization independent of psychiatric and of medical comorbidity.

Results of 2 studies controlling for the effect of depression and anxiety disorders support the independent impact of somatoform syndromes on consultation rates at primary care physicians as well as at specialists, and inpatient admission rates.[34,40]

Taken together, evidence suggests higher rates of medical care utilization in patients with somatoform disorders. This behavior pattern is not only costly, but could be even a part of maladaptive coping strategies. If patients are anxious, doctors' repeated reassurance could reinforce patients' health seeking behavior, and could prevent the development of adequate self-control strategies of patients. Reasons for higher utilization rates may vary inter-individually (subjective need of further diagnostic work-up, search for medical treatment, reassurance seeking). Not only the existence or the number of symptoms, but a *lower decision threshold for doctor visits*, seems to contribute to increased health care utilization in somatization syndrome.[36] Increased health care utilization was also associated with *dissatisfaction with care*.[41] Dissatisfaction with care does not necessarily lead to cessation of health care seeking, but reinforces the process of seeking better care—a process that contribute to further increases of health care costs.

Increased health care costs and lower patient satisfaction with medical interventions can be additionally caused by low positive effects of doctor visits. It has been shown that patients with somatoform disorders experience less reassuring effects from doctor's explanations compared to depressive patients and healthy controls.[42] *Reassurance seeking* can be a major cause for health care utilization. Reassurance seeking behavior seems to be one of the common features of chronic symptom syndromes like chronic widespread pain, oro-facial pain, irritable bowel syndrome, and chronic fatigue.[43]

Avoidance Behavior and Reduced Activity Levels

Another behavioral feature that may be a candidate criterion of CSSD is avoidance behavior. Avoidance refers to a pattern of behavior that delays, or puts off, an undesirable situation or experience. Avoidance behavior has long been recognized as adaptive response to acute injury and somatic disturbances, but is viewed as a maladaptive response if it persists after the acute exacerbations, eg, after remission of an injury or infection. Current biopsychosocial models of somatoform disorders as well as of chronic pain suggest that inappropriate avoidance behavior contributes to disability and even to the maintenance of the disorder (eg, the 'disuse syndrome'/physical deconditioning, dysphoric affect, preoccupation with somatic symptoms, increased body sensitivity), increasing the likelihood of experiencing physical symptoms.[44,45]

Avoidance can be related to activities or stimuli that are directly (eg, physical activities) or indirectly associated (eg, social activities) with the somatic complaints. The degree of avoidance behavior can vary between a generalized reduction of physical and/or social activities (with almost no activities in severe cases leading to disuse and loss of positive reinforcement) or to a reduction in specific symptom provoking sensations, situations or activities (eg, avoiding the perception of unspecific bodily sensations, certain movements, or cues like health related information).

Though not identical constructs, impairment of activities may indirectly indicate avoidance behavior. The association between medically unexplained as well as medically explained symptoms with an overall reduction of physical activities has been shown in cross-sectional and in longitudinal studies.[33,46–48] Even in subthreshold hypochondriasis, reduced activity levels were reported[38]; about 75% of people with hypochondriacal concerns reported less than 1 hour of physical activity per week, which was significantly different from controls without illness worries. This is also in line with pain research, showing that a reduction of physical activity is one of the "yellow flags" predicting poor course and symptom persistence.[49] Another large prospective study (Early Developmental Stages of Psychopathology) revealed that adolescents and young adults with regular physical activity had a substantially lower overall incidence of somatoform disorders (persistent pain, somatization, and undifferentiated somatoform disorders).[50] The latter finding is of interest as it indicates reduced physical activity to be a risk factor for developing a disabling somatic condition, not only for persistence of existing symptoms.

Recently, Chou and Shekelle[51] provided evidence for the predictive validity of fear-avoidance behavior in pain. Examining 20 prospective studies, they systematically reviewed the usefulness of individual risk factors for identifying patients more likely to develop persistent disabling low back pain. High level of maladaptive pain coping behaviors including fear-avoidance behavior, the presence of nonorganic symptom signs, high baseline functional impairment, presence of psychiatric comorbidities, and low general health status were the most powerful predictors of poor outcome 1 year later.

Little research has been done to study the fear-avoidance model in somatoform disorders other than pain conditions. In one recent study from our own group, the assessment variable 'avoidance of physical activities, that can provoke heart beat accelerations or sweating' proved to be the most powerful psychological variable in the prediction of health care utilization and disability in subjects with multiple somatic symptoms.[5] Therefore the concept of fear-avoidance should be further adapted to general somatoform conditions beyond pain.

In sum, these findings provide evidence of reduced general and physical activity levels in syndromes with medically unexplained symptoms, which could indicate avoidance behavior. Avoidance behavior may be the result of various 'pathways' in somatoform and pain disorders. First, pain intensity itself drives escape and avoidance, and contributes to the explanation of disability (for review, see Leeuw and colleagues[21]). Second, a catastrophizing coping style as described above can lead to avoidance. Finally, avoidance of activities may be triggered by fear. The concept of 'fear-avoidance' was introduced in the field of pain conditions, especially in chronic low back pain. It is assumed that fear of pain, fear of movement, fear of work-related activities, and fear of injury drive avoidance behavior and hinders recovery from symptoms.[44,49] This concept warrants further consideration as it points to the mediating role of cognitions and emotional reactions resulting in avoidance of physical demands, and of symptom-provoking actions or situations.

Further Aspects of Abnormal Illness Behavior

Other behavioral patterns have been suggested to characterize subjects with medically unexplained symptoms. An analysis of illness behavior[52] demonstrated various dimensions that may be relevant to somatoform disorders, and a scale was developed assessing 'the need for the verification of diagnosis,' 'the expression of symptoms,' 'the need for medication and treatment,' aspects of 'illness consequences' such as sick leave from work, reduction of social activities, and physical deconditioning, as well as 'body scanning' (attention focusing to bodily processes). Notably, these different aspects of illness behavior are only modestly interrelated.[52] Therefore, illness behavior can be characterized by very different behavioral facets between patients, indicating very different needs. One part of the problem of increased health care costs in somatization is the stereotypical reaction of health care providers to very different needs.

CONCLUSION

Somatic symptoms themselves do not justify being classified as a mental disorder according to DSM or ICD-10 section F, unless additional positive psychological features are present that characterize the disorder. Therefore the proposal of CSSD for DSM-5 including cognitive and affective criteria points in the right direction. However, the role of behavioral features (such as avoidance of potentially symptom-provoking situations, or the fear-avoidance concept) is not yet adequately addressed.

We found evidence that syndromes of somatization and pain conditions are associated with a broad range of cognitive characteristics (eg, somatic causal symptom attributions, catastrophizing, the self-concept of bodily weakness, low symptom tolerance), *and* a broad range of behavioral characteristics (eg, health care utilization associated with reassurance seeking, and avoidance behavior). Although cognitive, affective, and behavioral processes are often interrelated, they are not necessarily present at the same time and within the same individual. Rather, these features seem to vary considerably between affected subjects.

We therefore suggest operationalizing criterion B of the CSSD proposal: 'Excessive thoughts, feelings, and behaviors related to these somatic symptoms or associated health concerns' by providing *a range* of cognitive behavioral characteristics in addition to affective symptoms. Based on recent findings,[5] we suggest that the following psychological features aid in classifying people with clinically relevant somatic syndromes: (1) ruminations about physical complaints, worrying about health and illness issues; (2) catastrophizing of bodily sensations; (3) somatic illness attributions despite contradicting medical information; (4) self-concept of bodily weakness; 5) low symptom tolerance; immediate need for medical help; (6) avoidance of physical activity that could cause sweating or heart beat accelerations; (7) disuse of body parts because of complaints; 8) desperation because of symptoms, negative affectivity.

REFERENCES

1. Kroenke K, Mangelsdorff AD. Common symptoms in ambulatory care: incidence, evaluation, therapy and outcome. Am J Med 1989;86:262–6.
2. Hiller W, Rief W, Brähler E. Somatization in the population: from mild bodily misperceptions to disabling symptoms. Soc Psychiatry Psychiatr Epidemiol 2006;41:704–12.
3. Jackson JL, Kroenke K. Prevalence, impact, and prognosis of multisomatoform disorder in primary care: a 5-year follow-up study. Psychosom Med 2008;70:430–4.
4. Rief W, Rojas G. Stability of somatoform symptoms - implications for classification. Psychosom Med 2007;69:864–9.
5. Rief W, Mewes R, Martin A, et al. Are psychological features useful in classifying patients with somatic symptoms? Psychosom Med 2010;72:648–55.
6. American Psychiatric Association. Diagnostic and Statistical Manual for Mental Disorders DSM-IV. Washington: APA Press; 1994.
7. Duddu V, Chaturvedi SK, Isaac MK. Amplification and attribution styles in somatoform and depressive disorders–a study from Bangalore, India. Psychopathology 2003;36:98–103.
8. Henningsen P, Jakobsen T, Schiltenwolf M, et al. Somatization revisited - diagnosis and perceived causes of common mental disorders. J Nerv Ment Dis 2005;193:85–92.
9. Martin A, Korn H-J, Cebulla M, et al. Kausalattributionen von körperlichen Beschwerden bei somatoformen Störungen [Causal attributions about bodily sensations in somatoform disorders]. Zeitschrift für Psychiatrie, Psychologie und Psychotherapie 2007;55:31–41.

10. Nimnuan C, Hotopf M, Wessely S. Medically unexplained symptoms: an epidemiological study in seven specialities. J Psychosom Res 2001;51:361–7.
11. Rief W, Nanke A, Emmerich J, et al. Causal illness attributions in somatoform disorders: associations with comorbidity and illness behavior. J Psychosom Res 2004;57:367–71.
12. Hiller W, Cebulla M, Korn HJ, et al. Causal symptom attributions in somatoform disorder and chronic pain. J Psychosom Res 2010;68:9–19.
13. Groben S, Hausteiner C. Somatoform disorders and causal attributions in patients with suspected allergies: Do somatic causal attributions matter? J Psychosom Res 2011;70:229–38.
14. Taylor RE, Mann AH, White NJ, et al. Attachment style in patients with unexplained physical complaints. Psychol Med 2000;30:931–41.
15. Rief W, Broadbent E. Explaining medically unexplained symptoms:-models and mechanisms. Clin Psychol Rev 2007;27:821–41.
16. Riedl A, Maass J, Fliege H, et al. Subjective theories of illness and clinical and psychological outcome in patients with irritable bowel syndrome. J Psychosom Res 2009;67:449–55.
17. Schmaling KB, Fiedelak JI, Katon WJ, et al. Prospective study of the prognosis of unexplained chronic fatigue in a clinic-based cohort. Psychosom Med 2003;65:1047–54.
18. Dworkin RH, Hartstein G, Rosner HL, et al. A high-risk method for studying psychosocial antecedents of chronic pain: the prospective investigation of herpes zoster. J Abnorm Psychol 1992;101:200–5.
19. Frostholm L, Oernboel E, Christensen KS, et al. Do illness perceptions predict health outcomes in primary care patients? A 2-year follow-up study. J Psychosom Res 2007;62:129–38.
20. Hausteiner C, Bornschein S, Bubel E, et al. Psychobehavioral predictors of somatoform disorders in patients with suspected allergies. Psychosom Med 2009;71:1004–11.
21. Leeuw M, Goossens ME, Linton SJ, et al. The fear-avoidance model of musculoskeletal pain: current state of scientific evidence. J Behav Med 2007;30:77–94.
22. Quartana PJ, Campbell CM, Edwards RR. Pain catastrophizing: a critical review. Expert Rev Neurother 2009;9:745–58.
23. Seminovicz DA, Davis KD. Cortical responses to pain in healthy individuals depends on pain catastrophizing. Pain 2006;120:297–306.
24. Sullivan MJ, Rodgers WM, Wilson PM, et al. An experimental investigation of the relation between catastrophizing and activity intolerance. Pain 2002;100:47–53.
25. Rief W, Hiller W, Margraf J. Cognitive aspects in hypochondriasis and the somatization syndrome. J Abnorm Psychol 1998;107:587–95.
26. Barsky AJ, Ahern DK, Bailey ED, et al. Hypochondriacal patients' appraisal of health and physical risks. Am J Psychiatry 2001;158:783–7.
27. Barsky AJ, Coeytaux RR, Sarnie MK, et al. Hypochondriacal patient's beliefs about good health. Am J Psychiatry 1993;150:1085–9.
28. Hausteiner C, Huber D, Bornschein S, et al. Characteristics of oligosymptomatic versus polysymptomatic presentations of somatoform disorders in patients with suspected allergies. J Psychosom Res 2010;69:259–66.
29. Bass C, Murphy M. Somatoform and personality disorders: syndromal comorbidity and overlapping developmental pathways. J Psychosom Res 1995;39:403–27.
30. Mechanic D. The concept of illness behavior. J Chronic Dis 1962;15:189–94.
31. Pilowsky I. Abnormal illness behaviour. Br J Med Psychol 1969;42:347–51.
32. Pilowsky I. Abnormal Illness Behaviour. Chichester: Wiley & Sons; 1997.

33. Creed F, Barsky A. A systematic review of the epidemiology of somatisation disorder and hypochondriasis. J Psychosom Res 2004;56:391–408.
34. Barsky AJ, Orav J, Bates DW. Somatization increases medical utilization and costs independent of psychiatric and medical morbidity. Arch Gen Psychiatry 2005;62: 903–10.
35. Grabe HJ, Baumeister SE, John U, et al. Association of mental distress with health care utilization and costs: a 5-year observation in a general population. Soc Psychiatry Psychiatr Epidemiol 2009;44:835–44.
36. Mewes R, Rief W, Brähler E, et al. Lower decision threshold for doctor visits as a predictor of health care use in somatoform disorders and in the general population. Gen Hosp Psychiatry 2008;30:349–55.
37. Rief W, Martin A, Klaiberg A, et al. Specific effects of depression, panic, and somatic symptoms on illness behavior. Psychosom Med 2005;67:596–601.
38. Martin A, Jacobi F. Features of hypochondriasis and illness worry in the general population in Germany. Psychosom Med 2006;68:770–7.
39. Noyes R Jr, Carney CP, Hillis SL, et al. Prevalence and correlates of illness worry in the general population. Psychosomatics 2005;46:529–39.
40. de Waal MW, Arnold IA, Eekhof JA, et al. Follow up study on health care use of patients with somatoform, anxiety and depressive disorders in primary care. BMC Fam Pract 2008;9:5.
41. Noyes R Jr, Langbehn DR, Happel RL, et al. Health Attitude Survey. A scale for assesing somatizing patients. Psychosomatics 1999;40:470–8.
42. Rief W, Heitmüller AM, Reisberg K, et al. Why reassurance fails in patients with unexplained symptoms–an experimental investigation of remembered probabilities. PLoS Med 2006;3:e269.
43. Aggarwal VR, McBeth J, Zakrzewska JM, et al. The epidemiology of chronic syndromes that are frequently unexplained: do they have common associated factors? Int J Epidemiol 2006;35:468–76.
44. Asmundson GJG, Norton PJ, Norton GR. Beyond pain: the role of fear and avoidance in chronicity. Clin Psychol Rev 1999;19:97–119.
45. Rief W, Nanke A. Somatization disorder from a cognitive-psychobiological perspective. Curr Opin Psychiatry 1999;12:733–8.
46. Gureje O, Simon GE, Ustun TB, et al. Somatization in cross-cultural perspective: A World Health Organization study in primary care. Am J Psychiatry 1997;154:989–95.
47. Harris AM, Orav EJ, Bates DW, et al. Somatization increases disability independent of comorbidity. J Gen Intern Med 2009;24:155–61.
48. Kisely S, Simon G. An international study comparing the effect of medically explained and unexplained somatic symptoms on psychosocial outcome. J Psychosom Res 2006;60:125–30.
49. Vlaeyen JWS, Linton SJ. Fear-avoidance and its consequences in chronic musculoskeletal pain: a state of the art. Pain 2000;85:317–32.
50. Ströhle A, Höfler M, Pfister H, et al. Physical activity and prevalence and incidence of mental disorders in adolescents and young adults. Psychol Med 2007;37:1657–66.
51. Chou R, Shekelle P. Will this patient develop persistent disabling low back pain? JAMA 2010;303:1295–302.
52. Rief W, Ihle D, Pilger F. A new approach to assess illness behaviour. J Psychosom Res 2003;54:405–14.

Does Psychological Stress Cause Chronic Pain?

Afton L. Hassett, PsyD*, Daniel J. Clauw, MD

KEYWORDS
- Psychological stress • Chronic pain • Fibromyalgia
- Neuroendocrine

Seventeenth century philosopher Rene Descartes posed that a signal from a painful stimulus detected in the periphery would travel passively upward along a specific "hard wired" pathway to the brain to be sensed as pain. Variations on this theory were widely held until 1965 when Melzack and Wall challenged this approach to pain processing with the "Gate-Control" theory of pain.[1] They advanced the idea that peripheral sensory input is modulated in the dorsal horn of the spinal cord, and that spinal level influences play a major role in the determination of both the presence and severity of pain.

Several decades later, findings from functional brain imaging studies led to the realization that, in addition to this strong spinal control of pain, supraspinal influences also determine the presence and magnitude of pain. It is now clear that pain is controlled at a minimum of 3 levels in the central nervous system (ie, peripheral, spinal, and supraspinal), and at least 3 different dimensions of pain are sensed by cortical regions: sensory (pain location and degree of discomfort), affective (the emotional valence of pain), and cognitive (what is thought about the pain). Moreover, we now know that the pain experience (especially in chronic rather than acute pain) is the final product of a complex information processing network as opposed to signals relayed by specific pain fibers in nerves or specific pain pathways in the brain.

The wide acceptance of the Gate-Control theory of pain (even though the theory was only partially correct) opened the door to psychosomatic medicine as it pertains to pain. Yet, if the major objective of psychosomatic medicine is to elucidate the biological mechanisms whereby behaviors, cognitions, emotions, and social factors are translated into physical illness,[2] then the study of the psychosomatics of chronic pain may be more frustrating than fruitful. Although a multitude of behavioral experiments have shown that pain inflicted in experimental settings can be exacerbated or moderated by cognitive and emotional factors, the relationship between persistent psychological stress and the manifestation of chronic pain conditions is

The authors have nothing to disclose.
Department of Anesthesiology, Chronic Pain & Fatigue Research Center, University of Michigan Medical School, 24 Frank Lloyd Wright Drive, Lobby M, Ann Arbor, MI 48106, USA
* Corresponding author.
E-mail address: afton@med.umich.edu

less clear. With the observation that psychiatric comorbidity is prevalent in patients with chronic pain, many clinicians and researchers alike came to believe that psychological stress causes chronic pain. This view has been dogma for some time; however, actual research findings cast doubt on the veracity of this simple unidirectional relationship.

The psychosomatics of pain is a vast topic and certainly one too robust to do justice in the context of this article. However, an overview of a single, well-studied chronic pain condition, fibromyalgia, along with findings from research related to similar chronic pain conditions, helps illustrate the most up-to-date thinking about pain and its interface with thoughts and emotion. This review will attempt to address the fundamental question, "Does psychological stress cause chronic pain?"

FIBROMYALGIA AND PSYCHOLOGICAL STRESS

Fibromyalgia is a non-inflammatory chronic pain disorder characterized by widespread musculoskeletal pain and multiple tender points.[3] At least 2% of the general population meets American College of Rheumatology criteria for fibromyalgia, primarily women[3]; however, under the new clinical criteria that do not require performing a tender point count to diagnose this condition, more people are likely to be diagnosed, including more men.[4] In addition to chronic widespread pain, patients often describe persistent fatigue, non-restorative sleep, mood disturbance, anxiety and cognitive problems (eg, "fogginess" or difficulties with concentration and memory).[3] Further complicating the clinical picture, fibromyalgia rarely seems to occur in isolation. In addition to psychiatric comorbidity, patients with fibromyalgia are also more likely to experience one or more regional chronic pain conditions (eg, irritable bowel syndrome (IBS), interstitial cystitis, temporomandibular joint disorder, tension headaches).[5-7] For example, it has been estimated that between 32% and 70% of individuals with fibromyalgia will also meet criteria for IBS.[8,9] Moreover, fibromyalgia is present in a subset of patients having other inflammatory or peripherally-mediated chronic pain conditions (eg, rheumatoid arthritis, osteoarthritis).[10,11]

Because it has been clear for some time that fibromyalgia is not an autoimmune disorder characterized by widespread inflammation or tissue damage causing pain (and, thus, the original diagnostic label "fibrositis" was abandoned in favor of "fibromyalgia"), psychological and psychiatric causes for this condition have been extensively studied. In fact, turning to psychological stress as a causal factor has a long tradition in medicine when the condition under study is not thoroughly understood. Rheumatoid arthritis, Lyme disease, inflammatory bowel disease, and peptic ulcer disease are all examples of diseases once thought to be psychiatric in nature.

Significant comorbidity with mood and anxiety disorders has been observed in patients with fibromyalgia.[12-14] Studies have shown that about 20% of fibromyalgia patients, as well as those in the community, will meet criteria for having a comorbid current major depressive disorder,[13-16] while a lifetime diagnosis of a major mood disorder has been observed in up to 74%.[12,15] The co-occurrence of depression and pain has been well explored—an average of 65% of patients with depression will report one or more pain complaints, while anywhere from 5% to 85% of pain patients will report depression (rates vary contingent upon the condition and study methodology).[17] Similarly, comorbid anxiety disorders have been reported in 10% to 25% of fibromyalgia patients evaluated in tertiary care.[13,14,16] Again, pain is commonly observed in patients with anxiety disorders, and these patients tend to experience pain differently and have an increased awareness of symptoms.[18]

Beyond psychiatric comorbidity, other psychological factors associated with poor outcomes (eg, greater pain and disability) have been reported in fibromyalgia, including pain catastrophizing,[19,20] an external locus of control,[21] high levels of negative affect,[22] low levels of positive affect,[22,23] passive coping,[19] and avoidance behavior.[24] The presence and severity of these psychological factors occur along a continuum ranging from a high incidence of personality disorders[14] on one extreme to psychological resilience on the other. Studies have clearly identified large sub-groups of fibromyalgia patients with no psychiatric comorbidity, high levels of positive affect, and significantly better functional outcomes.[22,25,26] Decades of research focused on psychopathological factors in fibromyalgia can be summarized in a single statement: most fibromyalgia patients do not have an identifiable current Axis I or II psychiatric diagnosis, and no single psychiatric or psychological factor accounts for the pain or behavior of most fibromyalgia patients.

THE EVIDENCE FOR PSYCHOLOGICAL STRESS CAUSING FIBROMYALGIA AND RELATED CONDITIONS

Several lines of "evidence" have been put forward as proof that psychological stress causes or, at the very least, triggers fibromyalgia. Such evidence would include: (1) high levels of distress are commonly observed among these patients; (2) abnormalities of the stress response systems of patients with fibromyalgia have been reported; and (3) a general feeling of "stress" is experienced by clinicians who care for them. Even though this narrative is enticing, it is simply inaccurate. The research linking psychological stress to these illnesses is predominantly cross-sectional and limited by sample characteristics; moreover, the relationship between distress and disease is much more complex than initially imagined.

The high rates of psychological stress observed in many case-control studies in fibromyalgia and other similar chronic pain conditions are partially due to the fact that many of these studies were performed in tertiary care settings. The high level of healthcare-seeking behavior likely differentiates these patients from others in primary care or in the general population. For example, the data are quite clear that individuals with fibromyalgia seen in tertiary care settings are more likely to have psychiatric co-morbidity than those evaluated in primary care settings or population-based studies.[12,27] Along the same lines, women with these disorders who are assessed in clinical settings are much more likely to report childhood physical or sexual abuse than are controls, or those who meet criteria for these disorders but have never sought healthcare.[28] Another caveat regarding the link between these conditions and previous traumatic events relates to relying on self-report data of distant events and the very human effort to find cause for or meaning in illness and misfortune.[29]

Studies performed with individuals from the general population, rather than those seeking care, limit these biases. Several groups in the United Kingdom have performed just such population-based studies evaluating the psychological predictors of chronic widespread or regional pain. Because they target the temporal and longitudinal relationship between distress and pain (which can help identify cause and effect) rather than a cross-sectional relationship (which could be identifying distress due to pain rather than causing pain), these studies are of particular importance. Results from these studies have consistently demonstrated that individuals with high levels of baseline psychological stress are only moderately more likely to later develop chronic widespread or regional pain (OR 1.5–2).[30–33] Of interest, significantly more individuals without baseline psychological stress develop widespread or regional pain than those with high levels of baseline distress.[30] Unlike the modest relationship between psychological stress at baseline and pain at follow-up, these studies reported stronger relationships between the number and severity of somatic symptoms at baseline and the subsequent development of pain (OR 3–9). Therefore, it seems that the tendency to experience somatic symptoms (often characterized as "somatization" but now felt to have a strong biological basis due to augmented sensory processing) is typically a more powerful predictor of future pain in longitudinal studies than psychological stress.[34]

Several other relationships between pain and psychological stress have been described in these United Kingdom population-based studies. For example, having chronic pain at baseline strongly predicted having future psychological stress (OR 3–5).[33] These findings support the hypothesis that psychological stress is both an "effect" of pain, as well as a potential cause. Once again, this process was mediated by the tendency to report pain and other symptoms at baseline. Further, these same researchers, using a population-based approach, found that children whose medical records indicated that they were involved in an automobile accident, or institutionalized, were 1.5 to 2 times more likely to develop chronic widespread pain 42 years later.[35] This appears to be among the first studies that show that various types of early life trauma are, in fact, a risk factor for developing chronic pain, even after eliminating the potential effect of recall bias. Finally, these same investigators have also demonstrated that the stress response system functioning at baseline (ie, hypothalamic-pituitary-adrenal [HPA] axis) is a predictor of the development of chronic widespread pain independent of psychological factors.[36]

The catastrophic terrorist attacks of 9/11 provided another window into the complex relationship between psychological stress and pain. Based on the hypothesis that psychological stress is a major trigger of pain, it would be anticipated that levels of pain among both patients with fibromyalgia and others exposed to these highly stressful events would increase.[37] Yet, in studies performed prior to and immediately after the attacks, no increase in pain or related symptoms was observed. There was neither an increase in somatic symptoms among people in the general population living in New York City,[38] nor an increase in pain levels in patients being followed with fibromyalgia in Washington, DC in the month before and month after the attacks.[39] It seems reasonable to conclude that this type of acute psychological stress that is associated with a strong sense of social support (ie, the intense patriotism surrounding the terrorist attack) may not engender the same consequences as the daily interpersonal hassles that lack this attribute and have been found to increase pain and other somatic symptoms in some situations.[40]

THE RELATIONSHIP BETWEEN STRESS RESPONSE SYSTEM DYSFUNCTION AND CHRONIC PAIN

Abnormalities in both stress responses systems, the HPA axis and the autonomic nervous system, have been reported in fibromyalgia and more broadly in chronic pain states.[41–44] However, these "abnormalities" are really not abnormal in that the group means for measures of these parameters may differ between patients and controls, but these values are not outside the normal range. There is always tremendous overlap between individuals within the patient and control groups. Further, the nature of the abnormality identified is inconsistent, with some studies describing hypoactivity and others finding hyperactivity of both the HPA axis and sympathetic nervous system.

Inconsistencies are likely the product of confounding variables common to this population, such as the presence of physical deconditioning, obesity, sleep disturbance, chronic pain, psychiatric comorbidity (especially mood disorders and anxiety disorders like post-traumatic stress disorder) and/or a history of childhood sexual abuse. Most early studies of HPA axis and autonomic function in fibromyalgia failed to control for these factors. Recent studies suggest that these factors may be more powerful drivers of stress response function than whether or not an individual has fibromyalgia. For example, early life stressors are increasingly being shown to significantly and permanently alter HPA axis functioning and the magnitude and direction of the perturbance may be determined by the age at which the stress occurs.[45,46] Further, salivary cortisol levels co-vary with pain levels, and cerebrospinal fluid levels of corticotrophin-releasing factor (CRF) have been found to be more closely related to an individual's level of pain or history of an early life trauma than to his or her status as an individual with fibromyalgia or a healthy control.[47] Lastly, a recent study found that HPA axis alterations in fibromyalgia patients occurred exclusively in those with co-morbid major depressive disorder.[48]

Regarding autonomic nervous system functioning, heart rate variability (baseline assessment and in response to tilt-table testing) has been extensively evaluated in patients with fibromyalgia. Consistent and reproducible findings support the notion that, in comparison to controls, those with fibromyalgia have lower baseline heart rate variability (HRV), which is indicative of poor autonomic function.[49,50] However, the link between changes in HRV and fibromyalgia and similar chronic pain conditions requires critical examination. Again, these studies have demonstrated considerable overlap between patients and controls in many HRV parameters, and it is highly likely that these "abnormalities" reflect subtle changes in autonomic function due to co-morbid conditions such as physical deconditioning. Prolonged diminished physical activity leads to deconditioning, which is characterized by predictable changes like a reduction in cardiac volume, a reduction in plasma volume, and/or marked tachycardia in response to standing or upright tilt-table testing.[51,52]

In addition, some of the changes noted in autonomic function in fibromyalgia and related chronic pain states may not be due to the chronic pain but, instead, represent a diathesis that puts individuals at risk of the subsequent development of pain. This hypothesis is supported by a number of longitudinal studies that follow individuals from pain-free to having pain. In one short experimental study, Glass and colleagues showed that a week of exercise cessation in healthy, regularly exercising adults caused many of these individuals to develop fibromyalgia-like symptoms.[53] The study found that a subgroup of these previously asymptomatic adults reported an increase in one or more symptoms including pain, fatigue, and mood, and that this sub-group had lower HPA axis (cortisol), autonomic (HRV), and immune system (NK cell-responsiveness to venipuncture) functioning at baseline (prior to cessation of exercise) than the healthy subjects who did not develop pain and other symptoms. Similar results were found in a subsequent study among healthy regularly exercising and sleeping individuals; disruption of their normal routine was associated with increased pain, fatigue, negative mood, and dyscognition, with sleep restriction producing even greater widespread pain and more severe symptoms than exercise deprivation.[53]

McBeth and colleagues have taken a different approach in assessing the link between baseline stress and HPA axis functioning. They measured HPA function in a large group of pain-free individuals and found that baseline HPA axis function affected the likelihood of subsequently developing chronic widespread pain.[54] They compared HPA axis function among 3 groups: individuals suffering from widespread pain, controls, and individuals considered to be at risk for developing widespread pain on the basis of physical symptom reporting and scores on a measure of illness behavior. In both the individuals with chronic pain and those "at risk," alterations in HPA axis function were observed and could not be explained by psychological stress. More importantly, this study showed that HPA axis dysfunction may actually precede the development of chronic pain.

These studies illustrate the need to examine both relationships between chronic pain and stress: (1) changes in the stress response system may lead to pain, and

(2) pain activates the stress response systems and leads to subsequent changes. In regard to the latter, levels of cortisol secretion and levels of cerebrospinal fluid (CRF) are correlated with momentary pain levels in fibromyalgia.[47,55] These studies also found that CRH levels were associated with other factors such as a self-reported history of physical or sexual abuse. Similar to the broader relationship between stress and pain, there are 3 potential explanations for the association between CRF and pain in fibromyalgia: (1) CRF may be involved in the generation of pain symptoms, (2) CRF is altered as a consequence of chronic stress caused by pain, and/or (3) CRF may be altered due to dysfunction of other central processes directly involved in the generation of fibromyalgia pain.

Thus, although it is possible that a stress response system dysfunction might cause pain or other symptoms seen in fibromyalgia and chronic pain states, these findings may also antedate the development of pain, or partially be due to the pain.

THE RELATIONSHIP BETWEEN PSYCHOLOGICAL FACTORS AND FIBROMYALGIA PAIN

The cardinal symptom of fibromyalgia is pain. Fortunately, pain is now better understood in light of tremendous advances in the basic neuroscience of pain taking place over the past 2 decades. For example, from the neurobiological perspective, there is more than one type of chronic pain. Some chronic pain that occurs because of peripheral nociceptive input (eg, due to damage or inflammation) may be adaptive and protective, whereas other pain that is "pathological" likely results from abnormal function of pain-processing pathways in the central nervous system (CNS).[56] In fact, based on a robust and growing body of research, many in the pain field now agree that chronic pain is a disease with similar CNS causes regardless of the location of the body it occurs in, or the specific "diagnosis" to which the pain is attributed.

An augmented processing of pain and sensory information in the central nervous systems has been demonstrated reliably in patients with fibromyalgia and other chronic pain syndromes (eg, IBS, interstitial cystitis, and temporomandibular joint disorder).[57–60] For example, although electrical, pressure, or thermal stimuli are not detectable at lower levels in fibromyalgia patients compared to healthy individuals, the objective intensity of these stimuli that leads to pain or unpleasantness is appreciably lower.[61,62] Further, those with fibromyalgia have a similar lower threshold for other sensory stimuli like noise.[63] These observations imply that, in some, hyperactive processing of any or all sensory stimuli, in addition to pain, could be at play. Because these findings have been observed even when stimuli are presented in a random and unpredictable fashion, it appears that psychological factors like hypervigilance may play only a minor role in modulating tenderness and augmented sensory processing.[59] Findings related to mechanical hyperalgesia (increased pain in response to pressure that would normally be painful) and/or allodynia (pain in response to normally non-painful stimuli) are arguably the most consistent biological findings in these conditions.[64,65] These same findings are not noted in individuals with psychiatric disorders such as depression.[66,67] The veracity of these findings showing objective evidence of augmented pain processing using experimental sensory testing was initially challenged (mostly due to the reliance on patient self-report of pain) but, subsequently, a plethora of functional neuroimaging studies have corroborated the presence of augmented central pain processing in this spectrum of illness.[68–71]

In the 1960s, several individuals proposed the existence of a "Pain Matrix," hypothesizing the existence of 3 separate domains of pain processing in the central nervous system—sensory, affective, and evaluative.[1] The sensory dimension includes the localization and severity of pain and involves the primary and secondary somatosensory cortices, thalamus, and posterior insula. The affective dimension of pain describes the emotional valence of pain and is ascribed to the anterior cingulate cortex, amygdala, and anterior insula. Lastly, the evaluative or cognitive dimension of pain involves the prefrontal cortex plus the affective areas noted above. We now know that no single brain region is specifically dedicated to pain processing, and that numerous brain regions—in addition to those historically thought to be part of the pain matrix—are activated during painful stimuli. Yet, this demarcation between sensory and affective processing, often referred to as "lateral" versus "medial" brain regions, is useful in elucidating the role that affect plays in pain processing.

Neuroimaging studies, especially those using functional MRI (fMRI), have greatly advanced our understanding of central pain augmentation in fibromyalgia and other similar conditions. Moreover, findings from these studies have largely borne out the validity of the pain matrix concept. Studies using fMRI have demonstrated that, compared to controls, fibromyalgia patients exhibit greater activity over many brain regions (eg, prefrontal, supplemental motor, insular, and anterior cingulate cortex) in response to both painful and non-painful stimuli.[70] Gracely and colleagues[68] were the first to show that, when fibromyalgia patients were exposed to painful pressures during a fMRI protocol (compared to controls), those with fibromyalgia demonstrated increased neural activations (ie, increases in the Blood-oxygen-level dependence [BOLD] signal) in both the primary and secondary somatosensory cortices and the insula and anterior cingulate. Pain-free controls subjected to greater pressures that evoked the same self-report pain ratings had similar neural activation patterns. These findings suggested that patients with fibromyalgia experience an increased gain or "volume control setting" in neural sensory processing systems. Thus, for those with fibromyalgia, the pain signal is amplified or augmented in the central nervous system. These results have been replicated many times subsequently in fibromyalgia, and have been similarly shown to be present in nearly every chronic pain state, even in conditions that heretofore had been considered to be primarily due to peripheral joint or tissue damage, such as osteoarthritis and chronic low back pain.[69,72,73]

Similarly, our understanding of how co-morbid psychological factors influence pain processing in fibromyalgia has been greatly enhanced by fMRI-based research. In a study evaluating the relationship between depression and enhanced evoked pain sensations, neither the presence of comorbid major depressive disorder nor the severity of sub-threshold depressive symptoms was associated with pain-testing results or the magnitude of neuronal activation in regions associated with the sensory dimension of pain (eg, primary and secondary somatosensory cortices).[67] In contrast, the presence of clinical depression was associated with the magnitude of pain-evoked neuronal activations in the amygdalae and contralateral anterior insula—regions associated with the affective dimension of pain. Interestingly, self-report pain intensity, as opposed to evoked pain, was significantly related to measures of both the sensory and affective dimensions of pain. These data support the central tenant of the pain matrix paradigm—the presence of parallel, independent neural pain-processing networks for the sensory and affective pain dimensions.

Studies using fMRI have also enabled us to better assess the effects of cognitive factors like catastrophizing on pain processing. Gracely and colleagues demon-strated that pain catastrophizing is associated with heightened neural activity in regions associated with pain anticipation (eg, cerebellum, medial frontal cortex), attention to pain (dorsal anterior cingulate gyrus, dorsolateral prefrontal cortex), the emotional dimension of pain (claustrum), and motor control.[74] Additional research may shed light on how pain processing is affected by other cognitive and affective characteristics, such as having an internal versus external locus of control or the differing effects of positive affect versus negative affect.

Lastly, a novel and noninvasive procedure known as proton magnetic resonance spectroscopy, or H-MRS, can be used to evaluate, *in vivo*, the relative concentration of specific brain metabolites. Using H-MRS, it has been demonstrated that patients with fibromyalgia have higher glutamate levels in the insula than do controls, and that dynamic changes in posterior insula glutamate levels are associated with changes in clinical pain.[75] Moreover, H-MRS studies have shown that changes in glutamate in the anterior insula are more closely related to changes in anxiety, while changes in glutamate in the posterior insula are more closely related to changes in the sensory dimension of clinical pain. These findings are consistent with the differential functions of the insula first suggested by Craig.[76]

When these results are taken together, the findings imply that psychological stress (ie, depression, anxiety) and pain are somewhat independently processed in the central nervous system. This is corroborated by clinical data showing that drugs that act as antidepressants and analgesics (eg, tricyclic compounds or serotonin-norepinephrine reuptake inhibitors) are equally effective analgesics in chronic pain patients whether or not depression is present.[77,78]

EVIDENCE SUPPORTS A DIATHESIS-STRESS MODEL FOR THE ETIOLOGY OF CHRONIC PAIN

Again, the role of psychological factors has played prominently in the quest to elucidate the etiology of fibromyalgia and other chronic pain conditions. However, research fails to support a simple unidirectional relationship between psychopathology and the development of chronic pain. Therefore, many in the field have adopted a diathesis-stress model for these disorders, as it takes in account the multiplicity of factors likely contributory to the pathogenesis of chronic pain. Such a model makes it possible to account for the varying degrees that genetic, environmental, and psychosocial factors contribute to a predisposition for disease, in this case chronic pain.

The initial support for genetic predisposition came from family studies in fibromyalgia.[79] Later, Arnold and colleagues expanded on these findings and demonstrated that first degree biological relatives of individuals with fibromyalgia display an 8-fold greater risk of developing fibromyalgia compared to individuals in the general population.[7] This study also showed that family members of fibromyalgia patients are more tender, and have more other types of chronic pain, than the family members of controls.[80-83] In contrast, this study showed that the odds for a major mood disorder in a family member of an individual with fibromyalgia are modest (estimated at 1.8).[7] This familial co-aggregation of conditions has been termed affective spectrum disorder[16] and, more recently, central sensitivity syndromes.[84] Although the nature of the relationship between mood disorders and fibromyalgia is not completely understood, these findings suggest that, although fibromyalgia is not caused by a mood disorder, mood disorders and fibromyalgia likely share common causal factors (especially genes controlling the synthesis, activity, or breakdown of neurotransmitters that control both pain and mood, and the ability to be triggered by various types of biological stressors).[7,83]

Over the last 10 years, researcg has greatly advanced our understanding of the genetics of pain. For example, just as there is variability in pain sensitivity between strains of rodents, there is great variability in pain sensitivity in humans.[85,86] We have learned that genes responsible for catechol-O-methyltranferase (COMT), GTP cyclohydrolase 1 (GCH1), voltage-gated sodium channels Nav1.7,1.8,1.9, and potassium channels (KCNS1) all exert significant control over human pain perception.[87–93] This new appreciation has contributed to a wider acceptance of chronic pain as being a disease of the central nervous system.[56] It seems that where pain arises in the body is likely not as important as the individual's genetically determined level of pain sensitivity. Evidence that an increased risk for developing fibromyalgia is specifically associated with certain genetic polymorphisms is starting to emerge. The serotonin transporter, serotonin 5-HT2A receptor polymorphism T/T phenotype, and dopamine 4 receptor, and COMT polymorphisms are all seen in higher frequency in fibromyalgia compared to controls.[94] This genetic vulnerability, combined with the neuroplastic changes that can occur in the central nervous system, likely lead to the augmented pain and other sensory processing observed in these conditions. However, many of the genetic polymorphisms implicated in augmented pain processing are the same as those associated with mood and anxiety disorders. The resultant alterations in monoamines likely contribute to both the experience of increased pain and affective disturbances.

MANY TYPES OF STRESSORS TRIGGER CHRONIC PAIN IN FIBROMYALGIA AND RELATED CONDITIONS

A diathesis-stress model for fibromyalgia and other similar chronic pain conditions presupposes that, in addition to genetic polymorphisms, environmental factors can contribute to the vulnerability of an individual to a given condition and can also act as triggers to set the disease process in motion. Many lines of research have shown that a whole host of external factors, in addition to psychological stress, are capable of triggering fibromyalgia. In addition to catastrophic events such as war or terrorism, and particularly manmade disasters,[95] automobile accidents have been linked with the development of fibromyalgia.[35,96] However, traumatic events are not necessarily the most potent triggers.

Both peripheral pain syndromes like osteoarthritis and systemic diseases like rheumatoid arthritis and systemic lupus erythematosus, which result in regional or multifocal pain, have a well-documented capacity to precede or "trigger" the subsequent development of chronic widespread pain and fibromyalgia.[11] Also, there is compelling data implicating a number of infections, both viral and bacterial, in the triggering of fibromyalgia and related conditions.[97,98] Epstein Barr virus, Lyme disease, brucellosis, Ross River virus, Q fever, hepatitis C virus (HCV), as well as human immunodeficiency virus (HIV), are among those pathogens implicated.

Interestingly, infections may more reliably trigger fibromyalgia than will psychological stress; however, there is scant evidence that persistent symptoms are the result of persistent infection. Because the symptoms of fibromyalgia seem to overlap considerably with those associated with viral or atypical infections, considerable research has explored various pathogens. Numerous attempts to show clear serological evidence of increased rates of ongoing infection in these patients have resulted in mixed findings.[99] Not even in chronic fatigue syndrome patients, whose clinical manifestations are arguably most reminiscent of EBV infection, does there seem to be appreciable support for chronic infection with this virus.[100]

Individuals with documented infections with the Lyme spirochete can subsequently develop diffuse arthralgias and myalgias and fatigue, as well as cognitive difficulties such as impaired concentration and memory—thus, symptomatically, it closely resembles fibromyalgia. Many patients evaluated in Lyme disease specialty centers who are suffering from fibromyalgia have been diagnosed as cases of "chronic Lyme disease" and have received months or years of antibiotic treatment.[14,101] This occurs despite the fact that rigorous studies assessing patients suffering from chronic Lyme disease have failed to show that these patients respond to antibiotic treatment directed against *Borrelia burgdorferi*, the pathogen causing Lyme disease. Approximately 8% of patients suffering from Lyme disease and receiving adequate antibiotic treatment will go on to develop fibromyalgia within 1 to 3years.[102] Symptom persistence after Lyme disease treatment could be seen as a test case for revealing the relationship between fibromyalgia and infection. Effective antimicrobial treatment against Lyme disease is available, which is not the case in many other infectious agents that have been tied to fibromyalgia. Because a subset of Lyme disease patients treated with adequate antibiotic therapy manifests fibromyalgia post-infection, it seems quite possible that infection triggers a chain of events that, once initiated, will persist without the necessity of an ongoing infection.

The most compelling study exploring the underlying mechanisms operative in infections triggering these illnesses analyzed the long-term consequences of infection with 3 different pathogens (ie, Ross River Virus [the cause of epidemic polyarthritis], Coxiella Burnetii [cause of Q fever], and EBV) and the development of chronic fatigue syndrome.[103] The authors followed patients suffering from acute infections with these vastly different pathogens over 12 months and monitored them for the development of musculoskeletal pain, fatigue, cognitive dysfunction, and mood disturbances. At 12 months, 12% of patients developed this symptom complex. Despite the fact that these infections cause markedly different acute presentations, a highly stereotypical syndrome characterized by pain, fatigue, and memory difficulties occurred at remarkably similar rates after each infection. Demographic or microbiological factors during the acute infection did not predict the development of this symptom complex.[103,104] Further, none of the psychological factors—which included the presence of a pre-morbid or current psychiatric disorder, neuroticism—or locus of control significantly predicted the development of chronic symptoms. However, although psychological stress *per se* did not predict persistent or new symptoms after infection, the presence and severity of somatic symptoms during the acute infection was again closely associated with the subsequent development of chronic symptoms.

Quite remarkably, relationships between any number of acute infections and the development of chronic regional pain and other somatic symptoms have been noted. For example, Halvorson and colleagues noted, in a meta-analysis summarizing findings from 8 different studies, that approximately 10% of patients with an episode of acute infectious gastroenteritis caused by nearly any viral or bacterial pathogen will develop post-infectious IBS.[105] Correspondingly, acute urinary tract infection often precedes the development of interstitial cystitis/painful bladder syndrome.[106] As a whole, findings from these studies suggest that many forms of acute infection are capable of triggering widespread or regional pain (usually in the area of the body initially affected by pain), along with symptoms like fatigue, memory, and mood disturbances.

Across studies, it appears that there is a 10% risk of the post-infectious manifestation of this symptom complex, although the reason for this consistency is not known. Potentially, genetic factors could predispose individuals to this vulnerability. Perhaps the lack of specificity in regard to the trigger effect of infection may be related to an underlying genetic predisposition that is activated similarly across pathogens. This and/or any number of maladaptive behavioral responses could contribute to the expression of these symptoms (eg, cessation of routine exercise or sleep).

SUMMARY

Given the evidence compiled thus far, it is reasonable to conclude that, in some cases, psychological stressors can cause chronic pain, but perhaps less reliably than other types of stressors like physical trauma and infectious disease. Conversely, the experience of chronic pain seems quite capable of causing psychological stress and/or dysfunction of the stress response systems. Most importantly, the data show that a simple unidirectional relationship between the two does not exist. Interestingly, studies using neuroimaging techniques suggest that psychological stress (eg, depression and anxiety) and pain are processed fairly independently in the central nervous system.[67] Studies that support this observation include clinical trials demonstrating that antidepressant drugs with analgesic effects work equally well in pain patients with and without depression.[78] However, genetic and family studies suggest a shared heritable component between mood disorders and chronic pain. Although causation is not clear, suffice it to say that it is likely that the degree to which psychological stress affects pain and, conversely, pain affects psychological stress is largely mediated by personal factors such as cognitive and affective style, behaviors and habits, social support, cultural context, and other uniquely individual characteristics.

REFERENCES

1. Melzack R, Wall PD. Pain mechanisms: a new theory. Science 1965;150:971–9.
2. Lane RD, Waldstein SR, Critchley HD, et al. The rebirth of neuroscience in psychosomatic medicine, Part II: clinical applications and implications for research. Psychosom Med 2009;71:135–51.
3. Wolfe F, Smythe HA, Yunus MB, et al. The American College of Rheumatology 1990 Criteria for the Classification of Fibromyalgia. Report of the Multicenter Criteria Committee. Arthritis Rheum 1990;33:160–72.
4. Wolfe F, Clauw DJ, Fitzcharles MA, et al. The American College of Rheumatology preliminary diagnostic criteria for fibromyalgia and measurement of symptom severity. Arthritis Care Res (Hoboken) 2010;62:600–10.
5. Aaron LA, Burke MM, Buchwald D. Overlapping conditions among patients with chronic fatigue syndrome, fibromyalgia, and temporomandibular disorder. Arch Intern Med 2000;160:221–7.
6. Hudson JI, Hudson MS, Pliner LF, et al. Fibromyalgia and major affective disorder: a controlled phenomenology and family history study. Am J Psychiatry 1985;142:441–6.
7. Arnold LM, Hudson JI, Hess EV, et al. Family study of fibromyalgia. Arthritis Rheum 2004;50:944–52.
8. Sperber AD, Atzmon Y, Neumann L, et al. Fibromyalgia in the irritable bowel syndrome: studies of prevalence and clinical implications. Am J Gastroenterol 1999;94:3541–6.
9. Veale D, Kavanagh G, Fielding JF, et al. Primary fibromyalgia and the irritable bowel syndrome: different expressions of a common pathogenetic process. Br J Rheumatol 1991;30:220–2.
10. Wolfe F, Michaud K. Severe rheumatoid arthritis (RA), worse outcomes, comorbid illness, and sociodemographic disadvantage characterize ra patients with fibromyalgia. J Rheumatol 2004;31:695–700.
11. Clauw DJ, Katz P. The overlap between fibromyalgia and inflammatory rheumatic disease: when and why does it occur? J Clin Rheumatol 1995;1:335–42.
12. Arnold LM, Hudson JI, Keck PE, et al. Comorbidity of fibromyalgia and psychiatric disorders. J Clin Psychiatry 2006;67:1219–25.
13. Epstein SA, Kay G, Clauw D, et al. Psychiatric disorders in patients with fibromyalgia. A multicenter investigation. Psychosomatics 1999;40:57–63.

14. Hassett AL, Radvanski DC, Buyske S, et al. Psychiatric comorbidity and other psychological factors in patients with "chronic Lyme disease". Am J Med 2009;122: 843–50.

15. Raphael KG, Janal MN, Nayak S, et al. Psychiatric comorbidities in a community sample of women with fibromyalgia. Pain 2006;124:117–25.

16. Hudson JI, Goldenberg DL, Pope HG Jr, et al. Comorbidity of fibromyalgia with medical and psychiatric disorders. Am J Med 1992;92:363–7.

17. Bair MJ, Robinson RL, Katon W, et al. Depression and pain comorbidity: a literature review. Arch Intern Med 2003;163:2433–45.

18. Culpepper L. Generalized anxiety disorder and medical illness. J Clin Psychiatry 2009;70 (Suppl 2):20–4.

19. Hassett AL, Cone JD, Patella SJ, et al. The role of catastrophizing in the pain and depression of women with fibromyalgia syndrome. Arthritis Rheum 2000;43:2493–500.

20. Edwards RR, Bingham CO III, Bathon J, et al. Catastrophizing and pain in arthritis, fibromyalgia, and other rheumatic diseases. Arthritis Rheum 2006;55:325–32.

21. Shuster J, McCormack J, Pillai Riddell R, et al. Understanding the psychosocial profile of women with fibromyalgia syndrome. Pain Res Manag 2009;14:239–45.

22. Hassett AL, Simonelli LE, Radvanski DC, et al. The relationship between affect balance style and clinical outcomes in fibromyalgia. Arthritis Rheum 2008;59:833–40.

23. Zautra AJ, Fasman R, Reich JW, et al. Fibromyalgia: evidence for deficits in positive affect regulation. Psychosom Med 2005;67:147–55.

24. Karsdorp PA, Vlaeyen JW. Active avoidance but not activity pacing is associated with disability in fibromyalgia. Pain 2009;147:29–35.

25. Giesecke T, Williams DA, Harris RE, et al. Subgrouping of fibromyalgia patients on the basis of pressure-pain thresholds and psychological factors. Arthritis Rheum 2003;48:2916–22.

26. Turk DC, Okifuji A, Sinclair JD, et al. Pain, disability, and physical functioning in subgroups of patients with fibromyalgia. J Rheumatol 1996;23:1255–62.

27. Raphael KG, Janal MN, Nayak S. Comorbidity of fibromyalgia and posttraumatic stress disorder symptoms in a community sample of women. Pain Med 2004;5: 33–41.

28. Finestone HM, Stenn P, Davies F, et al. Chronic pain and health care utilization in women with a history of childhood sexual abuse. Child Abuse Negl 2000;24:547–56.

29. Hudson JI, Pope HG Jr. Does childhood sexual abuse cause fibromyalgia? Arthritis Rheum 1995;38:161–3.

30. McBeth J, Macfarlane GJ, Benjamin S, et al. Features of somatization predict the onset of chronic widespread pain: results of a large population-based study. Arthritis Rheum 2001;44:940–6.

31. Papageorgiou AC, Silman AJ, Macfarlane GJ. Chronic widespread pain in the population: a seven year follow up study. Ann Rheum Dis 2002;61:1071–4.

32. Croft P. The epidemiology of pain: the more you have, the more you get. Ann Rheum Dis 1996;55:859–60.

33. McBeth J, Macfarlane GJ, Silman AJ. Does chronic pain predict future psychological distress? Pain 2002;96:239–45.

34. McLean SA, Clauw DJ. Predicting chronic symptoms after an acute "stressor"—lessons learned from 3 medical conditions. Med. Hypotheses 2004;63:653–8.

35. Jones GT, Power C, Macfarlane GJ. Adverse events in childhood and chronic widespread pain in adult life: results from the 1958 British Birth Cohort Study. Pain 2009;143:92–6.

36. McBeth J, Silman AJ, Gupta A, et al. Moderation of psychosocial risk factors through dysfunction of the hypothalamic-pituitary-adrenal stress axis in the onset of chronic widespread musculoskeletal pain: findings of a population-based prospective cohort study. Arthritis Rheum 2007;56:360–71.
37. Hassett AL, Sigal LH. Unforeseen consequences of terrorism: medically unexplained symptoms in a time of fear. Arch Intern Med 2002;162:1809–13.
38. Raphael KG, Natelson BH, Janal MN, et al. A community-based survey of fibromy-algia-like pain complaints following the World Trade Center terrorist attacks. Pain 2002;100:131–9.
39. Williams DA, Brown SC, Clauw DJ, et al. Self-reported symptoms before and after September 11 in patients with fibromyalgia. JAMA 2003;289:1637–8.
40. Affleck G, Urrows S, Tennen H, et al. Sequential daily relations of sleep, pain intensity, and attention to pain among women with fibromyalgia. Pain 1996;68:363–8.
41. Demitrack MA, Crofford LJ. Evidence for and pathophysiologic implications of hypothalamic-pituitary-adrenal axis dysregulation in fibromyalgia and chronic fatigue syndrome. Ann N Y Acad Sci 1998;840:684–97.
42. Crofford LJ, Pillemer SR, Kalogeras KT, et al. Hypothalamic-pituitary-adrenal axis perturbations in patients with fibromyalgia. Arthritis Rheum 1994;37:1583–92.
43. Qiao ZG, Vaeroy H, Morkrid L. Electrodermal and microcirculatory activity in patients with fibromyalgia during baseline, acoustic stimulation and cold pressor tests. J Rheumatol 1991;18:1383–9.
44. Vaeroy H, Qiao ZG, Morkrid L, et al. Altered sympathetic nervous system response in patients with fibromyalgia (fibrositis syndrome). J Rheumatol 1989;16:1460–5.
45. Heim C, Nater UM, Maloney E, et al. Childhood trauma and risk for chronic fatigue syndrome: association with neuroendocrine dysfunction. Arch Gen Psychiatry 2009;66:72–80.
46. Penza KM, Heim C, Nemeroff CB. Neurobiological effects of childhood abuse: implications for the pathophysiology of depression and anxiety. Arch Womens Ment Health 2003;6:15–22.
47. McLean SA, Williams DA, Harris RE, et al. Momentary relationship between cortisol secretion and symptoms in patients with fibromyalgia. Arthritis Rheum 2005;52:3660–9.
48. Wingenfeld K, Nutzinger D, Kauth J, et al. Salivary cortisol release and hypothalamic pituitary adrenal axis feedback sensitivity in fibromyalgia is associated with depression but not with pain. J Pain 2010;11:1195–202.
49. Cohen H, Neumann L, Shore M, et al. Autonomic dysfunction in patients with fibromyalgia: application of power spectral analysis of heart rate variability. Semin Arthritis Rheum 2000;29:217–27.
50. Martinez-Lavin M, Hermosillo AG, Rosas M, et al. Circadian studies of autonomic nervous balance in patients with fibromyalgia: a heart rate variability analysis. Arthritis Rheum 1998;41:1966–71.
51. Joyner MJ, Masuki S. POTS versus deconditioning: the same or different? Clin Auton Res 2008;18:300–7.
52. Dorfman TA, Rosen BD, Perhonen MA, et al. Diastolic suction is impaired by bed rest: MRI tagging studies of diastolic untwisting. J Appl Physiol 2008;104:1037–44.
53. Glass JM, Lyden AK, Petzke F, et al. The effect of brief exercise cessation on pain, fatigue, and mood symptom development in healthy, fit individuals. J Psychosom Res 2004;57:391–8.

54. McBeth J, Chiu YH, Silman AJ, et al. Hypothalamic-pituitary-adrenal stress axis function and the relationship with chronic widespread pain and its antecedents. Arthritis Res Ther 2005;7:R992–1000.

55. McLean SA, Williams DA, Stein PK, et al. Cerebrospinal fluid corticotropin-releasing factor concentration is associated with pain but not fatigue symptoms in patients with fibromyalgia. Neuropsychopharmacology 2006;31:2776–82.

56. Woolf CJ. What is this thing called pain? J Clin Invest 2010;120:3742–4.

57. Munakata J, Naliboff B, Harraf F, et al. Repetitive sigmoid stimulation induces rectal hyperalgesia in patients with irritable bowel syndrome. Gastroenterology 1997;112: 55–63.

58. Maixner W, Fillingim R, Booker D, et al. Sensitivity of patients with painful temporo-mandibular disorders to experimentally evoked pain. Pain 1995;63:341–51.

59. Petzke F, Clauw DJ, Ambrose K, et al. Increased pain sensitivity in fibromyalgia: effects of stimulus type and mode of presentation. Pain 2003;105:403–13.

60. Clauw DJ, Schmidt M, Radulovic D, et al. The relationship between fibromyalgia and interstitial cystitis. Journal of Psychiatric Research 1997;31:125–31.

61. Lautenbacher S, Rollman GB, McCain GA. Multi-method assessment of experimental and clinical pain in patients with fibromyalgia. Pain 1994;59:45–53.

62. Mense S, Hoheisel U, Reinert A. The possible role of substance P in eliciting and modulating deep somatic pain. Progress in Brain Research 1996;110:125–35.

63. Geisser ME, Glass JM, Rajcevska LD, et al. A psychophysical study of auditory and pressure sensitivity in patients with fibromyalgia and healthy controls. J Pain 2008; 9:417–22.

64. Geisser ME, Gracely RH, Giesecke T, et al. The association between experimental and clinical pain measures among persons with fibromyalgia and chronic fatigue syndrome. Eur J Pain 2007;11:202–7.

65. Harris RE, Gracely RH, McLean SA, et al. Comparison of clinical and evoked pain measures in fibromyalgia. J Pain 2006;7:521–7.

66. Normand E, Potvin S, Gaumond I, et al. Pain inhibition is deficient in chronic widespread pain but normal in major depressive disorder. J Clin Psychiatry 2011; 72:219–24.

67. Giesecke T, Gracely RH, Williams DA, et al. The relationship between depression, clinical pain, and experimental pain in a chronic pain cohort. Arthritis Rheum 2005;52:1577–84.

68. Gracely RH, Petzke F, Wolf JM, et al. Functional magnetic resonance imaging evidence of augmented pain processing in fibromyalgia. Arthritis Rheum 2002;46: 1333–43.

69. Giesecke T, Gracely RH, Grant MA, et al. Evidence of augmented central pain processing in idiopathic chronic low back pain. Arthritis Rheum 2004;50:613–23.

70. Cook DB, Lange G, Ciccone DS, et al. Functional imaging of pain in patients with primary fibromyalgia. J Rheumatol 2004;31:364–78.

71. Naliboff BD, Derbyshire SW, Munakata J, et al. Cerebral activation in patients with irritable bowel syndrome and control subjects during rectosigmoid stimulation. Psychosom Med 2001;63:365–75.

72. Mayer EA, Naliboff BD, Craig AD. Neuroimaging of the brain-gut axis: from basic understanding to treatment of functional GI disorders. Gastroenterology 2006;131: 1925–42.

73. Gwilym SE, Keltner JR, Warnaby CE, et al. Psychophysical and functional imaging evidence supporting the presence of central sensitization in a cohort of osteoarthritis patients. Arthritis Rheum 2009;61:1226–34.

74. Gracely RH, Geisser ME, Giesecke T, et al. Pain catastrophizing and neural responses to pain among persons with fibromyalgia. Brain 2004;127(Pt 4):835–43.
75. Harris RE, Sundgren PC, Pang Y, et al. Dynamic levels of glutamate within the insula are associated with improvements in multiple pain domains in fibromyalgia. Arthritis Rheum 2008;58:903–7.
76. Craig AD. How do you feel? Interoception: the sense of the physiological condition of the body. Nat Rev Neurosci 2002;3:655–66.
77. Fishbain D. Evidence-based data on pain relief with antidepressants. Ann Med 2000;32:305–16.
78. Arnold LM. Duloxetine and other antidepressants in the treatment of patients with fibromyalgia. Pain Med 2007;8(Suppl 2):S63–74.
79. Hudson JI, Pope HG Jr. The relationship between fibromyalgia and major depressive disorder. Rheum Dis Clin North Am 1996;22:285–303.
80. Buskila D, Neumann L, Hazanov I, et al. Familial aggregation in the fibromyalgia syndrome. Semin Arthritis Rheum 1996;26:605–11.
81. Kato K, Sullivan PF, Evengard B, et al. Chronic widespread pain and its comorbidities: a population-based study. Arch Intern Med 2006;166:1649–54.
82. Hudson JI, Arnold LM, Keck PE Jr, et al. Family study of fibromyalgia and affective spectrum disorder. Biol Psychiatry 2004;56:884–91.
83. Raphael KG, Janal MN, Nayak S, et al. Familial aggregation of depression in fibromyalgia: a community-based test of alternate hypotheses. Pain 2004;110: 449–60.
84. Yunus MB. Central sensitivity syndromes: a new paradigm and group nosology for fibromyalgia and overlapping conditions, and the related issue of disease versus illness. Semin Arthritis Rheum 2008;37:339–52.
85. Mogil JS, Wilson SG, Bon K, et al. Heritability of nociception II. 'Types' of nociception revealed by genetic correlation analysis. Pain 1999;80:83–93.
86. Mogil JS, Wilson SG, Bon K, et al. Heritability of nociception I: responses of 11 inbred mouse strains on 12 measures of nociception. Pain 1999;80:67–82.
87. Costigan M, Belfer I, Griffin RS, et al. Multiple chronic pain states are associated with a common amino acid-changing allele in KCNS1. Brain 2010;133:2519–27.
88. Tegeder I, Adolph J, Schmidt H, et al. Reduced hyperalgesia in homozygous carriers of a GTP cyclohydrolase 1 haplotype. Eur J Pain 2008;12:1069–77.
89. Tegeder I, Costigan M, Griffin RS, et al. GTP cyclohydrolase and tetrahydrobiopterin regulate pain sensitivity and persistence. Nat Med 2006;12:1269–77.
90. Amaya F, Wang H, Costigan M, et al. The voltage-gated sodium channel Na(v)1.9 is an effector of peripheral inflammatory pain hypersensitivity. J Neurosci 2006;26: 12852–60.
91. Nackley AG, Tan KS, Fecho K, et al. Catechol-O-methyltransferase inhibition increases pain sensitivity through activation of both beta2- and beta3-adrenergic receptors. Pain 2007;128:199–208.
92. Diatchenko L, Anderson AD, Slade GD, et al. Three major haplotypes of the beta2 adrenergic receptor define psychological profile, blood pressure, and the risk for development of a common musculoskeletal pain disorder. Am J Med Genet B Neuropsychiatr Genet 2006;141:449–62.
93. Diatchenko L, Slade GD, Nackley AG, et al. Genetic basis for individual variations in pain perception and the development of a chronic pain condition. Hum Mol Genet 2005;14:135–43.
94. Buskila D, Sarzi-Puttini P, Ablin JN. The genetics of fibromyalgia syndrome. Pharmacogenomics 2007;8:67–74.

95. Clauw DJ, Engel CC Jr, Aronowitz R, et al. Unexplained symptoms after terrorism and war: an expert consensus statement. J Occup Environ Med 2003;45:1040–8.
96. McLean SA, Clauw DJ, Abelson JL, et al. The development of persistent pain and psychological morbidity after motor vehicle collision: integrating the potential role of stress response systems into a biopsychosocial model. Psychosom Med 2005;67: 783–90.
97. Ortega-Hernandez OD, Shoenfeld Y. Infection, vaccination, and autoantibodies in chronic fatigue syndrome, cause or coincidence? Ann N Y Acad Sci 2009;1173: 600–9.
98. Ablin JN, Buskila D, Clauw DJ. Biomarkers in fibromyalgia. Curr Pain Headache Rep 2009;13:343–9.
99. Buchwald D, Goldenberg DL, Sullivan JL, et al. The "chronic, active Epstein-Barr virus infection" syndrome and primary fibromyalgia. Arthritis Rheum 1987;30: 1132–6.
100. Whelton CL, Salit I, Moldofsky H. Sleep, Epstein-Barr virus infection, musculoskeletal pain, and depressive symptoms in chronic fatigue syndrome. J Rheumatol 1992;19:939–43.
101. Hassett AL, Radvanski DC, Buyske S, et al. Role of psychiatric comorbidity in chronic Lyme disease. Arthritis Rheum 2008;59:1742–9.
102. Dinerman H, Steere AC. Lyme disease associated with fibromyalgia. Ann Intern Med 1992;117:281–5.
103. Hickie I, Davenport T, Wakefield D, et al. Post-infective and chronic fatigue syndromes precipitated by viral and non-viral pathogens: prospective cohort study. BMJ 2006;333:575.
104. Vollmer-Conna U, Cameron B, Hadzi-Pavlovic D, et al. Postinfective fatigue syndrome is not associated with altered cytokine production. Clin Infect Dis 2007;45: 732–5.
105. Halvorson HA, Schlett CD, Riddle MS. Postinfectious irritable bowel syndrome—a meta-analysis. Am J Gastroenterol 2006;101:1894–9.
106. Warren JW, Howard FM, Cross RK, et al. Antecedent nonbladder syndromes in case-control study of interstitial cystitis/painful bladder syndrome. Urology 2009;73: 52–7.

Can Neural Imaging Explain Pain?

Stuart W.G. Derbyshire, PhD

KEYWORDS

• Pain • Neural imaging • Placebo • Nocebo • Chronic pain

An enduring medical challenge is why some people seem to be more pain sensitive than others and whether such sensitivity is related to pain that persists despite the absence of obvious tissue damage or disease. Differences in sensitivity and pain in the absence of injury or disease undermine the intuitive link between objective damage and subjective experience. If one person feels more pain from a given stimulus or feels pain without a stimulus, then the pain must, at least in part, derive from something unique to the person rather than the world outside. The pain is being constructed by the person's mind or brain and involves processes associated with the thoughts and behavior of the person or with the sensory integration performed by their brain. The problem of how pain might be inflated or created by brain–mind mechanisms is a core concern of psychosomatic medicine and has been investigated through the use of sensitive neural imaging techniques since they became available toward the end of the 1980s.

Twenty years ago, there were a handful of imaging papers examining brain responses to somatic noxious stimulation.[1–5] These studies demonstrated involvement of both the "lateral" and "medial" systems in processing an acute noxious stimulus. Lateral spinothalamic pathways transmit information to primary sensory cortex (S1), which is believed to code for the intensity, duration, and location of noxious stimuli. Medial spinothalamic pathways transmit information to limbic cortices, including the anterior cingulate cortex, which are believed to code the motivational and affective qualities associated with noxious stimulation. After these early studies, there has been an exponential rise in the number of functional imaging studies using noxious stimulation (for reviews, see references Lane and colleagues[6] and Vogt[7]).

Fig. 1 summarizes reported activations on the lateral and medial surface of the brain. Each circle was plotted according to the reported coordinates in the original reports. The procedure follows previous reviews and the figure adapted from a previous report to include noxious cold as well as noxious heat.[6] Fig. 1 illustrates that pain experience results in widespread lateral cortical activity encompassing areas traditionally associated with sensory processing (S1 and secondary somatosensory

University of Birmingham, School of Psychology, Edgbaston B15 2TT, UK
E-mail address: s.w.derbyshire@bham.ac.uk

Psychiatr Clin N Am 34 (2011) 595–604
doi:10.1016/j.psc.2011.05.002
0193-953X/11/$ – see front matter © 2011 Elsevier Inc. All rights reserved.

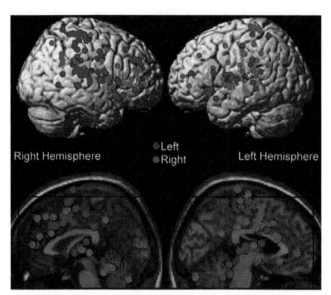

Fig. 1. Lateral (*top*) and medial (*bottom*) surface activation during noxious experience (adapted from the figure in Lane and colleagues[6]). The center of each reported rCBF increase is shown when the noxious stimuli was delivered to the left side of the body (*red circles*) or to the right side of the body (*blue circles*). There is extensive clustering of response in the primary and secondary somatosensory cortex, prefrontal cortex, anterior cingulate cortex, and thalamus (*Adapted from* Lane RD, Waldstein SR, Critchley H, et al. The rebirth of neuroscience in psychosomatic medicine, Part II: clinical applications and implications for research. Psychosom Med 2009;71:135–51; with permission.).

cortex, S2) as well as areas associated with cognition and the organization of behavior (prefrontal cortices). There is evident lateralization of responses in primary sensory cortex, which is consistent with the presumed role of localization and the known anatomy. **Fig. 1** also illustrates widespread activation on the medial surface with evident activation of the midcingulate region.[7] The midcingulate cortex (MCC) connects to dorsolateral prefrontal and motor cortices and is believed to be predominantly involved in the organization of behaviors to minimize stress or conflict. Intriguingly, there is evidence of laterality with left-sided noxious stimulation showing an evident bias toward right MCC and right-sided noxious stimulation a bias toward the left MCC. Although the usual interpretation of MCC activity includes affect, a lateralized pattern clearly suggests that some sensory coding may also be occurring.

In summary, a variety of functional imaging studies with noxious somatic stimuli have demonstrated reasonably consistent activation of S1, S2, the MCC, and the prefrontal cortex. These widespread activations are consistent with the understanding of pain as a complex, multidimensional experience involving sensory, affective, and cognitive components, broadly consistent with the idea of pain being a biopsychosocial phenomenon.[8–10]

More recent brain imaging studies have extended well beyond the mere association of noxious stimulation with brain activity. In 2010, studies have examined clinical pain,[11–15] emotional pain,[16,17] interactions of acute pain with a history of stress,[18,19] novel mechanisms of analgesia,[20–22] temporal summation,[23] associations of pain responses with individual differences,[24–27] interactions of acute pain with psychiatric disorder,[28] drug effects,[29–31] interactions of acute pain with mood,[32,33] empathic pain,[34,35] imagined pain,[36] and interactions of acute pain with age.[37] Other studies have also examined how acute pain was associated with pain ratings,[38,39] virtual pain,[40,41] the sensory and affective components of acute pain,[42] central sensitization,[43,44] descending inhibition,[45,46] acute pain responses in clinical pain patients,[47,48] gender differences,[49,50] interactions of acute pain with cognition,[51,52] and pain expectation.[53,54] That list is by no means exhaustive.

Reviewing all neural imaging studies pertaining to pain in a single article was once possible,[55] but is no longer. This review, therefore, focuses on 2 areas of particular interest: Efforts to enhance pain without a typical noxious stimulus and efforts to reduce pain without a typical analgesic or anesthetic. The review considers also broader issues and problems associated with pain imaging.

ENHANCING PAIN

Saint Teresa of Avila (Teresa de Cepeda y Ahumada) was born in Avila, Spain, in 1515. At the age of 16 she was sent to a Catholic convent school and eventually she entered the Carmelite Order as a nun. Teresa famously wrote of being visited by an angel who carried a spear circa 1560:

> In his hands I saw a long golden spear and at the end of the iron tip I seemed to see a point of fire. With this he seemed to pierce my heart several times so that it penetrated to my entrails. When he drew it out, I thought he was drawing them out with it and he left me completely afire with a great love for God. The pain was so sharp that it made me utter several moans; and so excessive was the sweetness caused me by this intense pain that one can never wish to lose it, nor will one's soul be content with anything less than God. It is not bodily pain, but spiritual, though the body has a share in it—indeed, a great share. *The life of Teresa of Jesus, The Autobiography of Teresa of Ávila.*[56(pp 164–5)]

Teresa's experience was captured by Bernini in his most magnificent marble sculpture, *The Ecstasy of Saint Teresa*, which can be found in the Cornaro Chapel, Santa Maria della Vittoria, Rome. The sculpture is shown in **Fig. 2** and it is clear that Bernini took considerable artistic license with Teresa's account. The smiling angel aims an arrow, not a spear, and he aims it rather lower than the heart. Bernini was clearly interested in the ecstasy part of Teresa's experience, but what is interesting for us is her insistence that the pain was felt not just spiritually but bodily; she had a physical manifestation of pain from the vision. Assuming she was not actually visited by an angel, the pain she felt presumably derived from her own mental activity.

Rather more recently, a builder was reported entering a British emergency room having jumped down onto a 15-cm (6-inch) nail that passed clean through his boot and, presumably, also his foot inside the boot.[57] The boot and nail are shown in **Fig. 3**. From what can be seen in **Fig. 3**, it is not surprising that the builder entered in considerable pain and required sedation and opioid analgesia. Once calm, however, the boot was carefully removed to reveal that the nail had passed directly between the toes, leaving his foot entirely uninjured. As with Saint Teresa, the pain felt presumably derived from his mental activity.

These two anecdotes illustrate that pain can be generated in the complete absence of what might be typically considered a noxious stimulus, which suggests that neuropsychological mechanisms alone might be sufficient to drive at least some types of pain. Understanding those mechanisms might provide insight into a variety painful disorders that occur without obvious disease or injury.[58] Studying hallucinating nuns or

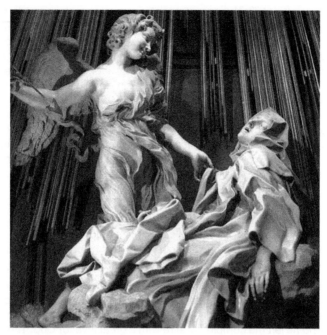

Fig. 2. The *Ecstasy of Saint Teresa* is the central sculptural group in white marble set in an elevated shrine in the Cornaro Chapel, Santa Maria della Vittoria, Rome. The sculpture was designed and completed by Bernini in 1652.

coaxing people to jump onto nails, however, are not practical options for the laboratory.

Laboratory techniques to generate pain in the absence of injury have included hypnotic suggestion of pain without a noxious stimulus[59,60]; manipulations of visual

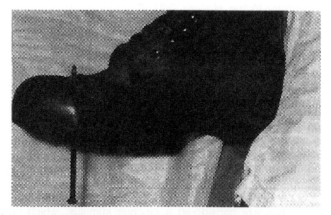

Fig. 3. The boot and nail as it penetrated the boot while worn by a 29-year-old builder. The nail passed directly through the builder's toes without causing any tissue damage but the builder expressed considerable pain and distress before the boot was removed (*From* Fisher JP, Hassan DT, O'Connor N. Minerva. Brit Med J 1995;310:70; with permission.).

feedback so as to be incongruous with motor movements, which is sometimes experienced as painful[61-63]; presentation of pain images, which induces pain in some[35,64-65]; difficult-to-detect stimuli that sometimes results in pain being reported when the stimulus is not delivered[66,67]; the presentation of noxious stimuli in a virtual environment[40,41]; and manipulations of expectancy so that the participant expects a strong noxious stimulus that is not delivered and then experiences pain.[54] In general, these procedures produce pain reports that are not easily discriminable from pain reports based on delivery of typically noxious stimuli.

Use of these techniques in combination with functional imaging has revealed activation of the pain neuromatrix, including anterior cingulate, and primary and secondary somatosensory cortices.[54,60,64] Although the precise mechanisms remain to be revealed, these studies demonstrate that areas of the pain neuromatrix do not just passively respond to noxious stimuli but, under the right circumstances, actively create a noxious experience. Patients suffering pain without any known injury or disease might, therefore, be suffering a problem associated with pain generated directly by the neuromatrix.[68]

REDUCING PAIN

Publication of gate control theory[69] firmly established that noxious information does not force itself onto the brain to create pain, but instead noxious information gains access to the brain only under certain circumstances and then creates pain only under certain circumstances. There is no dedicated line system from the periphery to the brain that dictates pain; the central nervous system unravels various sources of noxious and non-noxious inputs to produce a final experience. Part of that unraveling involves descending inhibitory control from the brain[20,70] and studies have demonstrated that descending inhibitory control can be reliably activated in the laboratory using additional noxious stimuli.[71] Similar inhibition of pain, however, has also been demonstrated with placebo[21] and with the offset of a strong noxious stimulus.[20,46,72]

Broadly speaking, placebo interventions that manipulate pain related expectancy seem to influence a neocortical network involving prefrontal and rostral anterior cingulate regions[21,73] and there is some evidence that these neocortical responses may be dysfunctional in some chronic patients suffering pain without any known injury or disease.[45] In patients with fibromyalgia, for example, the rostral anterior cingulate cortex does not respond to noxious pressure even though other regions of the pain neuromatrix seem to more readily respond to noxious pressure.[45] Presumably, the rostral anterior cingulate cortex is involved in pain analgesia that is dysfunctional in patients with fibromyalgia. To an extent, studies demonstrating active involvement of the neocortex in pain analgesia associated with placebo mirror the studies demonstrating involvement of the neocortex in pain enhancement, which might be viewed as nocebo studies.[54,59,60]

In contrast, pain reduction associated with a drop in a noxious stimulus, known as "offset analgesia," seem to involve brainstem regions including the periaqueductal gray and rostral ventral medulla.[46,72] Stimulation of these regions is known to produce analgesic responses,[74] whereas damage to these regions can cause pain.[71,75] It is therefore possible that patients suffering pain without any known injury or disease have unseen damage in these regions of the brain that typically provide ongoing inhibition of noxious information.

DESCRIBING PAIN AND EXPLAINING PAIN

It is an obvious hope that neural imaging will help us to understand pain and thus bring us closer to novel and effective interventions. The need for effective intervention is especially pressing for patients who suffer pain without identifiable injury, disease, or other pathology, such as fibromyalgia or nonspecific low back pain. Such patients are often described as suffering a "functional disorder." These disorders are common in the general population with estimates of chronic sufferers ranging from 5% to 20%.[76,77] Treatment of the functional disorders is difficult and physicians and patients often reach for multiple treatments, sequentially or in combination, to achieve symptom relief. Unfortunately, this strategy often results in failure. In many cases, physicians are left frustrated and patients dissatisfied with chronic, unremitting symptoms. Because the brain is the final common pathway for pain experience, and pain is a central symptom of many functional disorders, it is generally believed that a better understanding of brain activity during pain will provide an improved mechanistic understanding of pain with the possibility of better treatment approaches for functional disorders and other chronic pain problems.[78]

To date that hope has not been realized. In part, investigations are still new and there is a need for further information and better detail regarding the neural mechanisms underpinning chronic pain. But it is also in part because neural imaging data do not, in themselves, provide an explanation for the behavioral phenomenon being explored. Knowing that the rostral anterior cingulate cortex, for example, is associated with placebo analgesia does not provide an explanation for the placebo effect or obviously point toward a new treatment. Such studies provide information regarding the location of effects, but do not provide information regarding the mechanism of action. Indeed, there is a danger of being lulled into thinking that brain activity is the explanation and thus being distracted from the necessary work of trying to understand what is driving brain activity.

Further knowledge about the brain, what it does during noxious stimulation, and what it does when someone reports pain experience will continue to be interesting, but we lose something when we boil pain down to the brain. We lose the situation within which pain takes place and the conception of sensation as a subjective experience along with more subtle and complex notions of how social and psychological factors impinge on the experience. Neural activation is an important part of the story and provides a rich description of what happens during pain but neural activation is not, in itself, an explanation of pain.

REFERENCES

1. Talbot JD, Marret S, Evans AC, et al. Multiple representations of pain in human cerebral cortex. Science 1991;251:1355–8.
2. Jones APK, Brown WD, Friston KJ, et al. Cortical and subcortical localization of response to pain in man using positron emission tomography. Proc R Soc Lond 1991;244:39–44.
3. Casey KL, Minoshima S, Berger KL, et al. Positron emission tomographic analysis of cerebral structures activated specifically by repetitive noxious heat stimuli. J Neurophysiol 1994;71:802–7.
4. Coghill RC, Talbot JD, Evans AC, et al. Distributed processing of pain and vibration by the human brain. J Neurosci 1994;14:4095–8.
5. Derbyshire SWG, Jones AKP, Devani P, et al. Cerebral responses to pain in patients with atypical facial pain measured by positron emission tomography. J Neurol Neurosurg Psychiat 1994;57:1166–73.
6. Lane RD, Waldstein SR, Critchley H, et al. The rebirth of neuroscience in psychosomatic medicine, part II: clinical applications and implications for research. Psychosom Med 2009;71:135–51.

7. Vogt B. Pain and emotion interactions in subregions of the cingulate cortex. Nature Rev Neurosci 2005;6:533–44.
8. Keefe FJ, Dunsmore J, Burnett R. Behavioral and cognitive-behavioral approaches to chronic pain: Recent advances and future directions. J Consult Clin Psychol 1992; 60:528–36.
9. Drossman DA. Gastrointestinal illness and the biopsychosocial model. J Clin Gastroenterol 1996;22:252–4.
10. Turk DC, Rudy TE. Cognitive factors and persistent pain: a glimpse into Pandora's box. Cognit Ther Res 1992;16:99–122.
11. Buavanendran A, Ali A, Stoub TR, et al. Brain activity associated with chronic cancer pain. Pain Physician 2010;13:E337–42.
12. Gustin SM, Schwarz A, Birbaumer N, et al. NMDA-receptor antagonist and morphine decrease CRPS-pain and cerebral pain representation. Pain 2010;151:69–76.
13. Walton KD, Dubois M, Llinas RR. Abnormal thalamocortical activity in patients with complex regional pain syndrome (CRPS) type I. Pain 2010;150:41–51.
14. Napadow V, La Count L, Park K, et al. Intrinsic brain connectivity in fibromyalgia is associated with chronic pain intensity. Arthritis Rheum 2010;62:2545–55.
15. Malinen S, Vartiainen N, Hlushchuk Y, et al. Aberrant temporal and spatial brain activity during rest in patients with chronic pain. Proc Natl Acad Sci U S A 2010;107: 6493–7.
16. Reisch T, Deifritz E, Esposito F, et al. An fMRI study on mental pain and suicidal behavior. J Affect Disord 2010;126:321–5.
17. Dewall CN, Macdonald G, Webster GD, et al. Acetaminophen reduces social pain: behavioral and neural evidence. Psych Sci 2010;21:931–7.
18. Strigo IA, Simmons AN, Mathews SC, et al. Neural correlates of altered pain response in women with posttraumatic stress disorder from intimate partner violence. Biol Psychiatry 2010;68:442–50.
19. Hohmeister J, Kroll A, Wollgarten-Hadamek I, et al. Cerebral processing of pain in school-aged children with neonatal nociceptive input: an exploratory fMRI study. Pain 2010;150:257–67.
20. Baliki MN, Geha PY, Fields HL, et al. Predicting value of pain and analgesia: nucleus accumbens response to noxious stimuli changes in the presence of chronic pain. Neuron 2010;66:149–60.
21. Petrovic P, Kalso E, Petersson KM, et al. A prefrontal non-opioid mechanism in placebo analgesia. Pain 2010;150:59–65.
22. Rottman S, Jung K, Vohn R, et al. Long-term depression of pain-related cerebral activation in healthy man: an fMRI study. Eur J Pain 2010;14:615–24.
23. Tran TD, Wang H, Tandon A, et al. Temporal summation of heat pain in humans: evidence supporting thalamocortical modulation. Pain 2010;150:93–102.
24. Piche M, Arsenault M, Rainville P. Dissection of perceptual, motor and autonomic components of brain activity evoked by noxious stimulation. Pain 2010;149:453–62.
25. Mobascher A, Brinkmeyer J, Thiele H, et al. The val158met polymorphism of human catechol-O-methyltransferase (COMT) affects anterior cingulate cortex activation in response to laser stimulation. Molecular Pain 2010;6:32.
26. Ziv M, Tomer R, Defrin R, et al. Individual sensitivity to pain expectancy is related to differential activation of the hippocampus and amygdala. Hum Brain Mapp 2010;31: 326–38.
27. Ploner M, Lee MC, Wiech K, et al. Prestimulus functional connectivity determines pain perception in humans. Proc Natl Acad Sci U S A 2010;107:355–60.

28. de la Fuente-Sandoval C, Favila R, Gomez-Martin D, et al. Functional magnetic resonance imaging response to experimental pain in drug-free patients with schizophrenia. Psychiatry Res 2010;183:99–104.

29. Scrivani S, Wallin D, Moulton EA. A fMRI evaluation of lamotrigine for the treatment of trigeminal neuropathic pain: pilot study. Pain Med 2010;11:920–41.

30. Mhuircheartaigh RN, Rosenorm-Lanng D, Wise R, et al. Cortical and subcortical connectivity changes during decreasing levels of consciousness in humans: a functional magnetic resonance imaging study using propofol. J Neurosci 2010; 30:9095–102.

31. Cosgrove KP, Esterlis I, McKee S, et al. Beta2* nicotinic acetylcholine receptors modulate pain sensitivity in acutely abstinent tobacco smokers. Nicotine Tob Res 2010;12:535–9.

32. Berna C, Leknes S, Holmes EA, et al. Induction of depressed mood disrupts emotion regulation neurocircuitry and enhances pain unpleasantness. Biol Psychiatry 2010; 67:1083–90.

33. Yahino A, Okamoto Y, Onoda K, et al. Sadness enhances the experience of pain via neural activation in the anterior cingulate cortex and amygdala: an fMRI study. Neuroimage 2010;50:1194–201.

34. Noll-Hussong M, Otti A, Laeer L, et al. Aftermath of sexual abuse history on adult patients suffering from chronic functional pain syndromes: an fMRI pilot study. J Psychosom Res 2010;68:483–7.

35. Osborn J, Derbyshire SW. Pain sensation evoked by observing injury in others. Pain 2010;148:268–74.

36. Gustin SM, Wrigley PJ, Henderson LA, et al. Brain circuitry underlying pain in response to imagined movement in people with spinal cord injury. Pain 2010;148: 438–45.

37. Cole LJ, Farrell MJ, Gibson SJ, et al. Age-related differences in pain sensitivity and regional brain activity evoked by noxious pressure. Neurobiol Aging 2010;31:494–503.

38. Baliki MN, Geha PY, Apkarian AV. Parsing pain perception between nociceptive representation and magnitude estimation. J Neurophysiol 2009;101:875–87.

39. Schoedel AL, Zimmermann K, Handwerker HO, et al. The influence of simultaneous ratings on cortical BOLD effects during painful and non-painful stimulation. Pain 2008;135:131–41.

40. Said Yekta S, Vohn R, Ellrich J. Cerebral activations resulting from virtual dental treatment. Eur J Oral Sci 2009;117:711–9.

41. Ushida T, Ikemoto T, Taniguchi S, et al. Virtual pain stimulation of allodynia patients activates cortical representation of pain and emotions: a functional MRI study. Brain Topography 2005;18:27–35.

42. Oshiro Y, Quevedo AS, McHaffie JG, et al. Brain mechanisms supporting discrimination of sensory features of pain: a new model. J Neurosci 2009;29:14924–31.

43. Gwilym SE, Keltner JR, Warnaby CE, et al. Psychophysical and functional imaging evidence supporting the presence of central sensitization in a cohort of osteoarthritis patients. Arthrit Rheum 2009;61:1226–34.

44. Lee MC, Zambreanu L, Menon DK, et al. Identifying brain activity specifically related to the maintenance and perceptual consequence of central sensitization in humans. J Neurosci 2008;28:11642–9.

45. Jensen KB, Kosek E, Petzke F, et al. Evidence of dysfunctional pain inhibition in Fibromyalgia reflected in rACC during provoked pain. Pain 2009;144:95–100.

46. Derbyshire SWG, Osborn J. Offset analgesia is mediated by activation in the region of the periaqueductal grey and rostral ventromedial medulla. Neuroimage 2009;47: 1002–6.

47. Pujol J, Lopexz-Sola M, Ortiz H, et al. Mapping brain responses to pain in fibromyalgia patients using temporal analysis of fMRI. PLoS ONE 2009;4:e5224.

48. Burgmer M, Pogatzki-Zahn E, Gaubitz M, et al. Altered brain activity during pain processing in fibromyalgia. Neuroimage 2009;44:502–8.

49. Henderson LA, Gandevia SC, Macefield VG. Gender differences in brain activity evoked by muscle and cutaneous pain: a retrospective study of single-trial fMRI data. Neuroimage 2008;39:1867–76.

50. Moulton EA, Keaser ML, Gullapalli RP, et al. Sex differences in the cerebral BOLD signal response to painful heat stimulation. Am J Physiol Reg I 2006;291:R257–67.

51. Seminowicz DA, Davis KD. Interactions of pain intensity and cognitive load: the brain stays on task. Cereb Cortex 2007;17:1412–22.

52. Seminowicz DA, Davis KD. Pain enhances functional connectivity of a brain network evoked by performance of a cognitive task. J Neurophysiol 2007;97:3651–9.

53. Berns GS, Chappelow J, Cekic M, et al. Neurobiological substrates of dread. Science 2006;312:754–8.

54. Koyoma T, McHaffie JG, Laurienti PJ, et al. The subjective experience of pain: where expectations become reality. Proc Nat Acad Sci U S A 2005;102:12950–5.

55. Derbyshire SWG. Exploring the pain "neuromatrix." Curr Rev Pain 2000;6:467–77.

56. Peers EA. The life of Teresa of Jesus, The autobiography of Teresa of Ávila [electronic text]. 1995. Available at: http://www.jesus.org.uk/vault/library/teresa_life.pdf. Accessed February 3, 2011.

57. Fisher JP, Hassan DT, O'Connor N. Minerva. Brit Med J 1995;310:70.

58. Wessely S, Nimnuan C, Sharpe M. Functional somatic syndromes: one or many? Lancet 1999;354:936–9.

59. Whalley MG, Oakley DA. Psychogenic pain: a study using multidimensional scaling. Contemp Hypn 2003;20:16–24.

60. Derbyshire SWG, Whalley MG, Stenger VA, et al. Cerebral activation during hypnotically induced and imagined pain. Neuroimage 2004;23:392–401.

61. McCabe CS, Cohen H, Blake DR. Somaesthetic disturbances in fibromyalgia are exaggerated by sensory–motor conflict: implications for chronicity of the disease? Rheumatol 2007;46:1587–92.

62. McCabe CS, Haigh RC, Halligan PW, et al. Simulating sensory-motor incongruence in healthy volunteers: implications for a cortical model of pain. Rheumatol 2005; 44:509–16.

63. Derbyshire SWG, Cameron AD, Lloyd DM, et al. A motor version of the rubber arm illusion: Does it hurt when it moves 'wrong'? The BackCare Journal 2010;Autumn: 24–9.

64. Giummarra MJ, Bradshaw JL. Synaesthesia for pain: Feeling pain with another. In: Pineda JA editor. The role of mirroring processes in social cognition. Totowa (NJ): Humana Press Inc.; 2008.

65. Fitzgibbon BM, Giummarra MJ, Georgiou-Karistianis N, et al. Shared pain: From empathy to synaesthesia. Neuroscience and Biobehavioral Reviews 2009;34: 500–12.

66. Kirwilliam SS, Derbyshire SWG. Increased bias to report heat or pain following emotional priming of pain-related fear. Pain 2008;137:60–5.

67. Brown RJ, Brunt N, Poliakoff E, et al. Illusory touch and tactile perception in somatoform dissociators. J Psychosom Res 2010;69:241–8.

68. Derbyshire SWG, Whalley MG, Oakley DA. Fibromyalgia pain and its modulation by hypnotic and non-hypnotic suggestion: an fMRI analysis. Eur J Pain 2009;13:542–50.
69. Melzack R, Wall PD. Pain mechanisms: a new theory. Science 1965;150:971–9.
70. Fields H. State-dependent opioid control of pain. Nature Rev Neurosci 2004;5:565–74.
71. Yarnitsky D, Crispel Y, Eisenberg E, et al. Prediction of chronic post-operative pain: pre-operative DNIC testing identifies patients at risk. Pain 2008;138:22–8.
72. Yelle MD, Oshiro Y, Kraft RA, et al. Temporal filtering of nociceptive information by dynamic activation of endogenous pain modulatory systems. J Neurosci 2009;29:10264–71.
73. Petrovic P, Dietrich T, Fransson P, et al. Placebo in emotional processing—induced expectations of anxiety relief activate a generalized modulatory network. Neuron 2005;46:957–69.
74. Hosobuchi Y, Adams JE, Linchitz R. Pain relief by electrical stimulation of the central gray matter in humans and its reversal by naloxone. Science 1977;197:183–6.
75. Bowsher D. Allodynia in relation to lesion site in central post-stroke pain. J Pain 2005;6:736–40.
76. Neumann L, Buskila D. Epidemiology of fibromyalgia. Curr Pain Headache Rep 2003;7:362–8.
77. Volinn E. The epidemiology of low back pain in the rest of the world. A review of surveys in low- and middle-income countries. Spine 1997;22:1747–54.
78. Borsook D, Becerra LR. Breaking down the barriers: fMRI applications in pain, analgesia and analgesics. Molecular Pain 2006;2:30.

Inflammation at the Intersection of Behavior and Somatic Symptoms

Michael R. Irwin, MD

KEYWORDS
- Fatigue • Sleep • Pain • Sickness behavior • Inflammation
- Somatization

Somatization refers to the persistence of multiple physical complaints that cannot be attributed to a medical illness. Increasing evidence suggests that activation of the proinflammatory cytokine network can lead to a constellation of behaviors, "sickness behavior," which might underlie the pathophysiology of certain psychiatric disorders.[1,2] In particular, depressive disorders, as well as somatoform disorders, share many components of "sickness behavior," including alterations in pain sensitivity such as exaggerated pain response (hyperalgesia), sleep disturbance, and fatigue.[3] It has recently been hypothesized that this overlap in symptoms between somatoform disorders and depression may be due to a common underlying biology, including activation of inflammatory biology dynamics.[3,4] In this review, we characterize inflammation, describe the connections between the immune system and the brain, and discuss the influence of proinflammatory cytokine activity on certain aspects of this constellation of behaviors that have been commonly referred to as "sickness behavior." In particular, we focus on 3 prominent behavioral complaints in somatic disorders: exaggerated pain sensitivity (hyperalgesia), sleep disturbance, and fatigue.[5] Within this conceptual frame linking inflammation with altered bodily perceptions, we consider the possibility that activation of proinflammatory cytokines, possibly acting in concert with stress, might lead to increased sensitization of the central nervous system. It is thought that such sensitization serves as a possible neuronal substrate for amplification of normal bodily sensations so that these perceptions lead to distress, complaints, and somatic symptoms, along with impairments in social, occupational, and health functioning.[6–8]

INFLAMMATORY CYTOKINES

Inflammatory cytokines are potent, low-molecular-weight proteins and glycoproteins that are secreted by white blood cells and assist in the development and proliferation

Cousins Center for Psychoneuroimmunology, UCLA Semel Institute for Neuroscience, 300 UCLA Medical Plaza, Room 3130, Los Angeles, CA 90095-7076, USA
E-mail address: mirwin1@ucla.edu

Psychiatr Clin N Am 34 (2011) 605–620
doi:10.1016/j.psc.2011.05.005
0193-953X/11/$ – see front matter © 2011 Elsevier Inc. All rights reserved.

of immune cell subsets, and in the promotion of nonspecific innate as well as adaptive immune responses. Examples of inflammatory cytokines are interleukin (IL)-1β, IL-2, IL-6, tumor necrosis factor (TNF)-α, and interferon (IFN)-γ, which together promote a variety of cell functions that stimulate and lead to an inflammatory cascade in response to infection or tissue injury. Although there are non-immune cells that can produce and express certain inflammatory cytokines (eg, adipocytes release IL-6), immune cells are the primary source of these cytokines. When released by tissue resident macrophages, inflammatory cytokines increase vascular permeability and cellular adhesion, allowing cells to leave the blood vessels and migrate to the site of infection. In turn, immune cell expression of endothelial adhesion molecules is induced, which promotes firm adhesion of the immune cell to endothelial cells so that these cells can migrate from the circulation to tissue. The migration of cells is further directed by inflammatory cytokines, which activate the expression of chemokines that assist in the adhesion process and guide cells to their proper destinations in tissues via chemical diffusion gradients. Finally, certain proinflammatory cytokines, including IL-6 and TNF-α, promote liver production and release of acute phase proteins such C-reactive protein (CRP), which acts a mediator of systemic inflammation. Together, these inflammatory cytokines and acute phase proteins induce additional systemic effects, including regulation of metabolic responses to pathogens with coordination of fever, for example, with additional effects on physiology as well as behavior. Hence, in this capacity, inflammatory cytokines function in a manner similar to neurotransmitters and hormones in mediating specific physiologic responses, which rely on receptor–ligand interactions with self (autocrine), local (paracrine), and distal (endocrine) effects.

COMMUNICATION PATHWAYS BETWEEN INFLAMMATORY CYTOKINES AND THE BRAIN

Inflammatory cytokines communicate with the brain through cellular, molecular, and/or neural mechanisms. Because cytokines are large proteins, they do not efficiently cross the blood–brain barrier via passive transport.[9] Nevertheless, in areas where the blood–brain barrier is not present (eg, circumventricular sites), circulating concentrations of cytokines can enter the central nervous system, and in so doing stimulate the release of central cytokines via activation of inflammatory mediators such as prostaglandins of the E2 series from macrophage-like cells that exist in the circumventricular organs.[2,10] Additionally, the cytokines that are produced in the circumventricular organs gradually diffuse into the brain side of the blood–brain barrier and recruit microglial cells in the brain parenchyma to form a cellular and molecular representation of the peripheral immune response. Second, peripheral cytokines can also communicate with the brain by binding to cerebral vascular endothelium. Again, binding of cytokines at receptor-dependent sites facilitates the release of active second messengers such as nitric oxide, which induces central cytokine activation. Third, cytokines can be actively transported across the blood–brain barrier via carrier-mediated mechanisms. Together, these communication pathways involving either macrophage-like cells residing in circumventricular organs, second-messenger activation, or active transport provide 3 overlapping cellular and molecular mechanisms by which the brain actively senses circulating cytokines and monitors changes in the composition of the internal milieu.[9]

Neural mechanisms also play a critical role in communication of the immune system with the brain. Afferent nerves innervate bodily sites, and at sites of inflammation, these afferent nerves become activated to promote the perception of the sensory components of inflammation (*calor* or heat and *dolor* or pain). Additionally, such activation of afferent nerves induces the expression of brain proinflammatory cytokines in response to peripheral inflammatory cytokines.[6] Indeed, a number of experimental findings support the role of afferent nerves in the immune-to-brain communication; bilateral section of the vagus nerve blocks inflammatory signaling from the abdominal cavity,[11,12] and a section of the trigeminal nerves does the same for oral inflammation.[13] Additionally, inflammatory signaling of afferent nerves such as the vagus occurs by receptor dependent binding of IL-1β, for example, on paraganglia that surround the terminals of the vagus. Moreover, circulating IL-1β is reported to stimulate vagal sensory activity,[14] which induces acetylcholine release from paraganglia neurons. Subsequently, activation of afferent vagal fibers sends neural impulses and signals the dorsal motor nucleus via the nucleus tractus solitarius, resulting in the production and release of proinflammatory cytokines in the brain.[6,15]

Counterregulatory neural mechanisms have also been defined that dampen peripheral inflammation, once central activation of inflammatory signaling occurs. Again, the vagus plays a critical role; activation of the efferent vagal pathway inhibits inflammation in the periphery at paraganglia sites via cholinergic mechanisms.[16] In summary, this neural pathway, or "inflammatory reflex," is a relatively fast-acting mechanism compared with the cellular pathways described.

INFLAMMATORY CYTOKINES AND SICKNESS BEHAVIOR: EVIDENCE FROM BASIC STUDIES

Studies in laboratory animals provide compelling evidence that administration of innate immune cytokines can induce a syndrome of "sickness behavior" that has many overlapping features with the somatic behavioral comorbidities commonly experienced by patients with somatoform disorder, including hyperalgesia, impaired sleep, and fatigue.[17,18] These effects of cytokines seem to be secondary to the capacity of peripheral cytokine signals to access the brain and activate inflammatory responses within the brain, which then interact with pathophysiologic pathways known to be involved in behavioral disorders.[1]

In response to peripheral inflammatory signaling, certain classes of brain cells, including microglial cells and astrocytes secrete cytokines.[19] Such endogenous expression of cytokines, and associated cytokine receptors, have been found throughout the brain, including the hypothalamus, basal ganglia, cerebellum, circumventricular sites, and brainstem nuclei.[20] Additionally, multiple cytokines are expressed in the brain, including each of the prominently described inflammatory cytokines such as IL-1β, TNF-α, IL-6, and IFN-γ. Each of these cytokines have been found to promote the release of neurotransmitters, including norepinephrine, dopamine, and serotonin,[19,20] implicating central inflammatory cytokines in the initiation or modulation of neurochemical cascades that directly affect behavior.

Inflammatory cytokines, via their interaction with central nervous system mechanisms, induce a constellation of behavioral responses, which was first described in animals as sickness behavior as a result of infection.[21] Sickness behavior includes disturbance in sleep–wake activity with alterations in measures of sleep continuity and architecture, decreases in daytime activity, as well as decreased interest in feeding, grooming, and socializing. Although the adaptive significance of these behaviors is not known, it is thought that these sickness behaviors allow the "sick" animals to more efficiently mobilize immune defenses against an unwanted pathogen.[22] Several lines of evidence support the role of inflammatory cytokines in driving these behavioral responses. Central or peripheral stimulation with cytokines (IL-1β or TNF-α) or endotoxin [lipopolysaccharide (LPS)] leads to decreased activity, hypersomnia, decreased feeding behavior, learning impairment, and social withdrawal.[23,24]

Conversely, antagonism of central cytokine activity via immunoneutralization or receptor-mediated blockade (eg, administration of IL-1 receptor antagonist) blocks the behavioral effects of peripheral immune activation. Further studies have found that the vagus nerve transduces the peripheral inflammatory signal to the brain; vagotomy has been found to attenuate sickness behavior responses but not to alter plasma levels or cytokine production by peritoneal macrophages.[11,25] Importantly, the vagal pathway seems to impact behavioral, but not necessarily febrile, response to inflammation.[26]

Coupled with regulation of behavioral responses to inflammatory challenge, inflammatory cytokines induce associated alterations in the regulation of the hypothalamic–pituitary–adrenal (HPA) axis. For example, first described as "endogenous pyrogen," IL-1β has been found to increase HPA axis function via the activation of corticotrophin-releasing factor in the paraventricular nucleus of the hypothalamus.[27] In turn, such HPA activation is thought to have counterregulatory effects and to dampen and control the inflammatory response, thus, defining a negative feedback loop.

INFLAMMATORY SIGNALING: THE ROLE OF STRESS

The physiologic linkages between inflammation and HPA axis activation suggest the possibility that stress, which is well known to have effects on HPA axis activation, might have a role in the pathophysiology of the immune-to-brain communication. Indeed, there seems to be a cross-sensitization between stressors and cytokines. Exposure to stress, for instance, sensitizes the peripheral as well as central cytokine responses. For example, after administration of a stressor such as inescapable electric shock, an immune challenge such as a dose of bacterial LPS is associated with an augmented inflammatory response as compared with a response in animals not previously exposed to stress.[28] Reciprocally, after IL-1 has been previously given, subsequent administration of inescapable electric shock induces an exaggerated HPA response for up to 2 to 3 weeks after the cytokine was given.[29] Additionally, sensitization can also occur when the same cytokine is administered twice at an interval of several days or weeks, and it affects both cytokine-sensitive neurotransmitter metabolism and pituitary–adrenal responsiveness to cyokines.[30]

Further data show that stressful stimuli have independent effects on inflammatory biology dynamics. Acute stressors activate inflammatory cytokines and their signaling pathways [eg, nuclear factor kappa B (NF-κB)] both in the periphery and in the brain.[31,32] In addition, data from rats indicate that stress can activate microglia in the brain and increase their sensitivity to immunologic stimuli such as LPS. Such activation of IL-1 in the brain reduces the expression of brain-derived neurotrophic factor (BDNF), which may have further effects on behavior; BDNF is believed to play a pivotal role in neuronal growth and development, learning, synaptic plasticity, and ultimately behavioral disorders.[33]

Activation of the sympathetic nervous system and the release of catecholamines that bind to α- and β-adrenergic receptors on relevant cells are thought to mediate the effects of stress on brain inflammatory pathways.[32,34] Conversely, activation of the parasympathetic nervous system via the release of acetylcholine seems to inhibit inflammatory signaling pathways (eg, NF-κB),[35] suggesting that sympathetic and parasympathetic pathways have opposing influences on inflammatory responses during stress.

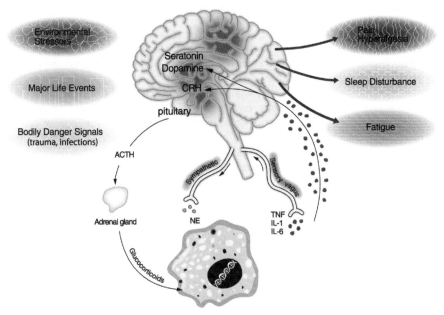

Fig. 1. Associations between environmental stress, life events, and trauma, activation of peripheral inflammation, and increases in central inflammatory signaling, which together are thought to contribute the occurrence of somatic symptoms of pain or hyperalgesia, sleep disturbance, and fatigue.

INFLAMMATION AND BEHAVIORAL SYMPTOMS IN HUMANS: GENERAL CONSIDERATIONS

Advances put forth from animal studies contrast with our limited understanding of the mechanistic role of inflammatory cytokine activity on sickness behavior-related symptoms (eg, hyperalgesia, sleep disturbance, and fatigue) in humans. Most of the evidence linking inflammatory immune activation and sickness behavior in humans is generated from naturalistic observations, which correlate elevated levels of cytokines with behavioral alterations. Nevertheless, there are also some experimental data showing that acute activation of proinflammatory cytokine activity and/or the acute and chronic administration of cytokines has a number of behavioral effects. Among the behavioral disturbances induced by cytokines, the induction of depressive symptoms is probably the most studied. Indeed, the administration of IFN-α, a potent inducer of inflammatory activity, leads to hallmark symptoms of depression, such as anhedonia and feelings of sadness, along with a range of other neurobehavioral changes, including disturbed sleep, fatigue, and loss of appetite.[36,37] Because these symptoms fully remit after cessation of cytokine therapy, it is thought that such inflammatory activity drives the onset of these symptoms.[20] Further, administration of immune challenges that provoke the activation of inflammatory responses leads to increases in feelings of fatigue and depressed mood.[38,39] Inflammation-driven changes in mood seem to be associated with neural changes such as reduced functional connectivity between the subgenual anterior cingulate cortex, amygdala, and medial prefrontal cortex,[40] as well as reduced ventral striatum activity in response to reward cues (**Fig. 1**).[38,39]

INFLAMMATION AND PAIN: TRANSLATION OF BASIC RESEARCH TO HUMANS

Pain is among the most prominent of the somatization symptoms, and such pain is characterized as pain for which there is no definable etiology in the body. Alternately, such pain is perceived as exaggerated, resulting from identifiable peripheral causes but in which sensations from the affected body region are grossly abnormal. For example, environmental stimuli that would not be normally perceived as painful are now perceived as such, whereas environmental stimuli that would typically be perceived as painful now evoke an amplified and/or persistent perception of pain.[41] Furthermore, in addition to perceptions of pain, simple environmental stimuli may evoke abnormal feelings of electric tingling or sensations that have other unusual and unpleasant qualities. This spontaneous pain, evoked by environmental stimuli or not, can occur frequently, at varying qualities, and throughout the body in varying locations. Increasingly, the immune system is thought to have a role in such pathologic pain states[41] and possibly in the occurrence of neuropathic pain found in somatization disorders, as well as in disorders that have an inflammatory basis.

Immune cells in and around peripheral nerves, and immune-like glial cells in spinal cord, are key players in both the creation and maintenance of pathologic pain states. Basic research has found that these immune cells, including macrophages, produce proinflammatory cytokines (eg, TNF-α, IL-1β, IL-6) after trauma; such increases of these cytokines parallel increases in pain perception.[42,43] Indeed, the magnitude of neuropathic pain correlates with both the number of activated macrophages and the number of IL-6–producing cells at the site of injury.[42]

Other experimental data from animals indicate a role of proinflammatory cytokines in the endogenous mediation of neuropathic pain. For example, experimental injection of proinflammatory cytokines onto or into peripheral nerves enhances pain responsivity.[44,45] In contrast, blockade of proinflammatory cytokine actions at the level of the sciatic nerve reduces neuropathic pain, as well as reducing immune cell recruitment and demyelination.[46] Likewise, neuropathic pain can be abrogated by treatments that decrease proinflammatory cytokines and/or increase anti-inflammatory cytokines such as IL-10.[47] Finally, in animals that lack the IL-6 gene (ie, IL-6 knockout mice), neuropathic pain does not seem to occur.[48]

Neuropathic pain or hyperalgesia often overlaps with other sickness behaviors, possibly owing to common underlying inflammatory biology. For example, immune activation in the periphery elicits hyperalgesia along with other sickness behaviors.[41] Similarly, administration of an immune challenge (eg, bacterial endotoxin) or doses of inflammatory cytokines signals pain responses,[6] in concert with provoking sickness behaviors.[6] In turn, pharmacologic blockade of TNF-α, for example, prevents sickness-induced hyperalgesia as well as other sickness behaviors. Importantly, central mechanisms mediate the action of proinflammatory cytokines on hyperalgesia. For example, peripheral administration of IL-1β elicits thermal hyperalgesia owing to the de novo production and release IL-1β within the brain, which can be antagonized by central administration of an endogenous antagonist of IL-1β (α-melanocyte–stimulating hormone).[49] Additionally, there is synergistic overlap between proinflammatory cytokines; TNF-α creates hyperalgesia by inducing the release of brain IL-1β,[50] and all 3 proinflammatory cytokines (TNF-α, IL-1β, IL-6) produce hyperalgesia via the release of prostaglandins,[51] substances repeatedly implicated in exaggerated pain states.

Translation of these basic studies to humans is limited, but this is clearly an issue that warrants serious consideration, given the prominent links between pain and inflammatory disorders, as well as chronic conditions such as metabolic disorder and obesity. Indeed, emerging data in humans support the notion that inflammation may contribute to hyperalgesia and neuropathic pain in cases where no known etiology can be readily identified. For example, among person with AIDS, more than 80% of these patients suffer from chronic pain, and of these, most suffer from vague and diffuse pains of unknown origin.[52,53] Although patients with AIDS suffer from pain from a variety of readily identifiable causes, including nerve damage, opportunistic cancers, and opportunistic infections from the disease as well as the drugs used in therapy, there is evidence that HIV-1 activation of spinal cord glia may in itself drive and/or perpetuate pain in these patients, creating pain for which there is no definable etiology in the body, as well as exaggerating pain resulting from identifiable peripheral causes. Indeed, the perception of pain is strongly amplified under the effect of proinflammatory mediators produced by activated glial cells in the spinal cord.[54] Additionally, glial activation is not restricted to the spinal cord, but also occurs in the brain in chronic inflammation associated, for instance, with progressive neurodegeneration,[55] obesity,[56] or aging. Together, it is hypothesized that the brain cytokine system becomes sensitized and responds to a greater extent to further activation of the peripheral innate immune system, which results in a more intense cytokine-induced sickness behavior (somatic amplification) and/or a delayed recovery from sickness.

INFLAMMATION AND SLEEP DISTURBANCE

Sleep complaints and associated daytime fatigue are thought to affect 30% to 40% of the general US population,[57] with 10% meeting criteria for chronic syndromal insomnia.[58] The prevalence of sleep complaints and syndromal insomnia is even higher among patients with medical disorders, and this is especially the case for those who suffer from chronic conditions with pain and/or underlying inflammation such as rheumatoid arthritis. Activation of inflammatory signaling can occur in the midst of sleep disturbance, and increases in inflammation have reciprocal effects on sleep, which together is thought to lead to a vicious cycle of sleep disturbance and inflammation, which perpetuates over time contributing to fatigue, and possibly depression. Hence, sleep disturbance might be viewed as principal behavioral culprit in the association between inflammation and multiple somatic symptoms.

Acute and chronic sleep disturbances are associated with immune alterations. Initial studies demonstrated that sleep loss results in decreases in innate immunity as reflected by decreases in the activity of natural killer cells.[59,60] However, sleep loss can also have activating effects on certain aspects of the immune system, leading to increases in increases in inflammatory markers such as IL-6, TNF-α, and CRP.[61,62] Furthermore, studies reveal that systemic increases in markers of inflammation are due to increased activation of cellular and genomic inflammatory mechanisms.[63] Partial night sleep deprivation, which is thought to mimic the kind of sleep loss often found in persons undergoing stress and/or suffering from a chronic medical disorder, is associated with increased monocyte production of IL-6 and TNF-α, as well as a greater than 3-fold increase in IL-6 messenger RNA and a 2-fold increase in TNF-α messenger RNA.[63] Monocytes are the primary immune cell source of proinflammatory cytokines. Interestingly, females show an exaggerated production of these cytokines after sleep loss,[64] which may be due to a greater activation of NF-κB in females as compared with males.[65] NF-κB is a transcription factor that has a critical role in initiating the inflammatory cascade, which leads to the production of cellular proinflammatory cytokines. An exaggerated activation of inflammatory signaling in females after sleep disruption has broad implications for understanding the increased risk of associated behavioral symptoms such as fatigue and depression in females, as well as a nearly 2-fold increase in the prevalence of disorders with an inflammatory basis (autoimmune disorders) in females compared with males.

Given these experimental data, it is not surprising that chronic sleep disturbance and clinical insomnia are associated with increases in inflammation as indexed by elevated levels of IL-6 and TNF-α.[66] In turn, such daytime elevations of proinflammatory cytokine seem to drive symptoms of fatigue; antagonism of TNF-α by pharmacologic blockade produces a partial improvement in symptoms of sleepiness, for example.[67]

The role of cytokines in the regulation of sleepiness raises the possibility that proinflammatory cytokines might also alter sleep during the night. Indeed, substantial evidence from animal studies reveal that IL-1β, TNF-α, and IL-6 all have a role in the homeostatic regulation of sleep.[68] For example, the central injection of IL-1β increases non–rapid eye movement (NREM) sleep time and suppresses rapid eye movement (REM) sleep.[69] Similarly, in animal models of infection, there are striking changes in sleep that parallel the alterations found after doses of proinflammatory cytokines, including increases in NREM sleep during times of usually high activity.[70] Interestingly, differences in sleep response to infection are partly attributed to genetic variants that contribute to differential increases in proinflammatory cytokines. In animals with genetic alleles that produce high levels of type 1 IFN-α and IFN-β, there are greater amounts of NREM sleep compared with animals with alleles associated with decreased production of these IFNs.[71] Such genetic variability has implications for understanding differences in the risk of sleep disturbance among populations who are exposed to inflammatory challenge.

In humans, studies that evaluate the effects of cytokines on the regulation of sleep are limited. Administration of endotoxin (*Salmonella abortus*, a LPS that stimulates proinflammatory cytokine production by macrophages) has been found to increase NREM stage 2 sleep, whereas slow-wave sleep and stages 3 and 4 are relatively unaffected.[72,73] In contrast, subcutaneous injection of IL-6 as well as IFN-α induce a reduction of slow-wave sleep, as well as REM sleep.[74,75] Finally, chronic IFN-α administration in patients with hepatitis C, who had no prior sleep disorder was associated with increases in wake after sleep onset, as well as decreases in slow-wave sleep and sleep efficiency.[76] Finally, Irwin and colleagues[77] demonstrated in a randomized, placebo-controlled study that neutralization of TNF-α activity was associated with a significant reduction of REM sleep in abstinent alcohol dependent patients, who have elevated amounts of REM sleep. Moreover, individual biologic variability in the degree of TNF antagonism, as reflected by circulating levels of soluble TNF receptor type II, correlated with declines in REM sleep.[77] Taken together, these data further support the hypothesis that circulating levels of TNF-α, as well as possibly other proinflammatory cytokines, may have a physiologic role in the regulation of NREM and REM sleep amounts in humans.

On a behavioral level, dysregulation in sleep may trigger fatigue,[78] and in turn chronic fatigue itself triggers sleep disturbance, possibly through alterations in sleep–wake activity chronobiology. Indeed, the co-occurrence of fatigue and sleep disorders is common, making it difficult to determine the causal symptom. Specific precipitating as well as perpetuating factors for sleep disturbance, and for fatigue, relate also to the presence and nature of a particular comorbid disorder, as well as the social and behavioral contexts and responses to initial dysregulation.

INFLAMMATION AND FATIGUE

Fatigue, which may be mostly viewed as "tiredness" or "lack of energy," has many components that might underlie its onset and persistence, including physiologic (eg, pain and anemia), psychological (eg, changes in mood), social/interpersonal, and chronobiological (eg, circadian rhythms disorders and sleep disruption) factors.[79] Peripherally related fatigue (fatigue associated with an inability for the musculature to transmit central nervous system signals) is the kind that is experienced more on a somatic level, whereas centrally related fatigue (which results in an inability to engage in or maintain voluntary activities) is the kind that includes the cognitive, motor, emotional, and social aspects of fatigue.[80] Fatigue is a common symptom of many other medical conditions and hence is a common somatic symptom found across disorders.

Basic research in animals has found that fatigue, as indexed by activity, can be elicited along with other sickness behaviors in association with immune activation, similar to findings with pain and sleep. In humans, the links between inflammation and fatigue are found across multiple medical comorbidities, with increases in inflammation correlating with fatigue among individuals with multiple sclerosis,[81] Sjögren syndrome,[82] and rheumatoid arthritis,[83] among others. Furthermore, among healthy persons, longitudinal studies have shown that plasma levels of the proinflammatory marker CRP predict the development of fatigue.[84] However, the most compelling evidence for an association between inflammation and fatigue has been most thoroughly generated in cancer populations. For example, a qualitative review examined the association between proinflammatory cytokines and fatigue in cancer patients before, during, and after treatment, and generally supported a finding of a positive association between inflammation and fatigue.[85] The reasons for such a prominent link between inflammation and fatigue in cancer populations is not fully understood, although tumors can secrete inflammatory cytokines and cancer treatments (radiation, chemotherapy) can induce inflammation. Indeed, chemotherapy-related alterations in proinflammatory cytokines, with reported increases in IL-6, IL-10, and serum soluble receptor 1 for TNF correlate with increases in symptom severity among non–small cell lung cancer patients[86] as well as breast cancer patients,[87] and these effects can be partially abrogated by the pharmacologic blockade of TNF-α.[88] Similar associations between inflammation and fatigue have also been found during radiation therapy in cancer patients, including in breast and prostate cancer patients undergoing radiation therapy.[89]

Similar to the sensitizing effects of cytokine on pain responses, it is possible that treatment-induced elevations in inflammatory markers sensitize peripheral and central mechanisms, which contribute to an amplification and/or perpetuation of inflammation and effects on fatigue symptoms. For example, even after chemotherapy and/or radiation treatments are over, fatigue lingers in about one third of survivors, with symptoms persisting for up to 10 years.[90] Those persons with persistent posttreatment fatigue have increased levels of a number of proinflammatory markers including plasma levels of IL-6, its soluble receptor, IL-1 receptor antagonist, CRP, soluble TNF receptor type II, and neopterin.[91,92] Additional studies suggest that underlying cellular and genomic activation of inflammatory biology dynamics drive these effects with increases in the cellular production of IL-6 and TNF-α found in fatigued versus-fatigued breast cancer survivors[92] and with an upregulation of the proinflammatory transcription factor NF-κB.[93] Again, genetic variants that contribute to variability in the expression of inflammation seem to be associated with differential risk of somatic symptoms, including fatigue; polymorphisms in inflammation-related genes are associated with increased risk of cancer-related fatigue.[94] Together, these data raise important questions about the development of treatments that specifically target inflammation for the treatment of fatigue, although such studies remain in development.

Treatment with TNF antagonists has, however, been associated with reductions in fatigue among individuals with inflammatory conditions such as psoriasis.[95]

Treatment Implications

The number of potential integrated mechanisms by which inflammatory cytokines might drive the onset of somatic symptoms, including the role of stress response pathways in initiating and perpetuating this cycle, suggests the opportunity for multiple targets and/or for efficacy of various treatments. To this end, there is limited evidence from randomized, controlled trials that both pharmacologic (anti-depressants) and nonpharmacologic (aerobic exercise, cognitive–behavioral therapy) treatments are able to attenuate some somatic symptoms such as sleep disturbance and fatigue, with possible attendant effects on inflammation. Little is known about whether inflammation mediates these outcomes, and treatments that specifically target activation of the brain cytokine system are not yet available.

Cognitive–behavioral, supportive, or insight-oriented treatments that target stress mechanisms may be especially relevant, given the potential role of stress-induced inflammation and altered regulation of inflammatory responses by the neuroendocrine system. Such behavioral strategies broadly vary, but are designed to reduce symptom severity. These approaches include relaxation training, enhancement of coping skills, graded exercise, and cognitive–behavioral therapy. Indeed, both cognitive–behavioral stress management and mindfulness-based stress reduction have been shown to alleviate psychological distress in certain patient populations (eg, breast cancer patients), while increasing lymphocyte proliferative responses and normalizing diurnal cortisol secretion.[96,97] There is also evidence that aerobic exercise can lead to reductions in inflammatory markers,[98] and that interventions that target both the mind and body (eg, a movement mediation, Tai chi) can mitigate age-related increases in inflammation among older adults.[99] Interestingly, recent studies using cognitive–behavioral therapy program, on the one hand, and Tai Chi on the other, found improvements in health functioning and physical activity, along with improvements in sleep and fatigue as compared with an active educational control condition.[100] However, the role of inflammatory mediators in driving these benefits has not been systematically investigated. For example, exercise interventions, which have shown beneficial effects on both fatigue and inflammatory markers,[98] have not evaluated whether decreases in inflammation mediate changes in fatigue outcomes. Likewise, a randomized, controlled trial of QiGong demonstrated decreases of fatigue and inflammation (as indexed by serum CRP levels),[101] but the mediating role of CRP was not assessed.

It is hypothesized that blockade of most upstream elements in the cytokine–central nervous system–behavior cascade may ameliorate complaints of pain, sleep disturbance, and fatigue; hence, it is also logical to consider biological treatments such as cytokine antagonists, anti-inflammatory agents, and drugs that disrupt cytokine signaling pathways (eg, NF-κB and p38 MAPK). Several trials have demonstrated that TNF-α blockade with etanercept can improve cancer-related fatigue, and other studies have found that administration of etanercept or another biological agent that block TNF-α [infliximab (Remicade)] can lessen daytime sleepiness and partially normalize sleep in rheumatoid arthritis patients, as well as those with alcohol dependence.[88,102,103]

Given evidence that inflammation can alter certain central nervous system neurotransmitters, including monoamines and serotonin pathways, pharmacologic agents that target these specific systems may benefit related symptom domains (eg, dopamine-active drugs for fatigue and psychomotor slowing). For example, dopaminergic agents such as methylphenidate (a psychostimulant) have been shown to treat fatigue in patients undergoing cancer treatments.[104]

Finally, drugs that enhance glucocorticoid-mediated negative feedback, through facilitation of glucocorticoid receptor function, may control corticotropin-releasing hormone overexpression and have additional action to inhibit inflammatory pathways.[105] Novel treatments supporting neuronal integrity/plasticity (neuroprotective agents), including drugs that stimulate the activity or signaling of relevant growth factors (eg, BDNF), may be especially important for future development, given the links of BDNF with pain responsivity.

SUMMARY

Many somatization symptoms, including pain, sleep disturbance, and fatigue, may represent activation of the central nervous system cytokine system in response to peripheral inflammatory signaling after stress, infectious challenge, or noninfectious trauma. Some clinical data show that activation of inflammatory signaling along with increases in the peripheral expression of proinflammatory cytokines correlates with, and possibly drives, the onset and persistence of these somatic symptoms. However, most data have been accumulated in healthy or chronic disease populations; there are limited findings linking these inflammation and symptoms of somatic distress in patients with somatoform disorders. One study found that patients with somatization, as well as those with major depression, had increases in circulating levels of IL-1 receptor antagonist as compared with healthy controls.[106] There are no other data, to our knowledge, that have systematically examined the associations between inflammation and somatic symptoms in patients with somatoform disorder. Moreover, no study has examined whether blockade of proinflammatory cytokine activity might improve symptoms of pain, sleep disturbance, and fatigue among patients with somatoform disorder.

REFERENCES

1. Miller AH, Maletic V, Raison CL. Inflammation and its discontents: the role of cytokines in the pathophysiology of major depression. Biol Psychiatry 2009;65: 732–41.
2. Dantzer R, O'Connor JC, Freund GG, et al. From inflammation to sickness and depression: when the immune system subjugates the brain. Nat Rev Neurosci 2008;9:46–56.
3. Dimsdale JE, Dantzer R. A biological substrate for somatoform disorders: importance of pathophysiology. Psychosom Med 2007;69:850–4.
4. Rief W, Barsky AJ. Psychobiological perspectives on somatoform disorders. Psychoneuroendocrinology 2005;30:996–1002.
5. Jain S, Shapiro SL, Swanick S, et al. A randomized controlled trial of mindfulness meditation versus relaxation training: effects on distress, positive states of mind, rumination, and distraction. Ann Behav Med 2007;33:11–21.
6. Watkins LR, Maier SF. The pain of being sick: implications of immune-to-brain communication for understanding pain. Annu Rev Psychol 2000;51:29–57.
7. Barsky AJ, Wyshak G, Klerman GL. The somatosensory amplification scale and its relationship to hypochondriasis. J Psychiatr Res 1990;24:323–34.
8. Black PH. Stress and the inflammatory response: a review of neurogenic inflammation. Brain Behav Immun 2002;16:622–53.
9. Quan N, Banks WA. Brain-immune communication pathways. Brain Behav Immun 2007;21:727–35.

10. Kronfol Z, Remick DG. Cytokines and the brain: implications for clinical psychiatry. Am J Psych 2000;157:683–94.
11. Bluthe RM, Michaud B, Kelley KW, et al. Vagotomy blocks behavioural effects of interleukin-1 injected via the intraperitoneal route but not via other systemic routes. Neuroreport 1996;7:2823–7.
12. Laye S, Bluthe RM, Kent S, et al. Subdiaphragmatic vagotomy blocks induction of IL-1 beta mRNA in mice brain in response to peripheral LPS. Am J Physiol 1995; 268:R1327–31.
13. Navarro VP, Iyomasa MM, Leite-Panissi CR, et al. New role of the trigeminal nerve as a neuronal pathway signaling brain in acute periodontitis: participation of local prostaglandins. Pflugers Arch 2006;453:73–82.
14. Ek M, Kurosawa M, Lundeberg T, et al. Activation of vagal afferents after intravenous injection of interleukin-1beta: role of endogenous prostaglandins. J Neurosci 1998; 18:9471–9.
15. Watkins LR, Maier SF. Implications of immune-to-brain communication for sickness and pain. Proc Nat Acad Sci U S A 1999;96:7710–3.
16. Tracey KJ. The inflammatory reflex. Nature 2002;420:853–9.
17. Capuron L, Ravaud A, Dantzer R. Timing and specificity of the cognitive changes induced by interleukin-2 and interferon-alpha treatments in cancer patients. Psychosom Med 2001;63:376–86.
18. Yirmiya R, Weidenfeld J, Pollak Y, et al. Cytokines, "depression due to a general medical condition," and antidepressant drugs. Adv Exp Med Biol 1999;461:283–316.
19. Camacho-Arroyo I, Lopez-Griego L, Morales-Montor J. The role of cytokines in the regulation of neurotransmission. Neuroimmunomodulation 2009;16:1–12.
20. Anisman H, Merali Z. Cytokines, stress, and depressive illness. Brain Behav Immun 2002;16:513–24.
21. Dantzer R. Cytokine-induced sickness behavior: mechanisms and implications. Ann N Y Acad Sci 2001;933:222–34.
22. Hart BL. Biological basis of the behavior of sick animals. Neurosci Biobehav Rev 1988;12:123–37.
23. Dinarello CA. Biology of interleukin 1. FASEB J 1988;2:108–15.
24. Gibertini M, Newton C, Friedman H, et al. Spatial learning impairment in mice infected with Legionella pneumophila or administered exogenous interleukin-1-beta. Brain Behav Immun 1995;9:113–28.
25. Bluthe RM, Michaud B, Kelley KW, et al. Vagotomy attenuates behavioural effects of interleukin-1 injected peripherally but not centrally. Neuroreport 1996;7:1485–8.
26. Konsman JP, Luheshi GN, Bluthe RM, et al. The vagus nerve mediates behavioural depression, but not fever, in response to peripheral immune signals; a functional anatomical analysis. Eur J Neurosci 2000;12:4434–46.
27. Berkenbosch F, VanOers J, DelRey A, et al. Corticotropin-releasing factor-producing neurons in the rat activated by interleukin-1. Science 1987;238:524–6.
28. Johnson JD, O'Connor KA, Deak T, et al. Prior stressor exposure sensitizes LPS-induced cytokine production. Brain Behav Immun 2002;16:461–76.
29. Tilders FJ, Schmidt ED, Hoogendijk WJ, et al. Delayed effects of stress and immune activation. Baillieres Best Pract Res Clin Endocrinol Metab 1999;13:523–40.
30. Anisman H, Merali Z, Hayley S. Sensitization associated with stressors and cytokine treatments. Brain Behav Immun 2003;17:86–93.
31. Pace TW, Mletzko TC, Alagbe O, et al. Increased stress-induced inflammatory responses in male patients with major depression and increased early life stress. Am J Psychiatry 2006;163:1630–3.

32. Bierhaus A, Wolf J, Andrassy M, et al. A mechanism converting psychosocial stress into mononuclear cell activation. Proc Natl Acad Sci U S A 2003;100:1920–5.
33. Barrientos RM, Sprunger DB, Campeau S, et al. BDNF mRNA expression in rat hippocampus following contextual learning is blocked by intrahippocampal IL-1beta administration. J Neuroimmunol 2004;155:119–26.
34. Johnson JD, Campisi J, Sharkey CM, et al. Catecholamines mediate stress-induced increases in peripheral and central inflammatory cytokines. Neuroscience 2005;135: 1295–307.
35. Pavlov VA, Tracey KJ. The cholinergic anti-inflammatory pathway. Brain Behav Immun 2005;19:493–9.
36. Capuron L, Gumnick JF, Musselman DL, et al. Neurobehavioral effects of interferon-alpha in cancer patients: phenomenology and paroxetine responsiveness of symptom dimensions. Neuropsychopharmacology 2002;26:643–52.
37. Capuron L, Ravaud A, Dantzer R. Early depressive symptoms in cancer patients receiving interleukin 2 and/or interferon alfa-2b therapy. J Clin Oncol 2000;18: 2143–51.
38. Eisenberger NI, Berkman ET, Inagaki TK, et al. Inflammation-induced anhedonia: endotoxin reduces ventral striatum responses to reward. Biol Psychiatry 2010;68: 748–54.
39. Eisenberger NI, Inagaki TK, Mashal NM, et al. Inflammation and social experience: an inflammatory challenge induces feelings of social disconnection in addition to depressed mood. Brain Behav Immun 2010;24:558–63.
40. Harrison NA, Brydon L, Walker C, et al. Inflammation causes mood changes through alterations in subgenual cingulate activity and mesolimbic connectivity. Biol Psychiatry 2009;66:407–14.
41. Watkins LR, Hutchinson MR, Milligan ED, et al. "Listening" and "talking" to neurons: implications of immune activation for pain control and increasing the efficacy of opioids. Brain Res Rev 2007;56:148–69.
42. Cui JG, Holmin S, Mathiesen T, et al. Possible role of inflammatory mediators in tactile hypersensitivity in rat models of mononeuropathy. Pain 2000;88:239–48.
43. Okamoto K, Martin DP, Schmelzer JD, et al. Pro- and anti-inflammatory cytokine gene expression in rat sciatic nerve chronic constriction injury model of neuropathic pain. Exp Neurol 2001;169:386–91.
44. Sorkin LS, Doom CM. Epineurial application of TNF elicits an acute mechanical hyperalgesia in the awake rat. J Peripher Nerv Syst 2000;5:96–100.
45. Zelenka M, Schafers M, Sommer C. Intraneural injection of interleukin-1beta and tumor necrosis factor-alpha into rat sciatic nerve at physiological doses induces signs of neuropathic pain. Pain 2005;116:257–63.
46. Ma W, Quirion R. Targeting invading macrophage-derived PGE2, IL-6 and calcitonin gene-related peptide in injured nerve to treat neuropathic pain. Expert Opin Ther Targets 2006;10:533–46.
47. George A, Marziniak M, Schafers M, et al. Thalidomide treatment in chronic constrictive neuropathy decreases endoneurial tumor necrosis factor-alpha, increases interleukin-10 and has long-term effects on spinal cord dorsal horn met-enkephalin. Pain 2000;88:267–75.
48. Ramer MS, Murphy PG, Richardson PM, et al. Spinal nerve lesion-induced mechanoallodynia and adrenergic sprouting in sensory ganglia are attenuated in interleukin-6 knockout mice. Pain 1998;78:115–21.
49. Oka T, Oka K, Hosoi M, et al. Inhibition of peripheral interleukin-1 beta-induced hyperalgesia by the intracerebroventricular administration of diclofenac and alpha-melanocyte-stimulating hormone. Brain Res 1996;736:237–42.

50. Oka T, Wakugawa Y, Hosoi M, et al. Intracerebroventricular injection of tumor necrosis factor-alpha induces thermal hyperalgesia in rats. Neuroimmunomodulation 1996;3:135–40.

51. Yabuuchi K, Nishiyori A, Minami M, et al. Biphasic effects of intracerebroventricular interleukin-1 beta on mechanical nociception in the rat. Eur J Pharmacol 1996;300:59–65.

52. Breitbart W, McDonald MV, Rosenfeld B, et al. Pain in ambulatory AIDS patients. I: Pain characteristics and medical correlates. Pain 1996;68:315–21.

53. Hewitt DJ, McDonald M, Portenoy RK, et al. Pain syndromes and etiologies in ambulatory AIDS patients. Pain 1997;70:117–23.

54. Watkins LR, Hutchinson MR, Ledeboer A, et al. Norman Cousins Lecture. Glia as the "bad guys": implications for improving clinical pain control and the clinical utility of opioids. Brain Behav Immun 2007;21:131–46.

55. Bluthe RM, Michaud B, Delhaye-Bouchaud N, et al. Hypersensitivity of lurcher mutant mice to the depressing effects of lipopolysaccharide and interleukin-1 on behaviour. Neuroreport 1997;8:1119–22.

56. O'Connor JC, Satpathy A, Hartman ME, et al. IL-1beta-mediated innate immunity is amplified in the db/db mouse model of type 2 diabetes. J Immunol 2005;174:4991–7.

57. Hossain JL, Shapiro CM. The prevalence, cost implications, and management of sleep disorders: an overview. Sleep Breath 2002;6:85–102.

58. Ohayon MM. Epidemiology of insomnia: what we know and what we still need to learn. Sleep Med Rev 2002;6:97–111.

59. Irwin M, McClintick J, Costlow C, et al. Partial night sleep deprivation reduces natural killer and cellular immune responses in humans. FASEB J 1996;10:643–53.

60. Irwin M, Mascovich A, Gillin JC, et al. Partial sleep deprivation reduces natural killer cell activity in humans. Psychosom Med 1994;56:493–8.

61. Shearer WT, Reuben JM, Mullington JM, et al. Soluble TNF-alpha receptor 1 and IL-6 plasma levels in humans subjected to the sleep deprivation model of spaceflight. J Allergy Clin Immunol 2001;107:165–70.

62. Meier-Ewert HK, Ridker PM, Rifai N, et al. Effect of sleep loss on C-reactive protein, an inflammatory marker of cardiovascular risk. J Am Coll Cardiol 2004;43:678–83.

63. Irwin MR, Wang M, Campomayor CO, et al. Sleep deprivation and activation of morning levels of cellular and genomic markers of inflammation. Arch Intern Med 2006;166:1756–62.

64. Irwin MR, Carrillo C, Olmstead R. Sleep loss activates cellular markers of inflammation: sex differences. Brain Behav Immun 2010;24:54–7.

65. Irwin MR, Wang M, Ribeiro D, et al. Sleep loss activates cellular inflammatory signaling. Biol Psychiatry 2008;64:538–40.

66. Irwin M. Effects of sleep and sleep loss on immunity and cytokines. Brain Behav Immun 2002;16:503–12.

67. Vgontzas AN, Zoumakis E, Lin HM, et al. Marked decrease in sleepiness in patients with sleep apnea by etanercept, a tumor necrosis factor-alpha antagonist. J Clin Endocrinol Metab 2004;89:4409–13.

68. Krueger JM, Takahashi S, Kapάs L, et al. Cytokines in sleep regulation. Adv Neuroimmunol 1995;5:171–88.

69. Krueger JM, Walter J, Dinarello CA, et al. Sleep promoting effects of endogenous pyrogen (interleukin-1). Am J Physiol 1984;246:R994–9.

70. Toth LA, Verhulst SJ. Strain differences in sleep patterns of healthy and influenza-infected inbred mice. Behav Genet 2003;33:325–36.

71. Toth LA. Strain differences in the somnogenic effects of interferon inducers in mice. J Interferon Cytokine Res 1996;16:1065–72.
72. Pollmächer T, Schuld A, Kraus T, et al. Experimental immunomodulation, sleep, and sleepiness in humans. Ann N Y Acad Sci 2000;917:488–99.
73. Mullington J, Korth C, Hermann DM, et al. Dose-dependent effects of endotoxin on human sleep. Am J Physiol Regul Integr Comp Physiol 2000;278:R947–55.
74. Späth-Schwalbe E, Lange T, Perras B, et al. Interferon-alpha acutely impairs sleep in healthy humans. Cytokine 2000;12:518–21.
75. Spath-Schwalbe E, Hansen K, Schmidt F, et al. Acute effects of recombinant human interleukin-6 on endocrine and central nervous sleep functions in healthy men. J Clin Endocrinol Metab 1998;83:1573–9.
76. Raison CL, Rye DB, Woolwine BJ, et al. Chronic interferon-alpha administration disrupts sleep continuity and depth in patients with hepatitis C: association with fatigue, motor slowing, and increased evening cortisol. Biol Psychiatry 68:942–9.
77. Irwin MR, Olmstead R, Valladares EM, et al. Tumor necrosis factor antagonism normalizes rapid eye movement sleep in alcohol dependence. Biol Psychiatry 2009;66:191–5.
78. Thomas KS, Motivala S, Olmstead R, et al. Sleep depth and fatigue: role of cellular inflammatory activation. Brain Behav Immun 25:53–8.
79. Hwang SS, Chang VT, Kasimis BS. A comparison of three fatigue measures in veterans with cancer. Cancer Invest 2003;21:363–73.
80. Ryan JL, Carroll JK, Ryan EP, et al. Mechanisms of cancer-related fatigue. Oncologist 2007;12(Suppl 1):22–34.
81. Heesen C, Nawrath L, Reich C, et al. Fatigue in multiple sclerosis: an example of cytokine mediated sickness behaviour? J Neurol Neurosurg Psychiatry 2006;77:34–9.
82. Harboe E, Tjensvoll AB, Vefring HK, et al. Fatigue in primary Sjogren's syndrome—a link to sickness behaviour in animals? Brain Behav Immun 2009;23:1104–8.
83. Davis MC, Zautra AJ, Younger J, et al. Chronic stress and regulation of cellular markers of inflammation in rheumatoid arthritis: implications for fatigue. Brain Behav Immun 2008;22:24–32.
84. Cho HJ, Seeman TE, Bower JE, et al. Prospective association between C-reactive protein and fatigue in the Coronary Artery Risk Development in Young Adults Study. Biol Psychiatry 2009;66:971–8.
85. Schubert C, Hong S, Natarajan L, et al. The association between fatigue and inflammatory marker levels in cancer patients: a quantitative review. Brain Behav Immun 2007;21:413–27.
86. Wang XS, Shi Q, Williams LA, et al. Inflammatory cytokines are associated with the development of symptom burden in patients with NSCLC undergoing concurrent chemoradiation therapy. Brain Behav Immun 2010;24:968–74.
87. Mills PJ, Ancoli-Israel S, Parker B, et al. Predictors of inflammation in response to anthracycline-based chemotherapy for breast cancer. Brain Behav Immun 2008;22:98–104.
88. Monk JP, Phillips G, Waite R, et al. Assessment of tumor necrosis factor alpha blockade as an intervention to improve tolerability of dose-intensive chemotherapy in cancer patients. J Clin Oncol 2006;24:1852–9.
89. Bower JE, Ganz PA, Tao ML, et al. Inflammatory biomarkers and fatigue during radiation therapy for breast and prostate cancer. Clin Cancer Res 2009;15:5534–40.
90. Bower JE, Ganz PA, Desmond KA, et al. Fatigue in breast cancer survivors: occurrence, correlates, and impact on quality of life. J Clin Oncol 2000;18:743–53.

91. Bower JE, Ganz PA, Aziz N, et al. Fatigue and proinflammatory cytokine activity in breast cancer survivors. Psychosom Med 2002;64:604–11.

92. Collado-Hidalgo A, Bower JE, Ganz PA, et al. Inflammatory biomarkers for persistent fatigue in breast cancer survivors. Clin Cancer Res 2006;12:2759–66.

93. Bower JE, Ganz PA, Irwin MR, et al. Fatigue and gene expression in human leukocytes: Increased NF-kappaB and decreased glucocorticoid signaling in breast cancer survivors with persistent fatigue. Brain Behav Immun 2011;25:147–50.

94. Collado-Hidalgo A, Bower JE, Ganz PA, et al. Cytokine gene polymorphisms and fatigue in breast cancer survivors: early findings. Brain Behav Immun 2008;22:1197–200.

95. Tyring S, Gottlieb A, Papp K, et al. Etanercept and clinical outcomes, fatigue, and depression in psoriasis: double-blind placebo-controlled randomised phase III trial. Lancet 2006;367:29–35.

96. Carlson LE, Speca M, Patel KD, et al. Mindfulness-based stress reduction in relation to quality of life, mood, symptoms of stress, and immune parameters in breast and prostate cancer outpatients. Psychosom Med 2003;65:571–81.

97. Cruess DG, Antoni MH, McGregor BA, et al. Cognitive-behavioral stress management reduces serum cortisol by enhancing benefit finding among women being treated for early stage breast cancer. Psychosom Med 2000;62:304–8.

98. Nicklas BJ, Hsu FC, Brinkley TJ, et al. Exercise training and plasma C-reactive protein and interleukin-6 in elderly people. J Am Geriatr Soc 2008;56:2045–52.

99. Irwin MR, Olmstead R. Mitigating cellular inflammation in older adults. Am J Geriatr Psychiatry 2011, in press.

100. Irwin MR, Olmstead R, Motivala SJ. Improving sleep quality in older adults with moderate sleep complaints: a randomized controlled trial of Tai Chi Chih. Sleep 2008;31:1001–8.

101. Oh B, Butow P, Mullan B, et al. Impact of medical Qigong on quality of life, fatigue, mood and inflammation in cancer patients: a randomized controlled trial. Ann Oncol 21:608–14.

102. Madhusudan S, Foster M, Muthuramalingam SR, et al. A phase II study of etanercept (Enbrel), a tumor necrosis factor alpha inhibitor in patients with metastatic breast cancer. Clin Cancer Res 2004;10:6528–34.

103. Madhusudan S, Muthuramalingam SR, Braybrooke JP, et al. Study of etanercept, a tumor necrosis factor-alpha inhibitor, in recurrent ovarian cancer. J Clin Oncol 2005;23:5950–9.

104. Schwartz AL, Thompson JA, Masood N. Interferon-induced fatigue in patients with melanoma: a pilot study of exercise and methylphenidate. Oncol Nurs Forum 2002;29:E85–90.

105. Raison CL, Miller AH. When not enough is too much: the role of insufficient glucocorticoid signaling in the pathophysiology of stress-related disorders. Am J Psychiatry 2003;160:1554–65.

106. Rief W, Pilger F, Ihle D, et al. Immunological differences between patients with major depression and somatization syndrome. Psychiatry Res 2001;105:165–74.

Simulated Illness: The Factitious Disorders and Malingering

Cheryl B. McCullumsmith, MD, PhD*, Charles V. Ford, MD

KEYWORDS

- Factitious disorder • Malingering • Simulated illness
- Munchausen syndrome

INTRODUCTION

Consciously simulated illnesses fall into two diagnostic categories: factitious disorders and malingering, differentiated by both motivation for behavior and consciousness of that motivation. Factitious disorder behaviors are motivated by an unconscious need to assume the sick role, while malingering behaviors are driven consciously to achieve external secondary gains. Thus, factitious disorders are psychiatric disorders in the Diagnostic and Statistical Manual-IV text revision (DSM –IV TR), whereas malingering is listed as a condition not attributable to a mental illness. Diagnosis of factitious disorder depends first on detection of the conscious production of symptoms and then on delineation of the motivation behind the deception. This review will focus on the commonalities in detection of consciously simulated illnesses generally and on the difficulties in distinction between factitious disorder and malingering. The background and clinical presentations of factitious disorder and malingering have been extensively reviewed,[1-4] and will not be extensively covered in this review. This review will discuss current controversies in diagnosis and recent research providing further insights into the detection of simulated illnesses, and end with a discussion of ethical and legal issues associated with factitious disorder diagnoses.

Diagnosis

Factitious disorder diagnosis

Factitious disorder was introduced as a psychiatric diagnostic category in DSM-III in 1980, as a mid-way point between malingering and the somatization disorders,[5] characterized by "physical or psychological symptoms that are voluntarily initiated by

Department of Psychiatry and Behavioral Neurobiology, The University of Alabama at Birmingham, Eye Foundation Hospital - 3 FL, 1720 University Boulevard, Birmingham, AL 35294-0009, USA
* Corresponding author.
E-mail address: cmccs@uab.edu

Psychiatr Clin N Am 34 (2011) 621–641
doi:10.1016/j.psc.2011.05.013
0193-953X/11/$ – see front matter © 2011 Elsevier Inc. All rights reserved.

Box 1
Diagnostic criteria, existing and proposed, for factitious disorder

A: DSM-IV TR Criteria for Factitious Disorder

A. Intentional production or feigning of physical or psychological signs or symptoms.

B. The motivation for the behavior is to assume the sick role.

C. External incentives for the behavior (such as economic gain, avoiding legal responsibility, or improving physical wellbeing, as in Malingering) are absent.

Code based on type:

300.19 With Predominantly Psychological Signs and Symptoms: if psychological signs and symptoms predominate in the clinical presentation

300.19 With Predominantly Physical Signs and Symptoms: if physical signs and symptoms predominate in the clinical presentation

300.19 With Combined Psychological and Physical Signs and Symptoms: if both psychological and physical signs and symptoms are present but neither predominates in the clinical presentation

300.19 Factitious Disorder Not Otherwise Specified.

B. Proposed DSM-V Criteria for Factitious Disorder

1. A pattern of falsification of physical or psychological signs or symptoms, associated with identified deception.

2. A pattern of presenting oneself to others as ill or impaired.

3. The behavior is evident even in the absence of obvious external rewards.

4. The behavior is not better accounted for by another mental disorder such as delusional belief system or acute psychosis.

C. Rosenberg criteria for Munchausen by proxy (Rosenberg and Marino[124])

- Illness in a child which is simulated (faked) and/or produced by a parent or someone who is *in loco parentis*;

- Presentation of the child for medical assessment and care, usually persistently, often resulting in multiple medical procedures;

- Denial of knowledge by the perpetrator as to the etiology of the child's illness [at least before the deception is discovered]; and

- Acute symptoms and signs of the child abate when the child is separated from the perpetrator.

Excludes physical abuse only, sexual abuse only, and nonorganic failure to thrive only

---

the patient . . . (with) no apparent goal other than to assume the role of a patient.[6]" DSM-IV TR criteria for factitious disorder recognizes four sub-types differentiated by the type of symptom simulated (**Box 1,** A). Factitious disorder NOS largely consists of Munchausen by proxy, where one person, usually an adult caregiver, simulates or produces illness in someone else (proposed criteria in **Box 1,** C).

Since DSM-III, the diagnostic validity and appropriate classification of factitious disorder has been debated. Concerns have arisen over the difficulties inherent in objectively determining motivation for behavior in distinguishing between the sick role and secondary gain and in detecting production of psychological symptoms, as well as the lack of specific inclusion, exclusion criteria and outcomes data.[7] Some have argued that any deceptive behavior, including the conscious production of symptoms, should be categorized as malingering regardless of the motivation.[8,9] They argue that since individual patients use choice in their decision to deceive, giving

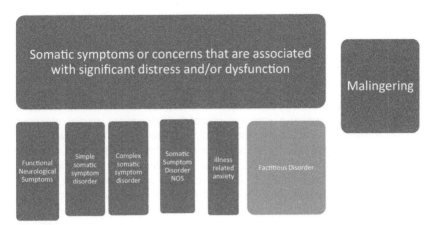

Fig. 1. Proposed DSM-V.

factitious disorder a psychiatric diagnosis removes personal responsibility for decep-tive behavior. Some consideration must be given to the degree of deception, as many clinicians have found patients commonly exaggerate symptoms to some degree in order to gain (some) desired outcome, be it an appointment, a medication, or a hospitalization. Indeed Menninger stated in 1935: "Every neurotic patient makes some use of their secondary gain from illness.. and to this extent every neurotic person is a malingerer." To further confuse matters, malingering, factitious disorder and other psychiatric disorders frequently co-exist in the same patient and may be shifting targets. In 1885, Weir Mitchell described "the curious progress from simula-tion, not consciously imitative, to conscious unresisted simulation, and at last dissimulation . . . of mimicry passing into well-sustained fraud."

Different diagnostic classifications have been proposed for factitious disorders. Kocalevent and colleagues[10] incorporate factitious disorders into a framework for autodestructive syndromes where the coalescing diagnostic feature is physical harm to self. Turner[11] has suggested new criteria for factitious disorder: criterion AR, 'lying or deliberate autobiographical falsification" and criterion BR, the behavior leads to self-harm. Krahn and colleagues[12] suggest that factitious disorder should be consid-ered a variant of somatoform disorders as in both conditions patients "organize their lives around seeking medical services in spite of having primarily a psychiatric condition." This latter model is being proposed in DSM-V, with factitious disorders recategorized as somatic symptom disorders (**Fig. 1**), with 2 types: factitious disorder imposed on self and factitious disorder imposed on other (criteria listed in **Box 1,** B). These new criteria for factitious disorder focus on observed phenomena and do not require determination of the patient's underlying motivation, other than the absence of obvious external rewards. A severity scale is proposed, from a score of 1 for reported or feigned symptoms to 4 when production of symptoms is life-threatening.

Malingering diagnosis

Malingering is defined in DSM-IV TR as the "intentional production of false or grossly exaggerated physical or psychological symptoms, motivated by external incentives such as avoiding military duty, avoiding work, obtaining financial compensation, evading criminal prosecution, or obtaining drugs." DSM-IV suggests that malingering should be suspected when there is a medicolegal context to the presentation, a marked discrepancy between the person's claimed stress of disability and the objective findings, lack of cooperation during the diagnostic evaluation and in complying with prescribed treatment regimen, or the presence of Antisocial Personality Disorder. However, these criteria have been found to be of little use in actually identifying individuals who are malingering, due to lack of specificity and objective findings. Further, malingering is a situationally dependent phenomenon and is not a stable description of a patient. Resnick[13] comments on potential subtypes of malingering: pure malingering involves complete fabrication, partial malingering involves exaggeration of existing symptoms, and false imputation occurs when an evaluee intentionally attributes symptoms to a cause that has little or no relationship to the development of the symptoms.[13] Rogers and Shuman[14] have suggested six signs of malingering: rare symptoms, improbable and absurd responses, indiscriminant symptom endorsement, unlikely symptom combinations, contradictory symptoms, and symptom severity. Diagnosis of malingering frustrates and even angers clinicians because clinicians are not trained as forensic lie detectors, but rather are trained to treat patient's presumed valid symptoms. Doctors want to make medical diagnoses, not document criminal or illegal actions.[5] Studies support that psychologists and psychiatrists may be no better at detecting lies than other professionals or the lay public, yet they are increasingly called upon to make these discriminations.[15]

Epidemiology

Factitious disorder epidemiology

Factitious disorders may account for as many as 5% of all physician visits.[16] Surveys of physicians have demonstrated perceived prevalence of 1.3% overall, with lower perceived factitious disorder among clinicians with larger practices and rates up to 15% among dermatologists and neurologists.[17]

Three distinct epidemiological categories of factitious disorder are reported in the medical literature: Munchausen syndrome, common factitious disorder, and Munchausen syndrome by proxy (MSbP). Munchausen syndrome was first described by Ascher in 1951 and consists of: (1) simulation of disease (2) pseudologia fantastica, or a kind of pathological lying with fantastic stories centering on the patient which often mix fact and fiction and (3) peregrination or wandering.[18] These patients often use aliases and travel from hospital to hospital, often crossing state lines. They are usually male, single, in their 40s, with antisocial personality disorder or significant cluster B traits. Although this syndrome is very dramatic and memorable, Munchausen syndrome likely encompasses a minority of factitious disorder cases. However, classic Munchausen syndrome patient characteristics were highly prevalent in a recent review of reported neurological cases of factitious disorder; this skewed distribution suggests that medically savvy women (who characterize the majority of factitious disorder in other populations) no longer choose to simulate neurological illnesses readily verifiable by radiological modalities.[5] Common factitious disorder is the most prevalent form of factitious disorder and occurs primarily in women in health care professions, who are stable and do not travel. In a large case series of factitious disorders at Mayo Clinic, Krahn and colleagues[19] found that 72% were women, of whom 65.7% had an affiliation with health related professions. These women typically have history of emotional deprivation and current sexual or relationship problems.[20] Although factitious disorder has often been reported to be associated with borderline personality disorder and posttraumatic stress disorder (PTSD),[21] few studies have been conducted prospectively. Fliege and colleagues[22] found that patients with factitious disorder were much less likely to meet criteria for anxiety, depressive, eating, or substance use disorders than patients with histories of overt self-harm. Structural brain problems may also exist: a recent case report describes a factitious anemia with a common factitious disorder presentation with prominent white matter changes on MRI.[23]

Munchausen syndrome by proxy has been reported as the cause of underlying symptoms in as many as 1.5% of infants brought to an Australian clinic because of apparent life-threatening episodes.[24] In a review of 451 cases of MSbP reported in the literature, Sheridan[25] found that over three quarters of perpetrators were mothers of victims under 5 years old with an average time from onset of symptoms until diagnosis of almost 22 months. During this time period, 6% of the children died and over 7% had permanent injuries. Shockingly, over 61% of siblings had had similar illnesses and 25% of the victims' siblings were dead. While many feel MSbP is overdiagnosed, others feel quite the opposite, that overdiagnosis of MSbP and subsequent efforts put forward into the establishment of MSbP diagnosis are often misplaced and lead to inappropriate assessment, with potentially lethal consequences.[26] Further, children and adolescents can also feign illness to assume the sick role without the knowledge of caregivers, thus having factitious disorder themselves.[27]

Malingering epidemiology
The adaptational model of malingering proposed by Rogers asserts that malingerers engage in a "cost-benefit analysis" during assessment: "Malingering is more likely to occur when (1) the context of the evaluation is perceived as adversarial, (2) the personal stakes are very high, and (3) no other alternatives appear to be viable."[28] Thus, individuals malinger based on their estimate of success in obtaining the desired external incentive. Consistent with this model, a review of 33,000 annual cases seen by neuropsychologists led to estimated base rates of malingering and symptom exaggeration ranging from 8% of medical and psychiatric cases (15% of depressive disorders) up to 30% of those seen for disability or workers compensation.[29] From a review of the literature, Larrabee[30] estimated the base rate of malingering to be 40% in cases where there was the potential for secondary gain.

Management and Treatment of Simulated Illness
Management of simulated disorders can be divided into two phases: the acute situation in the hospital, emergency room, or clinic and the chronic process of engaging the patient into therapeutic treatment (this for factitious disorder only). Management of factitious disorder in both phases must focus on negotiating the diagnosis with the patient and then engaging the patient into treatment by psychotherapy. Some authors support the use of direct confrontation with patients who feign illness.[31] In the case series review by Reich and Gottfried,[31] in 33/41 factitious disorder patients, when confronted with the diagnosis, thirteen acknowledged it and no patients signed out AMA or became suicidal. It should be noted that 39/41 of this sample were women and 28 were in medical fields. The authors stated that none of these patients were classic Munchausen syndrome, malingerers, or sociopaths, which likely contributed to their relative success. Other authors using confrontation have found a higher fraction of patients leaving against medical advice and lower acknowledgment rates.[32] Direct confrontation carries with it the risk of inefficacy and escalation and, perhaps, lawsuits. Evidence suggests the benefit of a more nuanced approach,[33] in lieu of direct confrontation, with three distinct but overlapping lines of approach. First, the clinician can provide inexact interpretations of psychological defense, where the stressors leading to illness simulation are identified and discussed with the patient, but not directly connected to the illness simulation. Second, the clinician can make therapeutic use of a double bind, by discussing a full range of

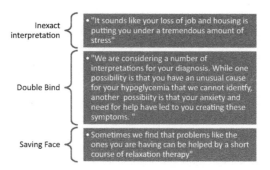

Fig. 2. Strategies for discussion of simulated symptoms.

possible diagnoses with the patient, including factitious disorder, and clearly establishing that the clinician is considering factitious disorder in the differential diagnosis. Third, the clinician can use treatment strategies and approaches that allow the patient to discard the factitious symptoms without losing face, such as biofeedback or hypnosis (Fig. 2). In their review, Eastwood and Bisson[34] found no evidence for efficacy of any specific treatment over another, when comparing initial confrontation versus nonconfrontational approaches, psychotherapy versus no psychotherapy, and psychotropic medication versus no medication. Lack of compliance among this patient population severely limited conclusions on efficacy.

Munchausen by proxy diagnoses carry additional medical and legal responsibilities, adding importance to the accuracy to this diagnosis. Once a diagnosis of Munchausen by proxy is established, management should involve the legal system and child protective services. It is therefore imperative that a complete investigation precedes the diagnosis. Bass and Jones[35] have examined case characteristics which suggested conditions where parental reunification with the child may be possible. These include: (a) acknowledgment of the fabrications; (b) an ability to work collaboratively with health and social services; (c) cessation of somatoform presentations to primary and tertiary care services; (d) reduction in frequency of any self-harming or substance misuse; (e) remaining in a stable relationship with social supports. As might be expected, better outcomes occur with development of a strong therapeutic alliance with the entire family.

In managing patients suspected of malingering, LeBourgeois[36] suggests wisely that clinicians follow the ABC's, where A is to avoid accusations of lying, B is to beware of countertransference, which is readily picked up by the sociopath and may inflame the interaction, C is to seek clarification, not confrontation, and "s" is to ensure that adequate security measures are present or readily available.

Detection of Simulated Illness

General

Detection of simulated illness by objective measures has been the subject of multiple case reports and review articles over the past century. Detection of simulated, or functional, neurological illness by physical examination has recently been reviewed by Stone and Carson[37] and other medical illness by Greer and colleagues.[38] Detection of simulated psychiatric illness using interviewing techniques with consideration of the usual presentation of psychiatric illnesses has been described in 2 papers by Resnick.[13,39] Laboratory tests including high performance liquid chromatography or scans can be used to diagnose purposeful creation of symptoms in many illnesses including thryotoxicoses,[40,41] hypoglycemia,[42,43] laxative abuse,[32,44] pheochromocytoma,[45] and Cushing's,[46] among others. Recent work describing brain activity during deceit are reviewed below. The distinction between factitious disorder and malingering still relies fundamentally on the determination of the patient's motivation for the simulation: an unconscious need for the sick role in factitious disorder or the secondary gain in malingering. Thus far, no objective measures can determine between these two motivations, leading to much frustration in diagnosis. We shall focus on recent work relative to detection of the simulation of illness generally and will apply these observations to both factitious disorder and malingering. Future research on these grounds may develop techniques to tease out differences between these two diagnoses. Two main areas of recent investigation into detection of simulated illness will be reviewed here: neuropsychological testing, and functional MRI studies.

Neuropsychological testing

The American Academy of Clinical Neuropsychology (AACN) published an extensive consensus statement in 2009 on the neuropsychological assessment of effort, response bias and malingering.[47] This document thoughtfully discusses considerations in defining terms, assessment methods for abilities, somatic and psychological issues and research evidence. Two main points for psychiatrists to consider from this review are (1) the difference between detection and diagnosis and (2) the strengths and limitations of neuropsychological tools in assessments.

Detection should be thought of as the determination of whether exaggeration of symptoms has occurred, whereas diagnosis of malingering or factitious disorder requires determination of intent. To this end, criteria for the diagnosis of malingered neurocognitive dysfunction have been proposed by Slick and colleagues,[48] including criteria for definite, probable, and possible malingered deficits. The criteria for definite malingered neurocognitive deficits include presence of a significant secondary gain, definitive neuropsychological testing evidence, and absence of psychiatric, neurological, or developmental factors that could fully account for the behaviors. The criteria for probable malingered neurocognitive deficits also include the presence of a significant secondary gain and absence of alternative explanatory factors, but less stringent neuropsychological testing evidence and/or the presence of inconsistencies in the patient's self report, either internally, with the medical record, or against known illness patterns. Possible malingered neuropsychological deficit cases meet criteria for either definite or probable malingered neurocognitive deficit except that other primary etiologies cannot be ruled out. All such diagnostic schemata require a comprehensive view of the patient, with consideration of a detailed history and the psychological, social, medical settings as well as specific examination findings. Criteria require validated, objective, reliable tests with good predictive value to determine a response bias indicative of malingering. The reader is referred to Iverson and Binder[49] or Lezak and colleagues[50] for a detailed review of neuropsychological assessment of malingering. Development of neuropsychological tests has taken two directions: use of information in existing neuropsychological batteries (embedded tests), and development of stand-alone tests designed specifically to detect deception (symptom validity tests, **Table 1**). Symptom validity testing (SVT) is used in neuropsychiatric assessment batteries to determine true responses from false ones; its theoretical basis has been reviewed by Bianchi and colleagues.[51] The AACN consensus statement supports the use of these stand-alone SVTs as screens, especially in conjunction with full neuropsychological assessment. Some of these SVTs, such as the test of memory malingering are specific to the skill being tested,

Table 1
Selected neuropsychological tests of use in detecting simulated illness

	Selected References	Time Required	Applicability
Selected Scales Extracted from Neuropsychological Batteries			
Meyers Index (from MMPI)	Meyers et al, 2002[63]		
Fake Bad Scale (From MMPI)	Lees-Haley, 1992[65]		
Reliable Digit Span	Jasinski et al, 2011[66]; Greve et al, 2010[67]		Suboptimal performance detection
PAI personality assessment inventory NIM subscale; MAL, RDF, CDF indices	Sullivan and King, 2010[125]; Hawes and Boccaccini, 2009[60]		Faking good and faking bad
WMS rarely missed index	Axelrod et al, 2010[54]		Suboptimal performance
Atypical response scale on Trauma Symptom inventory	Gray et al, 2010[68]		PTSD
Selected Independent Symptom Validity Tests (SVTs)			
Structured Inventory of Reported Symptoms (SIRS)	Edens et al, 2007[70]; Rogers et al, 2009[53]		Global scale, validated in forensic populations
Structured Inventory of Malingered Symptomatology (SIMS)	Smith and Burger, 1997[52]; Wisdom et al, 2010[126]	75 True/False questions	Global scale, validated in forensic populations
Symptom Checklist-90 (SCL-90-R)	Sullivan and King, 2010[125]	15 min Self-assessment	General psychiatric assessment tool; high scores may indicate malingering
TOMM (Test of Malingered Memory)	Gierok et al, 2005[127]	15 min	Memory
Rey 15-Item test	Reznek, 2005[128]	5 min	Memory Caution: should be used with other tests as it has low positive predictive value when used independently (Strauss et al)
Computerized Assessment of Response Bias	Green and Iverson, 2001[78]		Detection of suboptimal performance
Miller Forensic Assessment of Symptoms Test (M-FAST)	Miller, 2004[80]; Vitacco et al, 2008[73]	10 min	Psychiatric Illness
M-test	Beaber et al, 1985[129]; Hankins et al, 1993[130]	33 true false items	Psychosis Caution: low sensitivity in less educated populations and may be influenced by race (Rogers, 1997)

while others, such as the Structured Inventory of Malingered Symptomatology (SIMS)[52]; and Structured Inventory of Reported Symptoms[53] are more general. Some SVTs, like the SIMS and Structured Interview of Reported Symptoms (SIRS), were developed with a forensic population in mind, whereas others were developed to detect suboptimal performance on more routine neuropsychological assessment. There is controversy on the appropriate cutoffs for maximizing both sensitivity and specificity, especially in psychiatric illnesses where effort may not be optimal due to the illness itself; see Axelrod and colleagues.[54] To avoid labeling the truly ill as malingering, cut-off scores for these scales enhance specificity over sensitivity.[55] If several distinct symptom validity tests with high specificity are administered to the same patient, then the likelihood of detecting deception (as well as the sensitivity overall) increases.[30,56] Further, for some psychiatric illnesses, such as ADHD, SVTs have not been shown to discriminate simulation or malingering from true illness.[57] Although it has been correctly noted that malingering is context dependent and that these tests do not assess motivation for deception,[15] they might be incorporated into a thorough diagnostic evaluation to increase diagnostic accuracy. Neuropsychological testing has been reported to assist in difficult factitious disorder diagnoses such as individuals with Ganser syndrome.[58] Selected tests for feigned symptomatology are briefly described below.

Embedded Scales and Indices

Personality Assessment Inventory
Subscales within Personality Assessment Inventory (PAI) and indices drawn from the PAI for detection of malingering have been validated in inpatient psychiatric populations as well as forensic populations,[59] reviewed in Hawes and Boccaccini.[60] Two scales (Negative Impression Management and Positive Impression Management), and four indices drawn from the PAI (Malingering index, Defensiveness index, Cashel Discriminant Function,[61] and Rogers Discriminant Function[62]) are commonly used.

Meyers index
The Meyers index uses results from seven subscales of the MMPI[63] to detect malingering, originally in chronic pain patients. These findings have recently been replicated with a more commercially available abbreviated version of the Meyers index in traumatic brain injury and chronic pain patients.[64]

Fake bad scale
This scale is drawn from 43 questions on the MMPI found to correlate with malingering in a group of personal injury claimants.[65]

Reliable digit span
Poor performance on standard measures of memory using digit span have been shown to be reasonable measures of suboptimal performance in neuropsychological testing. Reliable digit span standards for suboptimal effort have been determined and are calculated by summing the longest string of digits repeated going both forward and backward over several trials.[66,67]

Atypical response scale of the trauma symptom inventory
This scale has shown validity in distinguishing genuine symptoms of PTSD from simulated PTSD.[68]

Stand Alone Symptom Validity Tests

Structured Inventory of Malingered Symptomatology

The Structured Inventory of Malingered Symptomatology (SIMS)[52] is 75 self-report, true–false items with five independent subscales, psychosis, neurologic impairment, amnestic disorders, low intelligence, and affective disorders and has well supported diagnostic accuracy.[69–73] SIMS was developed and validated in criminal and civil forensic settings[69,72,74]; it distinguishes between malingerers and normal controls; it might have difficulty distinguishing psychiatric patients from those with malingered symptomatology,[70] but see Merckelbach and Smith.[75] Coaching and knowledge of basic psychopathology have not been shown to diminish the efficacy of the SIMS.[76,77]

Computerized assessment of response bias

This computerized test has been used to detect poor effort or suboptimal performance in patients with mild traumatic brain injuries, pain disorders, fibromyalgia, and depression.[78]

Structured interview of reported symptoms

The SIRS is often used as the standard for malingering, especially in forensic cases. It consists of eight primary and five supplementary scales for the assessment of feigning, including a scale to assess defensiveness and is designed to detect 13 response styles commonly associated with feigning, and allows for classification as "feigning" (definite or probable) or "honest," as well as identification of inconsistent and other problematic response styles. It is well validated in the literature to distinguish between malingerers and normal controls, but might not distinguish psychiatric patients from those with malingered symptomatology.[70,79]

Miller Forensic Assessment of Symptoms Test

Miller Forensic Assessment of Symptoms Test (M-FAST) consists of twenty-five questions that can be administered in 10–15-min M-FAST scales to operationalize response styles and interview strategies that have been demonstrated to successfully identify individuals who are attempting to feign psychopathology. Scales include Reported versus Observed (symptoms), Extreme Symptomatology, Rare Combinations, Unusual Hallucinations, Unusual Symptom Course, Negative Image, and Suggestibility. It has been validated against the SIRS in forensic cases[73,80] and appears to have more efficacy at determination of feigned psychiatric than of feigned neurocognitive symptoms.[74]

Neuroimaging

Functional neuroimaging suggests that conscious production of symptoms involves different patterns of brain activity than either unconscious production or actual illness. Recent research has explored differences in brain activity when individuals are deceptive versus truthful. In most of these studies, normal subjects are asked to lie or to deceive an interviewer and brain activity is compared on functional MRI (fMRI) to when they are truthful.[81] While these studies involve small numbers of participants, taken overall, they suggest that deception is associated with increased activity in prefrontal cortex and anterior cingulate cortex; areas responsible for executive control.[82–85] The ventrolateral prefrontal cortex is believed to allow individuals to inhibit or modulate their responses when faced with different scenarios.[86,87] Knoch and colleagues[88] found that disruption of the function of the ventrolateral prefrontal cortex with low-frequency transcranial magnetic stimulation impaired abilities of subjects to prioritize social interests above their own immediate personal interests.

Furthermore, the increased activation of novel brain regions on fMRI correlated with an outwardly measurable physical sign of deception: increased response time during the lie. Increased response time has been previously associated with deceitful responses[89–91] and corroborate the time needed for extra cognitive processing occurring in other brain areas seen on fMRI during deception.

Recent fMRI work has focused on the area of simulated cognitive impairment, such as might be seen in factitious disorder or malingering. Browndyke and colleagues[92] instructed study participants performing memory tasks while in fMRI to "respond as though they were slightly injured in an automobile accident and to feign a memory impairment for financial gain, but not obviously so or risk detection and punishment for fraud." When the subject pretended to make a memory error, the inferior parietal and superior temporal lobes showed relative increased activity. When individuals pretended to not recognize familiar objects, they had additional dorsomedial frontal activation, whereas pretending to recognize an object that had not been seen activated bilateral ventrolateral frontal regions. Larsen and colleagues[93] found that when subjects were asked to feign memory impairment, they had areas of increased brain activity. Thus, different types of simulation (pretending not to recognize versus pretending to recognize) activated different brain regions. Increased brain activity in the dorsomedial frontal, temporal, and inferior parietal regions during simulated memory errors were associated with longer response times and additional peak strength in surrounding cortical regions compared to performing tasks truthfully.

Imaging studies find different areas of brain activation among those with conversion disorders than among those simulating weakness, suggesting true physiological differences underlying unconsciously versus consciously motivated processes.[94] fMRI studies demonstrate that patients with motor conversion symptoms had different areas of brain activation than patients who are feigning motor weakness.[95] Whereas patients with conversion disorder activated bilateral putamen and lingual gyri, left inferior frontal gyrus, and left insula and deactivated right middle frontal and orbitofrontal cortices, those simulating weakness activated the contralateral supplemental motor area and not the above areas. Electrophysiological testing has been used more recently to assist in the diagnosis of simulated and somatization disorders, especially movement disorders.[96,97] Psychogenic myoclonus shows pre-movement potentials indicative of voluntary movement.[96] Individuals with psychogenic movement disorders had significantly increased startle eye blink reflex in response to negative affective stimuli compared with controls, who normally show inhibition of this reflex.[98] Liepert and colleagues[99] found that imagining movements decreased cortical excitability in the affected limb motor conversion in disorder patients but increased in the unaffected limb compared to control. Theoretically, these electrophysiological findings could differentiate conversion disorder from factitious disorder or malingering.[97] However, it is unclear if patients with factitious disorder who have intentional production of symptoms for unconscious motivations would be discernible from malingering by imaging studies.

Development of neuroimaging studies that can detect deceit in individuals is fraught with methodological and ethical issues.[100] A number of critical issues must be addressed in order to develop and properly apply a functional brain imaging test diagnostically to an individual. Accuracy, sensitivity, and specificity of neuroimaging tests must be determined, just as with any other medical diagnostic test. Recent work suggests that study findings can be replicated in a different scanner and location.[100] However, subjects may use countermeasures to counteract fMRI changes on deception,[101] which could seriously limit the application of neuroimaging to factitious disorder or malingering diagnoses.

Ethical and Legal Issues in Factitious Disorders

Following the seminal article by Ascher,[18] there has been an ever-increasing number of reports and publications in regards to factitious illness. By the 1980s, it was apparent that these unique patients also create a variety of ethical and legal dilemmas for those who encounter them. Issues include rights to privacy/secrecy, confidentiality, involuntary treatment, litigation and whether patients with factitious behavior should be treated as patients or as miscreants. One recommendation by Ford and Abernathy[102] that has been widely adopted is that of management of complex ethical/legal issues by multidisciplinary task force discussions.[102,103] These ethical/legal issues continue to the present and are summarized below as individual topics although there is considerable overlap among them.

Right to privacy/secrecy

The earliest reports of factitious disorder frequently described activities such as secretly searching a patient's room looking for paraphernalia for the self-induction of disease and/or the performing various diagnostic tests, without the patient's knowledge, which would either prove or disprove the probability of factitious disease. Although these measures have been largely discounted as unethical, one such issue in reference to potential victims of Munchausen by proxy syndrome has remained contentious.

The diagnosis of Munchausen by proxy syndrome has, to a large extent, been determined by circumstantial evidence such as whether a child regains health after separation from the alleged perpetrator. One objective method of determining whether a parent might be actively producing disease in a child is through secret video surveillance. Hidden cameras placed in a child's hospital room can continuously monitor for illness producing behavior by parents or other visitors. Hospital personnel can immediately intervene if the child is in danger. This provides a "hard copy" of behavior to present to the courts. Covert video surveillance is in wide use in pediatric hospitals and, not surprisingly, many perpetrators have been identified.[104,105] However, this procedure is not without some risks in that damage can be done to the child prior to healthcare personnel intervention and, further, it is fraught with ethical/legal issues. Connelly[106] argues that covert video surveillance "expands the police role of medicine and as a consequence this practice may add to the erosion of public confidence in medicine." He goes on to state that parents have a right to some privacy with their children in that, "parental intimacy and quiet time with the child are part of the care considered to be in the best interest of the child." He also notes that the use of covert video surveillance interrupts the therapeutic alliance between caretakers and parents and creates an adversarial relationship. He poses the question for the medical community and society as to whether child abuse, such as in cases of Munchausen by proxy syndrome, is really a medical problem or a criminal issue. Further, there should be clarification between medical care and criminal surveillance, as well as the limits of physician responsibility in the police role. Arguments in favor of covert video surveillance have emphasized that if the child (or an impartial guardian) were to be aware of the circumstances permission would most certainly be granted and it is the child, not the parents, who is the patient. Court decisions have been mixed as to the admissibility of covert videotaped evidence of Munchausen by proxy syndrome. One decision by the District Court of Appeal of Florida holds that the perpetrator had a right to the expectation of privacy.[107]

Litigation: malpractice lawsuits
The initial concerns of legal/ethical issues with factitious disorder did not take into account another important phenomenon which has arisen, that is of litigation. Despite the fact that these patients create their own disease and lie to their physicians about symptoms, and what they know of causation, a large number of these persons have initiated malpractice suits against their physicians.[108–110] Eisendrath and McNeil[111] list three reasons as to why a lawsuit might be initiated; greed, rage (devaluation of the physician by a borderline patient), or an effort to change the center of attention from the hospital to the courtroom. One of the authors (C.V.F.), who has evaluated the medical records of a number of suspected factitious disorder plaintiffs at the request of defense attorneys, has found all three of the above motivations. It must be emphasized that when the primary issue becomes an effort to obtain a judgment of money, factitious illness should be redefined as malingering. The case below illustrates the complexity of these cases.

A 55-year-old Caucasian woman filed suit for malpractice by her surgeon. Following abdominal surgery, she had required repeated hospitalizations for an infected surgical wound. Of importance, the wound would always heal when an obstructive bandage was placed over it and become re-infected (polymicrobial) when sufficiently available to her hands. She denied any knowledge of why her wound would become re-infected.

Medical records obtained from another hospital indicated that following knee surgery she had a similar course of illness which was sufficiently severe to result in an amputation of a leg. During this hospitalization, a diagnosis of factitious infections was established.

During the testimony of an expert in factitious disorders, the woman sitting in a wheel chair dramatically waved the stump of her leg back and forth. It was clear that no surgical malpractice had occurred and the plaintiff's abdominal infections were most probably self-inflicted. The plaintiff's attorney, in an aggressive cross-examination, stated that the surgeon's failure to recognize factitious disorder was, in fact, malpractice and, therefore, it made little difference as to whether or not she had self-infected herself. The expert opined that a physician must assume that a patient is telling the truth and it was beyond a reasonable expectation of medical care that the surgeon should be a lie detector. The jury unanimously found in favor of the surgeon.

Follow-up data reported by Eisendrath and McNeil[111] indicated that factitious disorder patients who have been in litigation have a high rate of mortality. This suggests that issues in addition to greed may be reasons why these patients file lawsuits. There is an apparent increase of the number of plaintiffs with probable factitious illness who are pursuing lawsuits and all physicians should be alerted to this risk. Plastic surgeons may be at higher risk than other specialties.[112]

Confidentiality
To what extent can information about patients who seek medical care fraudulently be disseminated? In the past, "black lists" were proposed in order to alert other physicians as to the possibility of a patient with factitious behavior. In general, at least in the United States, this has been regarded as unethical, and yet failure to communicate information to other physicians does put the patient, him/herself, in risk for unnecessary medical interventions and, further, creates greater medical expenses. As demonstrated by Krahn and colleagues,[19] a review of past medical records from

other institutions may be essential to establish the diagnosis of factitious behavior. On the surface, the electronic medical record (EMR) should be an ideal manner by which such information can easily be transmitted from physician to physician and institution to institution. Van Dinter and Welsch[113] cross-references several data (eg, birth date) by computer search to discover that a patient with factitious disorder had been previously admitted to their hospital using different aliases. DeWitt and colleagues[114] utilized an Australian medical registry to find that their patient had been previously discharged from other hospitals with a diagnosis of Munchausen syndrome. The latter case solicited a vigorous response[115] which raised ethical issues in regard of the use of the EMR for these patients. They stated that the proposed systematic management of a somatizing patient would require a means of communication within the medical system that would have to override the patient's choice to withhold it. (It is not clear at this time as to the degree of control that a patient in the United States would have over his/her own EMR.) They also noted that this would stigmatize patients in a manner that might prevent appropriate evaluation and treatment of actual disease by inviting a problematic relaxation of clinical vigilance.

Involuntary treatment
There is little question that patients with factitious disorder do not ordinarily seek any type of psychiatric treatment. In fact, when detected, they usually refuse psychiatric referral and often move their base of operations to another healthcare system and/or city. Involuntary hospitalization, which might be appropriate for these self-destructive patients, has not been an option in the overwhelming number of jurisdictions where the standard for hospitalization is an imminent danger to one's self or to others. In one case in Oregon, the outpatient commitment of a patient with factitious disorder did result in lower medical costs and less iatrogenic morbidity[116]; similar cases, to the best of our knowledge, have not been reported. However, a unique form of commitment via the criminal legal system was described by Elmore.[117] In this situation, a patient with blatant factitious disorder and acting out behavior was diagnosed with Munchausen syndrome and Personality Disorder not otherwise specified. An interagency staff meeting including the local hospital emergency department staff, department of social services and police department representatives was conducted in order to coordinate responses to her. She continued severe acting out behavior and was charged with unlawful use of telephone calls to 911, was arrested and court ordered to attend alcohol and drug rehabilitation which she refused. Charges were then initiated for creating a disturbance in the emergency department. She was jailed, and then placed on house arrest using an ambulatory surveillance monitor, and was court ordered to outpatient treatment. She was no longer able to travel freely, or able to contact multiple physicians and emergency services. She subsequently made a quiet adjustment to her marital home doing much better than prior to her house arrest. The authors opined that over-solicitude or intimidation by a patient should not deter emergency staff in setting limits once an evaluation and diagnosis has been made; other agencies may be available to assist with containment of behavior.

In another case, a man who malingered psychosis was involuntarily psychiatrically hospitalized. It became apparent that his goal was not to seek hospitalization but rather to obtain disability. It was believed to be unlikely that he would seek psychiatric help of his own accord in the future because he had found the hospitalization significantly unpleasant.[118]

Factitious disorder and the internet

The increasing availability of resources on the internet has allowed increased sophistication in patients with factitious illness behavior and created new perplexing legal/ethical issues. The use of the internet support groups by persons misrepresenting themselves with various diseases was first noted by Feldman and Bibby.[119] Since that time, several papers have confirmed this type of behavior which, when detected, has become emotionally distressful for those persons in the support group who are genuinely sick. After one support group had a member, "Mr A", post repeated contradictory contributions accompanied by abusive and threatening posts to questions or doubts, a team of members of the support group set up a dedicated website to publicize their objections to this member's behavior. "Mr A" then took his accusers to court and asked the judge to close down the dedicated website as defamatory. The judge ruled that Mr A's medical records were the heart of the accusations and that cross-examination related to their contents would be allowed. Mr A then immediately withdrew his case and the judge dismissed the case with prejudice eliminating the plaintiff's right to sue the defendants again on the same charges. It was the opinion of Feldman and Peychers[120] that this legal outcome effectively ceded to the group the ability to expose individual's deceptions with minimal fear of being sued.

The internet can be used as a resource by patients with factitious illness to gain more sophisticated medical information which they can use to be more convincing in their simulation of disease. It is also possible to download medical summaries, radiographs, and other material which they may be presented as their own, in a fraudulent manner, when presenting themselves for medical care.[121–123] It is obvious with the ever-increasing importance and resources of the internet, clever patients who simulate diseases will have better information and tools with which to do it. The cunning of these fraudulent patients cannot be overestimated and we can only guess as to what future exploitation will occur with available expanding medical knowledge and the potential for abuse of the EMR.

Summary

The consciously simulated illnesses of factitious disorders and malingering pose many dilemmas for detection of symptoms, diagnostic categorization and definition as well as ethical and legal management. While DSM-IV TR criteria place factitious disorders diagnostically with somatization disorders, proposed DSM-V criteria would recategorize factitious disorders as somatic symptom disorders, with 2 types: factitious disorder imposed on self and factitious disorder imposed on other. Detection of simulated symptoms pathognomonic of both factitious disorder and malingering has relied on subjective criteria. However, research in the areas of neuropsychological testing and neuroimaging suggest that objective measures for detection of symptom simulation may soon be a tool to be used in conjunction with a thorough psychiatric evaluation placed in the full clinical context. Management of factitious disorder can be difficult, due to patient noncompliance and consideration of legal concerns. Technological advances have increased the accuracy of detecting patients with simulated illness. However, the legal and ethical issues associated with these patients remain complex and unresolved.

REFERENCES

1. Feldman MD, Ford CV. Patient or pretender: Inside the strange world of factitious disorders. New York: Wiley; 1994.
2. McDermott B, Feldman M. Malingering in the medical setting. Psychiatr Clin North Am;30:645–62.

3. Velazquez MD, Bolton J. Factitious disorder. Br J Hosp Med (Lond) 2006;67:548–9.
4. Eisendrath SJ, Young JQ. Factitious physical disorders. Oxford: John Wiley & Sons; 2005.
5. Kanaan RA, Wessely SC. The origins of factitious disorder. Hist Human Sci 2010; 23:68–85.
6. Hyler SE, Spitzer RL. Hysteria split asunder. Am J Psychiatry 1978;135:1500–04.
7. Rogers R, Bagby RM, Rector N. Diagnostic legitimacy of factitious disorder with psychological symptoms. Am J Psychiatry 1989;146:1312–4.
8. Ford CV. Factitious disorders: diagnosis or misbehavior. In: May M, Akiskal HS, Mezzick JE, et al, editors. Somatoform disorders. Oxford: John Wiley & Sons; 2005:354–7.
9. Bass C, Halligan PW. Illness related deception: social or psychiatric problem? J R Soc Med 2007;100:81–4.
10. Kocalevent RD, Fliege H, Rose M, et al. Autodestructive syndromes. Psychother Psychosom 2005;74:202–11.
11. Turner MA. Factitious disorders: reformulating the DSM-IV criteria. Psychosomatics 2006;47:23–32.
12. Krahn LE, Bostwick JM, Stonnington CM. Looking toward DSM-V: should factitious disorder become a subtype of somatoform disorder? Psychosomatics 2008;49: 277–82.
13. Resnick PJ. The detection of malingered psychosis. Psychiatr Clin North Am 1999;22:159–72.
14. Rogers R, Shuman DW. The mental state at the time of the offense measure: its validation and admissibility under Daubert. J Am Acad Psychiatry Law 2000;28: 23–8.
15. Drob SL, Meehan KB, Waxman SE. Clinical and conceptual problems in the attribution of malingering in forensic evaluations. J Am Acad Psychiatry Law 2009; 37:98–106.
16. Wallach J. Laboratory diagnosis of factitious disorders. Arch Intern Med 1994;154: 1690–96.
17. Fliege H, Grimm A, Eckhardt-Henn A, et al. Frequency of ICD-10 factitious disorder: survey of senior hospital consultants and physicians in private practice. Psychoso-matics 2007;48:60–4.
18. Asher R. Munchausen's syndrome. Lancet 1951;1(6650):339–41.
19. Krahn LE, Li H, O'Connor MK. Patients who strive to be ill: factitious disorder with physical symptoms. Am J Psychiatry 2003;160:1163–8.
20. Carney MW, Brown JP. Clinical features and motives among 42 artifactual illness patients. Br J Med Psychol 1983;56 (Pt 1):57–66.
21. Stern TA. Munchausen's syndrome revisited. Psychosomatics 1980;21:329–31, 335–6.
22. Fliege H, Lee JR, Grimm A, et al. Axis I comorbidity and psychopathologic correlates of autodestructive syndromes. Compr Psychiatry 2009;50:327–34.
23. Aouillé J, Rouillon F, Limosin F. Factitious anemia and magnetic resonance imaging abnormalities. Can J Psychiatry 2003;48:572–3.
24. Rahilly PM. The pneumographic and medical investigation of infants suffering appar-ent life threatening episodes. J Paediatr Child Health 1991;27:349–53.
25. Sheridan MS. The deceit continues: an updated literature review of Munchausen Syndrome by Proxy. Child Abuse Negl 2003;27:431–51.
26. Wrennall L. Munchausen Syndrome by Proxy/Fabricated and Induced Illness: does the diagnosis serve economic vested interests, rather than the interests of children? Med Hypotheses 2007;68:960–6.

27. Jaghab K, Skodnek KB, Padder TA. Munchausen's syndrome and other factitious disorders in children: case series and literature review. Psychiatry (Edgmont) 2006; 3:46–55.

28. Rogers R. Development of a new classificatory model of malingering. Bull the Am Acad Psychiatry Law 1990;18:323–33.

29. Mittenbert W, Patton C, Canyock EM, et al. Base rates of malingering and symptom exaggeration. J Clin Exp Neuropsychol 2002;24:1094–102.

30. Larrabee GJ. Aggregation across multiple indicators improves the detection of malingering: relationship to likelihood ratios. Clin Neuropsychol 2008;22:666–79.

31. Reich P, Gottfried LA. Factitious disorders in a teaching hospital. Ann Intern Med 1983;99:240–7.

32. Shelton JH, Santa Ana CA, Thompson DR, et al. Factitious diarrhea induced by stimulant laxatives: accuracy of diagnosis by a clinical reference laboratory using thin layer chromatography. Clin Chem 2007;53:85–90.

33. Eisendrath SJ. Factitious physical disorders: treatment without confrontation. Psychosomatics 1989;30:383–7.

34. Eastwood S, Bisson JI. Management of factitious disorders: a systematic review. Psychother Psychosom 2008;77:209–18.

35. Bass C, Jones DPH. Fabricated or induced illness: assessment of perpetrators and approaches to management. Psychiatry 2009;8:158–63.

36. LeBourgeois I. Psychiatric Times; April 15, 2007. Available at: www.psychiatrictimes.com. Accessed May 18, 2011.

37. Stone J, Carson A. Functional neurologic symptoms: assessment and management. Neurol Clin 2011;29:1–18.

38. Greer S, Chambliss L, Mackler L. Clinical inquiries. What physical exam techniques are useful to detect malingering? J Fam Pract 2005;54:719–22.

39. Resnick PJ. My favorite tips for detecting malingering and violence risk. Psychiatr Clin North Am 2007;30:227–32.

40. Ashawesh K, Murthy NP, Fiad TM. Severe hypercalcemia secondary to factitious thyrotoxicosis. Am J Med 2010;123:e1–2.

41. Abdel-Nabi H, Falko JM, Olsen J. The value of technetium Tc 99m pertechnetate thyroid scanning in the diagnosis of factitious thyrotoxicosis. Arch Intern Med 1982;142:644–5.

42. Yates C, Neoh S, Konpa A, et al. Factitious hypoglycaemia. Intern Med J 2009;39: e15–7.

43. Neal JM, Han W. Insulin immunoassays in the detection of insulin analogues in factitious hypoglycemia. Endocr Pract 2008;14:1006–10.

44. Roerig JL, Steffen KJ, Mitchell JE, et al. Laxative abuse: epidemiology, diagnosis and management. Drugs 2010;70:1487–503.

45. Chidakel AR, Pacak K, Eisenhofer G, et al. Utility of plasma free metanephrines in diagnosis of factitious pheochromocytoma. Endocr Pract 2006;12:568–71.

46. Kansagara DL, Tetrault J, Hamill C, et al. Fatal factitious Cushing's syndrome and invasive aspergillosis: case report and review of literature. Endocr Pract 2006;12: 651–5.

47. Heilbronner RL, Sweet JJ, Morgan JE, et al. American Academy of Clinical Neuropsychology Consensus Conference Statement on the neuropsychological assessment of effort, response bias, and malingering. Clin Neuropsychol 2009;23:1093–129.

48. Slick DJ, Sherman EM, Iverson GL. Diagnostic criteria for malingered neurocognitive dysfunction: proposed standards for clinical practice and research. Clin Neuropsychol 1999;13:545–61.

49. Iverson GL, Binder LM. Detecting exaggeration and malingering in neuroopsychological assessment. J Head Trauma Rehabil 2000;15:829–58.

50. Lezak M, Howieson D, Loring D, et al. Neuropsychological assessment: testing for response bias and incomplete effort. Oxford: Oxford University Press; 2004.

51. Bianchini KJ, Mathias CW, Greve KW. Symptom validity testing: a critical review. Clin Neuropsychol 2001;5:19–45.

52. Smith GP, Burger GK. Detection of malingering: validation of the Structured Inventory of Malingered Symptomatology (SIMS). J Am Acad Psychiatry Law 1997;25:183–9.

53. Rogers R, Payne JW, Berry DT, et al. Use of the SIRS in compensation cases: an examination of its validity and generalizability. Law Hum Behav 2009;33:213–24.

54. Axelrod BN, Barlow A, Paradee C. Evaluation of the WMS-III Rarely Missed Index in a naive clinical sample. Clin Neuropsychol 2010;24:95–102.

55. Larrabee GJ. Malingering scales for the Continuous Recognition Memory Test and the Continuous Visual Memory Test. Clin Neuropsychol 2009;23:167–80.

56. Vickery CD, Berry DT, Dearth CS, et al. Head injury and the ability to feign neuropsychological deficits. Arch Clin Neuropsychol 2004;19:37–48.

57. Loo Booksh R, Pella RD, Singh AN, et al. Ability of college students to simulate ADHD on objective measures of attention. J Atten Disord 2010;13:325–38.

58. Merckelbach H, Peters M, Jelicic M, et al. Detecting malingering of Ganser-like symptoms with tests: a case study. Psychiatry Clin Neurosci 2006;60:636–8.

59. Baity MR, Siefert CJ, Chambers A, et al. Deceptiveness on the PAI: a study of naïve faking with psychiatric inpatients. J Pers Assess 2007;88:16–24.

60. Hawes SW, Boccaccini MT. Detection of overreporting of psychopathology on the Personality Assessment Inventory: a meta-analytic review. Psychol Assess 2009;21:112–24.

61. Cashel ML, Rogers R, Sewell K, et al. The Personality Assessment Inventory (PAI) and the Detection of Defensiveness. Assessment 1995;2:333–42.

62. Rogers R, Sewell KW, Morey LC, et al. Detection of feigned mental disorders on the Personality Assessment Inventory: a discriminant analysis. J Pers Assess 1996;67:629–40.

63. Meyers JE, Millis SR, Volkert K. A validity index for the MMPI-2. Arch Clin Neuropsychol 2002;17:157–69.

64. Aguerrevere LE, Greve KW, Bianchini KJ, et al. Detecting malingering in traumatic brain injury and chronic pain with an abbreviated version of the Meyers Index for the MMPI-2. Arch Clin Neuropsychol 2008;23:831–8.

65. Lees-Haley PR. Efficacy of MMPI-2 validity scales and MCMI-II modifier scales for detecting spurious PTSD claims: F, F-K, Fake Bad Scale, ego strength, subtle-obvious subscales, DIS, and DEB. J Clin Psychol 1992;48:681–9.

66. Jasinski LJ, Berry DT, Shandera AL, et al. Use of the Wechsler Adult Intelligence Scale Digit Span subtest for malingering detection: a meta-analytic review. J Clin Exp Neuropsychol 2011;33:300–14.

67. Greve KW, Bianchini KJ, Etherton JL, et al. The Reliable Digit Span test in chronic pain: classification accuracy in detecting malingered pain-related disability. Clin Neuropsychol 2010;24:137–52.

68. Gray MJ, Elhai JD, Briere J. Evaluation of the Atypical Response scale of the Trauma Symptom Inventory-2 in detecting simulated posttraumatic stress disorder. J Anxiety Disord 2010;24:447–51.

69. Clegg C, Fremouw W, Mogge N. Utility of the Structured Inventory Malingered Symptomatology (SIMS) and the Assessment of Depression Inventory (ADI) in

screening for malingering among outpatients seeking to claim disability. J Forensic Psychiatry Psychol 2009;20:239–54.

70. Edens JF, Poythress NG, Watkins-Clay MM. Detection of malingering in psychiatric unit and general population prison inmates: a comparison of the PAI, SIMS, and SIRS. J Pers Assess 2007;88:33–42.

71. Heinze MC, Purisch AD. Beneath the mask: Use of psychological tests to detect and subtype malingering in criminal defendents. J Forensic Psychol Practice 2001;1:23–52.

72. Lewis JL, Simcox AL, Berry DTR. Screening for feigned psychiatric symptoms in a forensic sample by using the MMPI-2 and the Structured Inventory of Malingered Symptomatology. Psychol Assess 2002;14:170–6.

73. Vitacco MJ, Jackson RL, Rogers R, et al. Detection strategies for malingering with the Miller Forensic Assessment of Symptoms Test: a confirmatory factor analysis of its underlying dimensions. Assessment 2008;15:97–103.

74. Alwes YR, Clark JA, Berry DT, et al. Screening for feigning in a civil forensic setting. J Clin Exp Neuropsychol 2008;30:133–40.

75. Merckelbach H, Smith G. Diagnostic accuracy of the Structured Inventory of Malingered Symptomatology (SIMS) in detecting instructed malingering. Arch Clin Neuropsychol 2003;18:145–52.

76. Jelicic M, Peters MVJ, Leckie V, et al. Basic knowledge of psychopathology does not undermine the efficacy of the Structured Inventory of Malingered Symptamology (SIMS) to detect feigned psychosis. Neth J Psychol 2007;63:107–10.

77. Jelicic M, Merckelbach H, Candel I, et al. Detection of feigned cognitive dysfunction using special malinger tests: a stimulation study in naïve and coached malingerers. Int J Neurosci 2007;117:1185–92.

78. Green P, Iverson GL. Validation of the computerized assessment of response bias in litigating patients with head injuries. Clin Neuropsychol 2001;15:492–7.

79. Heinze M. The notion of subjectivity in psychopathology. Seishin Shinkeigaku Zasshi 2003;105:1026–36.

80. Miller HA. Examining the use of the M-FAST with criminal defendants incompetent to stand trial. Int J Offender Ther Comp Criminol 2004;48:268–80.

81. Spence SA, Hunter MD, Farrow TF, et al. A cognitive neurobiological account of deception: evidence from functional neuroimaging. Philos Trans R Soc Lond B Biol Sci 2004;359(1451):1755–62.

82. spence SA, Farrow TF, Hertford AE, et al. Behavioral and functional anatomical correlates of deception in humans. Neuroreport 2001;12:2849–53.

83. Langleben DD, Schroeder L, Maldjian JA, et al. Brain activity during simulated deception: an event-related functional magnetic resonance study. Neuroimage 2002;15:727–32.

84. Lee TM, Liu HL, Tan LH, et al. Lie detection by functional magnetic resonance imaging. Hum Brain Mapp 2002;15:157–64.

85. Ganis G, Kosslyn SM, Stose S, et al. Neural correlates of different types of deception: An fMRI investigation. Cerebral Cortex 2003;13:830–6.

86. Fellows LK, Farah MJ. Ventromedial frontal cortex mediates affective shifting in humans: evidence from a reversal learning paradigm. Brain 2003;126(Pt 8):1830–37.

87. Aron AR, Robbins TW, Poldrack RA. Inhibition and the right inferior frontal cortex. Trends Cogn Sci 2004;8:170–7.

88. Knoch D, Schneider F, Schunk D, et al. Disrupting the prefrontal cortex diminishes the human ability to build a good reputation. Proc Natl Acad Sci U S A 2009;106:20895–9.

89. Wertheimer M, King DB, Peckler MA, et al. Carl Jung and Max Wertheimer on a priority issue. J Hist Behav Sci 1992;28:45–56.

90. Vendemia JM, Buzan RF, Simon-Dack SL. Reaction time of motor responses in two-stimulus paradigms involving deception and congruity with varying levels of difficulty. Behav Neurol 2005;16:25–36.

91. Willison J, Tombaugh TN. Detecting simulation of attention deficits using reaction time tests. Arch Clin Neuropsychol 2006;21:41–52.

92. Browndyke JN, Paskavitz J, Sweet LH, et al. Neuroanatomical correlates of malingered memory impairment: event-related fMRI of deception on a recognition memory task. Brain Inj 2008;22:481–9.

93. Larsen JD, Allen MD, Bigler ED, et al. Different patterns of cerebral activation in genuine and malingered cognitive effort during performance on the Word Memory Test. Brain Inj 2010;24:89–99.

94. Garcia-Campayo J, Fayed N, Serrano-Blanco A, et al. Brain dysfunction behind functional symptoms: neuroimaging and somatoform, conversive, and dissociative disordes. Curr Opin Psychiatry 2009;22:224–31.

95. Stone J, Zeman A, Simonotto E, et al. FMRI in patients with motor conversion symptoms and controls with simulated weakness. Psychosom Med 2007;69:961–9.

96. Hallett M. Physiology of psychogenic movement disorders. J Clin Neurosci 2010; 17:959–65.

97. Gupta A, Lang AE. Psychogenic movement disorders. Curr Opin Neurol 2009;22: 430–6.

98. Seignourel PJ, Miller K, Kellinson I, et al. Abnormal affective startle modulation in individuals with psychogenic [corrected] movement disorder. Mov Disord 2007;22: 1265–71.

99. Liepert J, Hassa T, Tüscher O, et al. Electrophysiological correlates of motor conversion disorder. Mov Disord 2008;23:2171–76.

100. Kozel FA, Trivedi MH. Developing a neuropsychiatric functional brain imaging test. Neurocase 2008;14:54–8.

101. Ganis G, Rosenfeld JP, Meixner J, et al. Lying in the scanner: covert countermeasures disrupt deception detection by functional magnetic resonance imaging. Neuroimage 2011;55:312–9.

102. Ford CV, Abernathy V. Factitious illness: a multidisciplinary consideration of ethical issues. Gen Hosp Psychiatry 1981;3:329–36.

103. Meropol NJ, Ford CV, Zaner RM. Factitious illness: an exploration in ethics. Perspect Biol Med 1985;28:269–81.

104. Southall DP, Plunkett MC, Banks MW, et al. Covert video recordings of life-threatening child-abuse: lessons for child protection. Pediatrics 1997;100:735–60.

105. Hall DE, Eubanks L, Meyyazhagan LS, et al. Evaluation of covert video surveillance in the diagnosis of munchausen syndrome by proxy: lessons from 41 cases. Pediatrics 2000;105:1305–12.

106. Connelly R. Ethical issues in the use of covert video surveillance in the diagnosis of Munchausen syndrome by proxy: the Atlanta study:an ethical challenge for medicine. HEC Forum 2003;15:21–41.

107. David TA. Court OK's video cameras on suspected Munchausen victims. Nurs Law Regan Report 2009;49:1.

108. Lipsitt DR. The factitious patient who sues. Am J Psychiatry 1986;143:1482.

109. Eisendrath SJ, McNiel DE. Factitious disorders in civil litigation: twenty cases illustrating the spectrum of abnormal illness-affirming behavior. J Am Acad Psychiatry Law 2002;30:391–9.

110. Janofsky JS. The Munchausen syndrome in civil forensic psychiatry. Bull Am Acad Psychiatry Law 1994;22:489–97.

111. Eisendrath SJ, McNeil DE. Factitious physical disorders, litigation and mortality. Psychosomatics 2004;45:350–3.
112. Eisendrath SJ, Telischak KS. Factitious disorders: potential litigation risks for plastic surgeons. Ann Plast Surg 2008;60:64–9.
113. Van Dinter TG, Welch BJ. Diagnosis of Munchausen's syndrome by an electronic health record search. Am J Med 2009;122:e3.
114. DeWitt DE, Ward SA, Prabhu S, et al. Patient privacy versus protecting the patient and the health system from harm: a case study. Med J Aust 2009;191:213–6.
115. Robertson MD, Kerridge IH. Through a glass darkly: the clinical and ethical implications of Munchausen syndrome. Med J Aust 2009;191:217–9.
116. McFarland BH, Resnick M, Bloom JD. Ensuring continuity of care for a Munchausen patient through a public guardian. Hosp Community Psychiatry 1983;34:65–7.
117. Elmore JL. Munchausen syndrome: an endless search for self, managed by house arrest and mandated treatment. Ann Emerg Med 2005;45:561–3.
118. Waite S, Geddes A. Malingered psychosis leading to involuntary psychiatric hospitalization. Australas Psychiatry 2006;14:419–21.
119. Feldman MD, Bibby M. Virtual factitious disorders and Munchausen by proxy. West J Med 1998;168:537–9.
120. Feldman MD, Peychers MA. Legal issues surrounding the exposure of Munchausen by internet. Psychosomatics 2007;48:451–2.
121. Griffiths EJ, Kampa R, Pearce C, et al. Munchausen's syndrome by Google. Ann R Coll Surg Engl 2009;91:159–60.
122. Levenson JL, Chafe W, Flanagan P. Factitious ovarian cancer: feigning via resources on the internet. Psychosomatics 2007;48:71–3.
123. Caocci G, Pisu S, La Nasa G. A simulated case of chronic myeloid leukemia: the growing risk of Munchausen's syndrome by internet. Leuk Lymphoma 2008;49: 1826–8.
124. Rosenberg NM, Marino D. Frequency of suspected abuse/neglect in burn patients. Pediatr Emerg Care 1989;5:219–21.
125. Sullivan K, King J. Detecting faked psychopathology: a comparison of two tests to detect malingered psychopathology using a simulation design. Psychiatry Res 2010;176:75–81.
126. Wisdom NM, Callahan JL, Shaw TG. Diagnostic utility of the structured inventory of malingered symptomatology to detect malingering in a forensic sample. Arch Clin Neuropsychol 2010;25:118–25.
127. Gierok SD, Dickson AL, Cole JA. Performance of forensic and non-forensic adult psychiatric inpatients on the Test of Memory Malingering. Arch Clin Neuropsychol 2005;20:755–60.
128. Reznek L. The Rey 15-item memory test for malingering: a meta-analysis. Brain Inj 2005;19:539–43.
129. Beaber RJ, Marston A, Michelli J, et al. A brief test for measuring malingering in schizophrenic individuals. Am J Psychiatry 1985;142:1478–81.
130. Hankins GC, Barnard GW, Robbins L. The validity of the M test in a residential forensic facility. Bull Am Acad Psychiatry Law 1993;21:111–21.

Somatoform Disorders in Children and Adolescents

Mary Lynn Dell, MD, DMin[a,b,]*, John V. Campo, MD[c]

KEYWORDS

• Childhood mental disorders • Somatoform • Diagnosis
• Management

INTRODUCTION

Most review articles and book chapters covering somatoform disorders in children and adolescents begin similarly to those addressing adult somatoform illness, and with good reason.[1–5] The basic definitions and principles underlying these disorders apply, for the most part, to both children and adults. Medical practice in industrialized Western countries has evolved in cultures that view mind and body as separate, or at best incompletely integrated, aspects of individuals. *Physical illness* – essentially the subjective suffering and impairment of the affected individual – is viewed within the biomedical model as resulting from demonstrable physical and/or biochemical insults to the human body at the intracellular, intercellular, organ, organ system, or at gross anatomical levels called *disease*. A parallel system has developed to conceptualize *mental illness,* with its own systems of diagnosis, treatment, coding, reimbursement, and care.[6] Inherent to this dualistic view of physical and emotional or psychological illnesses, the notion has developed that maladies associated with demonstrable physiological insults or pathologies are both "real" and "legitimate," whereas those appearing to lack a definitive etiology are somehow contrived and thus "illegitimate," reflecting weakness of character or moral stature. Over time, the terms "hysterical" and "psychogenic" have given way to the currently less pejorative descriptors "functional" and "psychosomatic."[7] The term *somatization* now refers to an individual's subjective experience and description of physical symptoms for which clearly demonstrable physical pathology or injury does not exist or is not diagnosable by standard-of-care assessment procedures and techniques; the term may also be applied when the level of distress or disability is judged to be greater than what is

[a] Division of Child and Adolescent Psychiatry, University Hospitals Case Medical Center, 10524 Euclid Avenue, W.O. Walker Building, Suite 1155A, Cleveland, OH 44106, USA
[b] Child and Adolescent Psychiatry Consultation Liaison Service, Rainbow Babies and Children's Hospital, Cleveland, OH, USA
[c] Department of Psychiatry, Ohio State University and Nationwide Children's Hospital, Columbus, OH
* Corresponding author. Division of Child and Adolescent Psychiatry, University Hospitals Case Medical Center, 10524 Euclid Avenue, W.O. Walker Building, Suite 1155A, Cleveland, OH 44106.
E-mail address: Mary.Dell@UHhospitals.org

Psychiatr Clin N Am 34 (2011) 643–660
doi:10.1016/j.psc.2011.05.012
0193-953X/11/$ – see front matter © 2011 Elsevier Inc. All rights reserved.

typically associated with the clinical findings.[8,9] Somatization in children and adolescents is associated with functional impairment, iatrogenic injuries, and unnecessarily high health care expenditures.[10,11]

CHILD AND ADOLESCENT SOMATOFORM DISORDERS IN DSM-IV-TR

The DSM category of somatoform disorders is applicable to both adult and child populations. Existing diagnostic criteria permit no adjustments in number, quality, or duration of symptoms necessary for diagnosis in children. The essential feature of the seven DSM-IV-TR somatoform disorders, summarized below, is the presence of physical symptoms that are the focus of concern, but are not fully explained by a general medical condition, another psychiatric disorder, or a cause and effect relationship to a particular substance. In addition, symptoms must lead to noticeable and significant distress or impairment in social (family, friends) and occupational spheres of functioning, which for children primarily means school and academic difficulties. A somatoform disorder may be diagnosed if a general medical condition is present providing that the associated physical pathology does not appear to fully explain the nature or severity of associated symptoms or impairment. Similarly, somatoform disorders must be distinguished from other DSM diagnoses associated with the presence of a general medical condition. For example, the diagnosis of *Psychological Factors Affecting Medical Condition* is applicable in situations in which there is definite medical illness that has been diagnosed and its symptom expressions are exacerbated by associated psychosocial factors and stressors. In *Factitious Disorder with Predominantly Physical Signs and Symptoms*, physical symptoms are produced intentionally by the child or adolescent in order to assume the role of a medically ill patient; the motivation is internal psychological gain. Factitious Disorder by Proxy is diagnosed when a caregiver, typically a child's biological mother, intentionally reports erroneous medical history, fabricates signs and symptoms, or directly produces illness in the child presumably in pursuit of perceived psychological benefits associated with parenting an ill child. In *Malingering*, listed in DSM-IV-TR as a V Code (ie, a condition that may be a focus of clinical attention), the intentional reporting, simulation, or production of a medical symptom is motivated by an external incentive. Examples of incentives for adults may include avoiding military or financial obligations. Children and adolescents may feign illness deliberately to avoid school, to avoid or escape the juvenile justice system, or to obtain prescription drugs, such as opiate pain medications.[12]

Somatization Disorder

This is the descendant of *hysteria*, also known historically as *Briquet's syndrome* in honor of the French psychiatrist Pierre Briquet, credited with its description in the mid-nineteenth century.[13] Chronic in nature, symptoms must begin before age 30, and result in medical help seeking, with associated significant impairment in social and occupational functioning. Though required symptoms were honed for DSM-IV-TR, the symptom list is still substantial: pain symptoms involving at least four sites or four bodily functions; one neurological and two gastrointestinal complaints other than pain; and one sexual or reproductive symptom other than pain, such as erectile dysfunction in males or irregular menses in females. The lifetime prevalence of the disorder is estimated to be 0.2–2.0% in adult women but less than 0.2% in adult men. Family members who model somatic symptoms and childhood histories of sexual abuse are often reported by adults with the disorder. Though multiple somatic complaints without demonstrable illness or tissue damage have been estimated in 4–11% of adolescents,[14] very few school-age children have been found to meet full diagnostic criteria.[15] The relatively low rate of diagnosis in the pediatric population may be due to the multiple symptoms required for diagnosis and the need for at least one sexual or reproductive symptom.[16,17] Children of parents with somatization disorder are more susceptible to developing the disorder than those with no family history.[18,19]

Undifferentiated Somatoform Disorder

This is the somatoform diagnosis applied in the presence of medically unexplained physical complaints across multiple body sites and/or non-pain symptoms such as fatigue, urinary, and gastrointestinal symptoms in the absence of full diagnostic criteria for Somatization Disorder being met. The complaints with resulting impairment of social and occupational/academic functioning must be present for a minimum of six months; there are no parameters named for age of onset.[12] Neurasthenia, a malady consisting of fatigue and at least two other neuromuscular symptoms, is commonly cited as the prototypical illness in this category.[3,20] Undifferentiated somatoform disorder is the DSM-IV-TR diagnosis most commonly applied in the case of children and adolescents who manifest multiple *medically unexplained symptoms*, likely due to the relatively narrow diagnostic criteria for somatization disorder.[3]

Conversion Disorder

Conversion disorder, though appearing to be relatively common in tertiary medical centers and neurology clinics, is relatively rare in the general population of children and adolescents. It may nevertheless be the most common somatoform disorder in children and adolescents in some non-Western cultures such as India.[4] A diagnosis of conversion disorder is made when there are one or more symptoms or deficits neurological functioning, typically representing deficits of voluntary motor or sensory functioning. The clinical picture presents similarly to a neurological disorder or another general medical condition, and conversion symptoms have been described in the past as "pseudoneurologic". A psychological stressor or conflict is often identified that preceded the beginning or the exacerbation of the symptoms or the inconsistent physical findings. Unlike in factitious disorders or malingering, the patient does not appear to perceive any voluntary sense of control over the symptom or deficit. The symptoms are not limited to pain or sexual concerns and cause significant functional impairment. DSM-IV-TR specifies four types, including: (1) with motor symptom or deficit; (2) with sensory symptom or deficit; (3) with seizures or convulsions; and (4) with mixed presentation.[12] Motor symptoms may include gait disturbances, weakness, tremors or shaking, jerking, and other abnormal motor movements. Common sensory expressions include numbness and paresthesias in the extremities, typically inconsistent with dermatomal patterns, and deafness, blindness, and other vision and hearing issues. Seizure-like events, or non-epileptic seizures, may be difficult to differentiate from genuine epileptic events, with 5–37% of initial seizure work-ups by neurologists deemed to be non-epileptiform in nature.[21]

Conversion disorders have traditionally been understood from the psychodynamic perspective. In order to suppress or keep a conflict, distressing thought, emotion, or event from consciousness, it has been posited that the mind translates, or "converts," the disturbing thought or conflict into a physical expression or symptom.[22] Primary gain refers to the presumably intrapsychic gain associated with the symptom (ie, psychological distress is minimized when the conflict is expressed as a physical or sensory symptom). Secondary gain refers to the interpersonal or social reinforcement of a symptom, as in the attention and concern elicited from others or the ability to avoid unpleasant tasks or activities and school work. Such interpersonal reinforcers may promote or maintain symptom expression and make management more difficult. Parents and medical professionals may be more concerned about the presentation than the child. This placid reaction on the part of the patient, termed *la belle indifference*, has been considered in the past to be consistent with, but not necessarily diagnostic of, a conversion disorder.[23]

Pain Disorder

Pain and pediatric mental health have a complex relationship. Pain may be acute, chronic, intermittent, constant, and have many perceived qualities, such as sharp, stabbing, dull, burning, or achy. Numerous acute and chronic pediatric injuries and illnesses can damage tissues, or stimulate the release of chemicals that stimulate pain receptors and nerve fibers involved in pain processes. The inclusion of Pain Disorder in DSM-IV-TR is a reminder that emotional or psychiatric factors may be of significance in the onset, type, severity, and continuance of pain, especially when the pain itself leads to functional impairment. Individuals suffering from pain disorder seek clinical attention for the pain, which interferes with healthy functioning, and is not due to another primary Axis I disorder; psychological considerations often appear to be important in the initiation, severity, and maintenance of the pain. Three subtypes of pain disorder are described, including pain associated with psychological factors, pain associated with a general medical condition, and pain associated with both psychological factors and a general medical condition. If present, the general medical condition is coded on Axis III. Clinicians are asked to specify whether the condition is acute (ie, less than six months in duration), or chronic in nature, having lasted more than six months.[12] Although there is a burgeoning interest in multidisciplinary approaches to the recognition, alleviation, and management of pediatric pain,[24] scant literature is available regarding the use of the DSM-IV-TR pain disorder diagnosis in children and adolescents.

Hypochondriasis

This disorder exists when an individual believes or fears he or she has a serious medical illness and the belief is based in a misinterpretation or misunderstanding of physical symptoms. Though the beliefs are not delusional, they are severe enough to cause appreciable distress and functional impairment for at least six months.[12] Little data is available on hypochondriasis as a circumscribed diagnostic entity in children and adolescents, consistent with observations that hypochondriasis is relatively unusual in youth and appears to be more common in early to middle adulthood. There is some evidence to suggest that adolescent preoccupation with acquiring illnesses such as cancer or AIDS constitute minor or subclinical forms of hypochondriasis in teens.[25] Hypochondriacal individuals often seek out the sick role, see numerous medical providers, and are at risk for complications, even iatrogenic harms, from diagnostic and surgical procedures. Hypochondriasis has been associated with comorbid anxiety disorders, especially obsessive compulsive disorder.[26–28]

Body Dysmorphic Disorder

Individuals suffering from body dysmorphic disorder (BDD) are preoccupied with an imagined defect or flaw in their appearance. In cases where a slight physical blemish or abnormality does exist, the person's concern or distress is extreme and out of proportion. The preoccupation leads to distress and impairment in social, occupational, or other spheres of functioning, and cannot be explained by another Axis I disorder, such as an eating disorder.[12] Some experts argue that BDD should be classified as a subtype of obsessive-compulsive disorder.[29,30] Other common co-morbidities during the lifetimes of affected individuals include major depressive disorder, social phobias, substance use disorders, and personality disorders, especially avoidant personality disorder. BDD patients may have higher suicide rates than non-affected individuals, and until recently, the likelihood of childhood physical, sexual, and emotional abuse and neglect may have been under-appreciated.[31–35] Prevalence estimates range from 5% to 9% in various adult dermatology and cosmetic surgery populations.[36–38]

Literature on BDD in the pediatric population remains limited, though more plentiful than for some other somatoform disorders. Isolated case reports of adolescent BDD were the rule until a relatively recent case series was published in which patients under the age of 18 years comprised 10% of the sample.[39,40] Adolescents are particularly susceptible to preoccupations about the skin, especially acne lesions and scars on the face. Compulsive picking and self-mutilation, in efforts to rid or fix the flaws, are common, even employing knives and other implements to surgically correct perceived deformities or imperfections themselves. Parents may report that affected children need significant reassurance that they look all right, and spend great amounts of time in the bathroom in front of the mirror, dressing, or in other activities directed at repairing or hiding the offending flaw. As they become older, adolescents may seek out increasingly expensive and potentially risky medical and surgical treatments, with or without parental knowledge and approval. BDD is typically a chronic condition. Clinicians should have a high index of suspicion when encountering somatically preoccupied youth, particularly those seeking cosmetic treatments and surgery, so that the condition can be managed and the young person experience minimal harm.

Somatoform Disorder, Not Otherwise Specified

This last category is employed when somatoform complaints and impairment are present and of concern, but specific diagnostic criteria are not met for one of the DSM-IV-TR somatoform disorders already discussed. An example might be hypochondriacal worries and preoccupations of less than 6 months duration.[12]

MEDICALLY UNEXPLAINED SYMPTOMS: THE CLINICAL REALITY

As helpful as an organized diagnostic system such as the DSM-IV-TR is, pediatric somatoform symptoms and disorders defy many of our profession's most methodologically rigorous, evidence-based efforts at reliable description, diagnosis, and categorization. Somatic symptoms such as pain and fatigue are present in a variety of disorders, some classified as general medical conditions and others as mental disorders, essentially cutting across a variety of clinical situations and existing diagnostic categories. As mentioned previously, somatic symptoms and complaints in pediatric populations are difficult to assess. There are few population-based studies in this area, and few structured or standardized assessments in either the research or clinical arenas. Even when thorough histories and medical work-ups are completed with fully cooperative children and their parents, reviews of symptoms, their development, and degree of functional impairment often are not a "good fit" with the diagnostic criteria for the more specific somatoform disorder diagnoses in the DSM. Quite often the default diagnoses are undifferentiated somatoform disorder and somatoform disorder, not otherwise specified.[25,41,42] Therefore, the term *medically unexplained symptoms (MUS)* often describes the real-life clinical scenarios children and adolescents present to their medical care providers. Indeed, somatic complaints are common in community and general pediatric clinic surveys, with approximately half of all preschool and school aged children reporting a minimum of one physical complaint in the two weeks before queried, and close to 15% of youth in that same age group reporting a minimum of four symptoms during the same time frame.[15,43,44] Eleven percent of 12–16-year-old girls and 4% of same-aged boys participating in the Ontario Child Health Study reported bothersome, recurrent physical symptoms.[14] Other studies have confirmed multiple and recurrent somatic complaints in as many as 15% of adolescents surveyed.[10,45] In addition, 2% to 20% of children presenting to medical care providers report symptoms for which no physical etiology can be found.[46]

Common specific complaints in community samples of children and adolescents include, but are not limited to, headache, abdominal pain, fatigue, nausea and gastrointestinal symptoms other than pain, muscle soreness, back pain, blurry vision, and food intolerance.[4,15]

Headache

Weekly headaches are reported by approximately 10% to 30% of children and adolescents, and account for 1% to 2% of outpatient pediatric visits.[44,47–49] *Migraine headaches* are characterized by a pulsating quality, unilateral location, and severe pain, may involve photophobia, nausea, vomiting, and may be made worse by physical movement. A migraine headache may be preceded by an aura, visual scotoma, numbness, tingling, dysphasia, and transient motor weakness. Episodes must last at least one hour to receive the diagnosis of migraine headaches. In contrast, *tension type headaches* tend to be bilateral, chronic or episodic, non-pulsatile, mild to moderate in severity, and not exacerbated by physical activity.[50]

Gastrointestinal Issues

Functional abdominal pain is the most common type of medically unexplained pain in preschool children,[43] carries a prevalence of 7% to 25% in school aged children,[51–53] and constitutes 2% to 4% of pediatric visits.[54] Apley's original description of the syndrome of *recurrent abdominal pain* required three episodes of abdominal pain occurring over at least a three-month period that are serious enough to affect the activities and functioning of the child.[52,53] The gender ratio is equal until puberty, when the disorder becomes more common in females than males.[49,52] The episodes of abdominal pain are not typically accompanied by laboratory, radiographic, structural, or infectious manifestation.[55,56] Other gastrointestinal symptoms include nausea, vomiting, diarrhea, and bloating. *Irritable bowel syndrome* is perhaps the best known functional gastrointestinal disorder, and is essentially characterized by functional abdominal pain associated with relief with defecation and/or changes in the frequency or consistency of bowel movements.[57] *Cyclical vomiting syndrome* consists of stereotyped, recurrent episodes of vomiting that may lead to dehydration and other medical complications. These bouts of vomiting may be related to migraines.[58] Gastroenterologists have developed specific diagnostic criteria for pediatric functional gastrointestinal disorders, such as change in stool frequency, change in bowel character, and pain that is improved or relieved after defecation.

Fatigue

Fatigue is common in childhood, with close to 50% of adolescents reporting weekly and 15% reporting daily fatigue.[10,48,59] *Chronic fatigue syndrome* implies extreme fatigue lasting at least 6 months, plus musculoskeletal pain, sleep disturbance, and changes in concentration and short-term memory not accounted for by other medical or psychiatric conditions. Though chronic fatigue syndrome is receiving increased attention in lay circles, available studies suggest that the prevalence is less than 1% in adolescence.[59]

Other Medically Unexplained Symptoms and Entities

Children and adolescents also report and are diagnosed with other conditions familiar to pediatricians and child and adolescent psychiatrists even though there may be no accompanying demonstrable laboratory, radiographic, or physical findings. These include dyspnea, vocal cord dysfunction,[60] chest, back, and limb pain,[41] and complex regional pain syndrome (reflex sympathetic dystrophy).[61]

MEDICALLY UNEXPLAINED SYMPTOMS: ADDITIONAL CONSIDERATIONS
Genetics, Temperament, Family Factors

Children and adolescents with MUS are more likely than unaffected youth to have family members who report higher levels of somatic symptoms.[3,16,49] Recent evidence suggests a heritable genetic component, including polymorphisms in catecholamine-O-methyl transferase (COMT) with pain sensitivity,[62] the promoter region of the serotonin transporter gene associated with trait neuroticism and anxiety,[63,64] and in the gene coding for tryptophan hydroxylase that may influence somatic anxiety.[65]

Individuals with functional pain syndromes, anxiety and depression manifest greater neuroticism, harm avoidance, behavioral inhibition, and worry than unaffected peers.[66] From a family systems perspective, the child's MUS may enable the family to avoid conflict, especially dealing with parental marital issues. The child's symptoms may serve to communicate the family distress and need for help.[67–69] Children with MUS may have been exposed to parental illness, may have a family model for their illness or particular symptoms, and may be perceived to be medically vulnerable by their parents.[70–73]

Trauma and Life Events

Emotional, physical, and sexual abuse and neglect have been associated with MUS in childhood and adolescence, and with somatoform disorders in adulthood.[25,41,74]

Service Utilization

Children and adolescents with MUS historically have been managed by their primary care physicians with reassurance, education, frequent follow-up visits. While that approach may be beneficial for some patients, particularly lesser-affected individuals and their families, these youth may experience significant functional limitations, especially academically and socially. They are at risk of enduring unnecessary evaluations and/or risky and costly treatments, as well as seeing many physicians and having dispersed care with little to no continuity over time.[11,25,41,44,59,66,75]

ASSESSMENT OF MUS AND SOMATOFORM DISORDERS IN CHILDREN AND ADOLESCENTS

Though assessment must be flexible and individualized according to the particular child, family, context, and experience and resources of the medical team, some general principles are helpful to keep in mind in every situation. First of all, clinicians must approach the care of these patients and families with discipline and humility. Both qualities are necessary lest important questions be unasked or answers misunderstood and nuances unappreciated, or an actual, new, or rare medical finding be missed. Children may come to attention in pain, frightened, and vulnerable. Parents may be very worried, exhausted, frustrated, angry, and feel that their care of their child and their parenting skills are being judged. Both may be fearful about a life-threatening diagnosis. They may feel dismissed or not taken seriously by previous physicians.

Typically, the primary care physician conducts a medical work-up long before the child is referred to psychiatry. This work-up, which often merges into many subsequent appointments that blend both ongoing evaluation and various treatments, includes a medical history, physical examination, and appropriate laboratory, imaging, and other diagnostic testing determined to yield potentially helpful information for diagnosis and treatment.[76] Clinicians may struggle to find the balance between coordinating a thorough work-up without exposing the patient to harm or perpetuating a conviction that a somatoform symptom or disorder is caused by a discernible physical problem or disease.

Clinicians are wise to consider medical and psychiatric differential diagnoses applicable to any individual patient. Physical illnesses that may include or mimic common MUS include myopathies, HIV/AIDS, acute intermittent porphyria, various infections, Guillain-Barré syndrome, thyroid or parathyroid disease, migraines, multiple sclerosis, myasthenia gravis, systemic lupus erythematosis, cardiac arrhythmias, autonomic dysfunction, and seizures.[77]

Fundamentally, clinicians performing the psychiatric assessment of children with MUS and their families must remember that the symptoms are real to the patient, cause very real functional impairment and suffering, and are not in the patients' voluntary control. While medical disorders should be identified and treated appropriately, somatoform disorders are not total diagnoses of exclusion because they are most often associated with other positive diagnostic features, and can sometimes be comorbid with demonstrable medical pathologies.[78] The psychiatrist should review all records and take a thorough medical history. Occasionally underlying physical disease is missed or develops independently of the MUS over time; in addition, the MUS themselves may change. A comprehensive psychiatric history should include information about the MUS, family medical and psychiatric histories, questions about anxiety and depressive symptoms, and the possibility of recent or past trauma, physical, and sexual abuse. Attention should be given to temperament, medical illnesses, and caregiver separations in early childhood, school and academic histories, peer relationships, and any clues or insights into possible secondary gains for the child with MUS. Interviewers should be alert to and inquire about symptom models in family members and significant others in the child's life.[3,31] Of several assessment instruments, available literature cites two scales as being particularly helpful. The Children's Somatization Inventory is a 35-item self report measure with parent and child versions. It can be used with children 7 years and older, and its subscales of pseudoneurological, cardiovascular, gastrointestinal, and pain/weakness symptoms are akin to somatization disorder symptom categories.[2,75] The Functional Disability Inventory is a 15-item scale emphasizing the past two weeks and includes attention to school attendance.[2,79]

TREATMENT AND MANAGEMENT OF SOMATIZATION DISORDERS AND MEDICALLY UNEXPLAINED SYMPTOMS IN PEDIATRIC PATIENT POPULATIONS

The long term outcomes of pediatric psychosomatic symptoms and disorders run the gamut from transient conversion symptoms lasting a few days never to recur, to estimates that 25–50% of children with recurrent abdominal pain will continue to be symptomatic as adults, to the chronic and relentless courses of the unusual youths who meet full DSM-IV-TR diagnostic criteria for hypochondriasis or BDD.[2,56,74,80-83] Given the unpredictability and the tendency for medically unexplained symptoms to recur, even if concerns do not rise to the level of a discrete disorder, it is important that all contacts with care providers be empathic, honest, consistent, and incorporate multidisciplinary treatment modalities.[2]

Existing management approaches are based primarily on accumulated clinical experience, as there is a relative lack of evidence based treatment literature addressing pediatric somatoform complaints and disorders. Affected children and adolescents often present with complex medical and psychiatric issues, often experienced over long time periods, and may require multiple types of care from several health care professionals.[2] Elements of a practical management model for pediatric somatization include:

1. **Be Honest and Direct.** Emphasize collaboration between patient, family, and caregivers, identify shared goals, and focus on improved functioning instead of a complete cure or permanent remission of symptoms.

2. **Reassurance.** Reassuring children and their families that the MUS are not fatal or associated with tissue damage should be accomplished early on, but may not relieve anxiety and worry completely. Clinicians need to address anxiety and fears about the symptoms directly.

3. **Cognitive-behavioral interventions.** Studies have accrued in the past twenty years that demonstrate benefits of cognitive-behavioral therapy (CBT) for pediatric patients suffering from psychosomatic disorders. CBT as part of a multidisciplinary treatment plan has demonstrated success in the treatment of recurrent abdominal pain.[84-86] Specifically, pain complaints, school absences, and health services utilizations have been have been targeted by CBT. Additional studies are needed to demonstrate the efficacy and effectiveness of CBT, as well as the outcomes associated with combining CBT and other treatment modalities.

4. **Rehabilitative Approach.** This group of strategies emphasizes coping with one's symptoms and minimizing sick-role behaviors, even if the child's symptoms and disabilities have not fully remitted. Coping and overcoming difficult challenges with problem-focused strategies become treatment goals in and of themselves, shifting the focus away from cure to successful functioning and from vulnerability to setting personal goals. Treatment of conversion disorder fits very well with this approach, especially when additional treatments such as physical therapy are employed.[67,73,87]

5. **Behavioral and operant interventions.** The goals of these approaches are to reinforce the child for healthy behaviors and decrease reinforcements/incentives for maladaptive behaviors inherent to somatization. The treatment team works with the child and significant adults to minimize secondary gains from the pain or illness behaviors. Parent training is essential, given that parents of somatic children are often inherently anxious themselves and unwittingly reward or reinforce illness behaviors at relatively high rates. These approaches have shown promise in treating youth with conversion symptoms and headache.[25,41,88,89]

6. **Self-Management and Other Individual Strategies.** Biofeedback, hypnosis, and relaxation techniques can be effective treatments in somatoform disorders.[90-96] Imagery and relaxation have assisted in treatment of nausea, headaches, and back pain, and have the added advantage that patients can be taught to self-administer treatment as indicated.[97-100] Hypnosis has been reported to be effective for some pediatric patients with MUS.[22,101]

7. **Family and Group Interventions.** Family therapy may assist parents, siblings, and other family members in seeing and relating to the patient with MUS as vulnerable and chronically or severely ill. Gradually, the family may be enlisted in reinforcing desired wellness attitudes and behaviors, and coping with any residual impairments. Addressing other family conflicts and issues may be helpful for all members, as well as alleviating conflicts that may have contributed to the expression of MUS in the first place.[69,86,102–106] Group therapy for the treatment of pediatric somatoform disorders has not been studied rigorously, despite significant interest over the years.

8. **Communication.** Early and regular communication with other professionals involved in a child's life is essential to good functional outcomes. The treating psychiatrist should maintain open lines of communication with primary care physicians, nurses, and other specialists involved in the assessment and care of youth with MUS.[107–109] Close working relationships with school officials can strengthen coping and rehabilitative efforts, minimize school absenteeism, and help keep medical professionals, families, and the school working in a consistent fashion with the patient toward mutually common goals.[11]

9. **Aggressive Treatment of Comorbid Psychiatric Problems.** As already stated, somatization is strongly associated with comorbid Axis I disorders, particularly emotional disorders such as anxiety and depression.[11,25,41] Psychiatrists provide a crucial service to patients by monitoring vigilantly for these comorbidities, and recommending pharmacotherapy when indicated, as described below.

10. **Consider Psychopharmacologic Interventions.** Methodologically rigorous clinical trials of psychotropic medications in the treatment of pediatric somatoform disorders and MUS have not been accomplished to date. However, clinical experience, case series, and evidence extrapolated from adult studies attest that psychopharmacology can be helpful for these conditions, especially when accompanied by comorbid Axis I internalizing disorders such as anxiety and depression, and in cases of unexplained pain, gastrointestinal symptoms, and fatigue.

Antidepressants appear to be helpful for adults with somatoform disorders and MUS,[110,111] including those with functional pain syndromes such as headache, fibromyalgia, and irritable bowel syndrome.[112–115] The complex roles serotonin plays in anxiety and depression, as well as in the gut and pain pathways, suggests that the use of relevant antidepressants might be worthy of consideration in functional pain syndromes.[66,116,117] In an open study of citalopram for pediatric functional abdominal pain, significant improvement was noted in patient, parent and clinician ratings of abdominal pain, anxiety, and depression.[66] Pediatric gastroenterologists and general pediatricians who treat functional abdominal pain commonly follow adult experience and prescribe low dose tricyclic antidepressants for functional abdominal pain,[118] though it remains unclear if this approach will be proven to be efficacious and safe over time.

The selective serotonin reuptake inhibitor (SSRI) fluoxetine and the serotonergic tricyclic antidepressant clomipramine have been successful in the treatment of BDD in adults.[119,120] Reports indicate that serotonergic antidepressants can also be effective for adolescent body BDD, though no randomized clinical trials have been accomplished in pediatric populations.[121,122]

Acetaminophen, ibuprofen, the serotonin receptor agonists such as sumatriptan have been shown to be effective for pediatric migraines.[123] Intravenous prochlorperazine also holds promise.[124] Numerous medications have been studied for potential pediatric headache prophylaxis, including cyproheptadine, the beta-blocker propranolol, the antidepressants amitriptyline and trazodone, and the anticonvulsants divalproex sodium, topiramate, and levetiracetam.[123,125] While adult studies suggest that the selective serotonin-norepinephrine reuptake inhibitors venlafaxine and duloxetine are effective for functional pain and other somatic symptoms, these agents have not been adequately studied in pediatric populations.[126,127]

The long acting benzodiazepine clonazepam and the shorter acting lorazepam demonstrate clinical utility in somatoform disorder patients with significant anxiety components. These may be used in a time-limited manner, as a way to provide more immediate anxiety relief than can be accomplished by other agents, or as a psychopharmacologic bridge until SSRIs, for instance, can achieve therapeutic efficacy.[2,128]

Of course, complete informed consent for medication management must be obtained, including potential risks, benefits, and treatment alternatives for all medications. In addition, parents should be informed about the black box warnings for the increased risk of suicide in individuals under the age of 24 years treated with antidepressants, as well as the fact that no psychotropic medications are approved by the US Food and Drug Administration specifically for somatoform disorders or MUS. Medications requiring additional study include the role of psychotropics in the treatment of pediatric chronic fatigue syndrome, as well as the use of drugs such as buspirone and antipsychotics for anxiety and symptoms such as nausea and vomiting associated with somatoform disorders and MUS.[128]

11. *Monitor Outcome.* Patients and their families need to know that all domains of their lives are important and should be assessed for improved functioning, including home, interpersonal relationships, academic and social functioning at school, and use of health care services. In addition, many must be reassured that their physical conditions will be reassessed periodically for objective signs of disease, and if physiological findings come to light, they will receive adequate care and not be abandoned by their providers.[2]

TOWARD DSM-V

The categorical approach to psychiatric diagnosis used in the existing Diagnostic and Statistical Manual of Mental Disorders, 4th edition (DSM-IV), assumes discontinuity between normality and pathology, and has generated considerable dissatisfaction among both clinicians and researchers.[129] Few diagnostic categories in the DSM-IV have been associated with greater dissatisfaction than that of the somatoform disorders. Medically unexplained or "functional" somatic symptoms cut across several diagnostic categories in current psychiatric nosology beyond the somatoform disorders, most notably mood and anxiety disorders. In addition to the existence of "cross-cutting symptoms," specific challenges to the categorical approach championed in the DSM-IV include high observed rates of "comorbidity" across different disorders, the frequent use of "not otherwise specified" designations for patients who fail to meet full criteria within a category, and the lack of explanatory pathophysiology unique to a specific disorder or diagnosis. Because of these perceived limitations, consideration is now being given to combining dimensional assessments with the existing categorical approach in the DSM-V.

The DSM-V will likely drop the somatoform disorder category, but will include a category known as Somatic Symptoms Disorders and characterized by somatic symptoms or complaints associated with distress and/or dysfunction. Effort has been made to develop DSM-V diagnostic criteria that evidence an appreciation of developmental and lifespan considerations. Three new diagnoses under consideration for inclusion for DSM V are especially relevant to the existing category of somatoform disorders. The diagnosis of *Complex somatic symptom disorder (CSSD)* will require: (1) the presence of one or more somatic symptom(s) that are distressing and/or result in significant disruption of daily life; (2) excessive thoughts, feelings, and behaviors related to the somatic symptoms (including health anxiety); and (3) chronicity, with symptom duration of at least six months. The CSSD diagnosis will likely simplify the diagnostic approach currently applied in the DSM-IV to children and adolescents with multiple somatic symptoms. CSSD would be applied as a diagnosis to those patients currently categorized as suffering from somatization disorder, undifferentiated somatoform disorder, pain disorder, and hypochondriasis.[130] Another proposed DSM-V diagnosis of interest to pediatric workers is *Simple (or Abridged) Somatic Symptom Disorder*, which will likely prove useful in situations where a single somatic symptom of only one month duration causes distress or impairment that brings the youth to professional attention. A third diagnosis with anticipated benefits for child and adolescent psychosomatic medicine is *Illness Anxiety Disorder.* Though related to the DSM-IV-TR hypochondriasis designation, this category recognizes that children and adolescents can suffer significant disruption in normal functioning due to pronounced worry and anxiety about having or acquiring an illness, even if somatic symptoms are mild or not even present.

REFERENCES

1. Abbey SE, Wulsin L, Levinson JL. Somatization and somatoform disorders. In: Levinson JL, editor. Textbook of psychosomatic medicine: psychiatric care of the medically ill. 2nd edition. Arlington (VA): American Psychiatric Publishing, Inc.; 2011. p. 261–89.
2. Campo JV, Fritz G. A management model for pediatric somatization. Psychosomatics 2001;42:467–76.
3. Campo JV, Fritz GK. Somatoform disorders. In: Martin A, Volkmar FR, editors. Lewis's child and adolescent psychiatry: a comprehensive textbook. 4th edition. Philadelphia (PA): Lippincott Williams and Wilkins; 2007. p . 633–47.
4. DeMaso DR, Beasley PJ. The somatoform disorders. In: Klykylo WM, Kay JL, editors. Clinical child psychiatry. 2nd edition. West Sussex (UK): Wiley; 2005. p. 471–86.
5. Folks DG, Feldman MD, Ford CV. Somatoform disorders, factitious disorders, and malingering. In: Stoudemire A, Fogel BS, Greenberg DB, editors. Psychiatric care of the medical patient. 2nd edition. New York: Oxford University Press; 2000. p. 459–75.
6. Fabrega H Jr. The concept of somatization as a cultural and historical product of western medicine. Psychosom Med 1990;52:653–72.
7. Parsons T. Social structure and personality. New York: Free Press; 1964.
8. Kellner R. Psychosomatic syndromes and somatic symptoms. Washington, DC: American Psychiatric Press; 1991.
9. Lipowski Z. Somatization: the concept and its clinical application. Am J Psychiatry 1988;145:1358–68.
10. Belmaker E, Espinoza R, Pogrund R. Use of medical services by adolescents with non-specific somatic symptoms. Int J Adolesc Med Health 1985;1:150–6.
11. Campo JV, Jansen-McWilliams L, Comer DM, et al. Somatization in pediatric primary care: association with psychopathology, functional impairment, and use of services. J Am Acad Child Adolesc Psychiatry 1999;38:1093–101.

12. American Psychiatric Association. Diagnostic and statistical manual of mental disorders. 4th edition. Washington, DC: American Psychiatric Association; 2000.
13. Shorter E. From paralysis to fatigue: a history of psychosomatic illness in the modern era. New York: The Free Press; 1992.
14. Offord DR, Boyle MH, Szatmari P, et al. Ontario Child Health Study. II. Six-month prevalence of disorder and rates of service utilization. Arch Gen Psychiatry 1987;44: 832–6.
15. Garber J, Walker LS, Zeman J. Somatization symptoms in a community sample of children and adolescents: further validation of the children's somatization inventory. Psychol Assess 1991;3:588–95.
16. Kreichman A. Siblings with somatoform disorders in childhood and adolescence. J Am Acad Child Adolesc Psychiatry 1987;26:226–31.
17. Livingston R, Martin-Cannici C. Multiple somatic complaints and possible somatization disorder in prepubertal children. J Am Acad Child Psychiatry 1985;24:603–7.
18. Cloninger C, Reich T, Guze S. The multifactorial model of disease transmission: III. Familial relationship between sociopathy and hysteria (Briquet's syndrome). Br J Psychiatry 1975;127:23–32.
19. Livingston R. Children of people with somatization disorder. J Am Acad Child Adolesc Psychiatry 1993;32:536–44.
20. Wessely S. Old wine in new bottles: neurasthenia and 'ME'. Psychol Med 1990;20: 35–53.
21. Salmon P, Al-Marzooqui SM, Baker G, et al. Childhood family dysfunction and associated abuse in patients with nonepileptic seizures: towards a causal model. Psychosom Med 2003;65:695–700.
22. Roelofs K, Keijsers GPJ, Hoogduin KA, et al. Childhood abuse in patients with conversion disorder. Am J Psychiatry 2002;159:1908–13.
23. Spierings C, Poels P, Sijben N, et al. Conversion disorders in childhood: a retrospective follow-up study of 84 inpatients. Devel Med Child Neurol 1990;32:865–71.
24. Bursch B. Pediatric pain. In: Shaw RJ, DeMaso DR, editors. Textbook of psychosomatic medicine. Arlington (VA): American Psychiatric Publishing, Inc.; 2010. p. 141–54.
25. Fritz GK, Fritsch S, Hagino O. Somatization disorders in children and adolescents: a review of the past 10 years. J Am Acad Child Adolesc Psychiatry 1997;36:1329–38.
26. Barsky AJ. Hypochondriasis and obsessive-compulsive disorder. Psychiatr Clin North Am 1992;15:791–801.
27. Neziroglu F, Yaryura-Tobias JA, Walz J, et al. The effect of fluvoxamine and behavior therapy on children and adolescents with obsessive-compulsive disorder. J Child Adolesc Psychopharmacol 2000;10:295–306.
28. Noyes R Jr. The relationship of hypochondriasis to anxiety disorders. Gen Hosp Psychiatry 1999;27:8–17.
29. Chosak A, Marques L, Greenbert JL, et al. Body dysmorphic disorder and obsessive-compulsive disorder: similarities, differences and the classification debate. Expert Rev Neurother 2008;8:1209–18.
30. Phillips KA, Stout RL. Associations in the longitudinal course of body dysmorphic disorder with major depression, obsessive-compulsive disorder, and social phobia. J Psychiatr Res 2006;40:360–9.
31. Didie ER, Tortolani CC, Pope CG, et al. Childhood abuse and neglect in body dysmorphic disorder. Child Abuse Negl 2006;30:1105–15.
32. Gunstad J, Phillips KA. Axis I comorbidity in body dysmorphic disorder. Compr Psychiatry 2003;44:270–6.

33. Phillips KA. Body dysmorphic disorder. In: Oldham JM, Riba MB, editors. Somatoform and factitious disorders (Review of Psychiatry series, vol. 20, no. 3). Washington, DC: American Psychiatric Press; 2001, p. 67–94.

34. Phillips KA, Diaz SF. Gender differences in body dysmorphic disorder. J Nerv Ment Dis 1997;185:570–7.

35. Phillips KA, McElroy SL, Keck PE Jr, et al. Body dysmorphic disorder: 30 cases of imagined ugliness. Am J Psychiatry 1993;150:302–8.

36. Phillips KA. Body dysmorphic disorder: clinical aspects and treatment strategies. Bull Menninger Clin 1998;62(4 Suppl A):A33–48.

37. Uzun O, Basoglu C, Akar A, et al. Body dysmorphic disorder in patients with acne. Compr Psychiatry 2003;44:415–9.

38. Veale D, De Haro L, Lambrou C. Cosmetic rhinoplasty in body dysmorphic disorder. Br J Plast Surg 2003;56:546–51.

39. Phillips K, Atala K, Albertini R. Case study: body dysmorphic disorder in adolescents. J Am Acad Child Adolesc Psychiatry 1995;34:1216–20.

40. Phillips K, Menard W, Fay C, et al. Demographic characteristics, phenomenology, comorbidity, and family history in 200 individuals with body dysmorphic disorder. Psychosomatics 2005;46:317–25.

41. Campo JV, Fritsch SL. Somatization in children and adolescents. J Am Acad Child Adolesc Psychiatry 1994;33:1223–35.

42. Garralda ME. Practitioner review: assessment and management of somatization in childhood and adolescence. J Child Psychol Psychiatr 1999;40:1159–67.

43. Domenech-Llaberia E. Jane C, Canals J, et al. Parental reports of somatic symptoms in preschool children: prevalence and associations in a Spanish sample. J Am Acad Child Adolesc Psychiatry 2004;43:598–604.

44. Fichtel A, Larsson B. Psychosocial impact of headache and comorbidity with other pains among Swedish school adolescents. Headache 2002;42:766–75.

45. Silber TJ, Pao M. Somatization disorders in children and adolescents. Pediatr Rev 2003;24:255–64.

46. Goodman JE, McGrath PJ. The epidemiology of pain in children and adolescents: a review. Pain 1991;46:247–64.

47. Aro H. Life stress and psychosomatic symptoms among 14 to 16-year-old Finnish adolescents. Psychological Medicine 1987;17:191–201.

48. Larsson B. Somatic complaints and their relationship to depressive symptoms in Swedish adolescents. J Child Psychol Psychiatry 1991;32:821–32.

49. Oster J. Recurrent abdominal pain, headache and limb pains in children and adolescents. Pediatrics 1972;50:429–36.

50. Lipton RB, Bigal ME, Steiner TJ, et al. Classification of primary headaches. Neurology 2004;63:427–35.

51. Abu-Arafeh I, Russell G: Prevalence and clinical features of abdominal migraine compared with those of migraine headache. Arch Dis Child 1995;72:413–7.

52. Apley J, Naish N. Recurrent abdominal pains: a field study of 1,000 school children. Arch Dis Child 1958;33:165–70.

53. Scharff L. Recurrent abdominal pain in children: A review of psychological factors and treatment. Clin Psychol Rev 1997;17:145–66.

54. Starfield B, Gross E, Wood M, et al. Psychosocial and psychosomatic diagnoses in primary care of children. Pediatrics 1980;66:159–67.

55. Boyle JT. Recurrent abdominal pain: an update. Pediatr Rev 1997;18:310–20.

56. Campo JV, Di Lorenzo C, Chiappetta L, et al. Adult outcomes of pediatric recurrent abdominal pain: do they just grow out of it? Pediatrics 2001;108:E1.

57. Rasquin-Weber A, Hyman PE, Cucchiara S, et al. Childhood functional gastrointestinal disorders. Gut 1999;45(Suppl 2):II60–8.
58. Fleischer DR. Cyclic vomiting syndrome and migraine. J Pediatr 1999;134:533–5.
59. Garralda ME, Chalder T. Practitioner review: chronic fatigue syndrome in childhood. J Child Psychol Psychiatry 2005;46:1143–151.
60. Goldman J, Muers M. Vocal cord dysfunction and wheezing. Thorax 1991;46: 401–4.
61. Raja SN, Grabow TS. Complex regional pain syndrome I (reflex sympathetic dystrophy). Anesthesiology 2002;96:1254–60.
62. Diatchenko L, Slade GD, Nackley AG, et al. Genetic basis for individual variations in pain perception and the development of a chronic pain condition. Hum Mol Genet 2005;14:135–43.
63. Greenberg BD, Li Q, Lucas FR, et al. Association between the serotonin transporter promoter polymorphism and personality traits in a primarily female sample. Am J Med Genet 2000;96:202–16.
64. Lesch KP, Bengel D, Heils A, et al. Association of anxiety related traits with a polymorphism in the serotonin transporter gene regulatory region. Science 1996; 274:1527.
65. Du L, Bakish D, Hrdina PD. Tryptophan hydroxylase gene 218A/C polymorphism is associated with somatic anxiety in major depressive disorder. J Affect Disord 2001;65:37–44.
66. Campo JV, Bridge J, Ehmann M, et al. Recurrent abdominal pain, anxiety, and depression in primary care. Pediatrics 2004;113:817–24.
67. Maisami M, Freeman JM. Conversion reactions in children as body language: a combined child psychiatry/neurology team approach to the management of functional neurologic disorders in children. Pediatrics 1987;80:46–52.
68. Minuchin S, Rosman BL, Baker L. Psychosomatic families: anorexia nervosa in context. Cambridge (MA): Harvard University Press; 1978.
69. Mullins LL, Olson RA. Familial factors in the etiology, maintenance, and treatment of somatoform disorders in children. Fam Syst Med 1990;8:159–75.
70. Craig TK, Cox AD, Klein K. Intergenerational transmission of somatization behaviour: a study of chronic somatizers and their children. Psychol Med 2002;32:805–16.
71. Grattan-Smith P, Fairley M, Procopis P. Clinical features of conversion disorder. Arch Dis Child 1988;63:408–14.
72. Green M, Solnit AJ. Reactions to the threatened loss of a child: a vulnerable child syndrome. Pediatric management of the dying child, part III. Pediatrics 1964;34: 58–66.
73. Leslie SA. Diagnosis and treatment of hysterical conversion reactions. Arch Dis Child 1988;63:506–11.
74. Lieb R, Zimmermann P, Friis RH, et al. The natural course of DSM-IV somatoform disorders and syndromes among adolescents and young adults: a prospective-longitudinal community study. Eur Psychiatry 2002;17:321–31.
75. Walker LS, Garber J, Greene JW. Psychosocial correlates of recurrent childhood pain: a comparison of pediatric patients with recurrent abdominal pain, organic illness, and psychiatric disorders. J Abnorm Psychol 1993;102:248–58.
76. Kreipe RE. The biopsychosocial approach to adolescents with somatoform disorders. Adolesc Med Clin 2006;17:1–24.
77. Shaw RJ, Spratt EG, Bernard RS, et al. Somatoform disorders. In: Shaw RJ, DeMaso DR, editors. Textbook of pediatric psychosomatic medicine. Arlington (VA): American Psychiatric Publishing, Inc; 2010. p. 121–39.

78. De Gucht V, Fischler B. Somatization: a critical review of conceptual and methodological issues. Psychosomatics 2002;43:1–7.
79. Walker LS, Greene JW. The functional disability inventory: measuring a neglected dimension of child health status. J Pediatr Psychol 1991;16:39–58.
80. Dhossche D, van der Steen F, Ferdinand R. Somatoform disorders in children and adolescents: a comparison with other internalizing disorders. Ann Clin Psychiatry 2002;14:23–31.
81. Fearon P, Hotopf M. Relation between headache in childhood and physical and psychiatric symptoms in adulthood: national birth cohort study. BMJ 2001;12: 322(7295):1145.
82. Fichter MM, Kohlboeck G, Quadflieg N, et al. From childhood to adult age: 18-year longitudinal results and prediction of the course of mental disorders in the community. Soc Psychiatry Psychiatr Epidemiol 2009;44:792–803.
83. Saps M, Seshadri R, Sztainberg M, et al. A prospective school-based study of abdominal pain and other common somatic complaints in children. J Pediatr 2009;154:322–6.
84. Finney JW, Lemanek KL, Cataldo MF, et al. Pediatric psychology in primary health care: brief targeted therapy for recurrent abdominal pain. Behav Ther 1989;20:283–91.
85. Sanders MR, Rebgetz M, Morrison M, et al. Cognitive-behavioral treatment of recurrent nonspecific abdominal pain in children: an analysis of generalization, maintenance, and side effects. J Consult Clin Psychol 1989;57:294–300.
86. Sanders MR, Shepherd RW, Cleghorn G, et al. The treatment of recurrent abdominal pain in children: a controlled comparison of cognitive-behavioral family intervention and standard pediatric care. J Consult Clin Psychol 1994;62:306–14.
87. Schulman JL. Use of a coping approach in the management of children with conversion reactions. J Am Acad Child Adolesc Psychiatry 1988;27:785–8.
88. Dickes RA. Brief therapy of conversion reactions: an in-hospital technique. Am J Psychiatry 1974;131:584–6.
89. Treischmann RB, Stolov WC, Montgomery ED. An approach to the treatment of abnormal ambulation resulting from conversion reaction. Arch Phys Med Rehabil 1970;51:198–206.
90. Klonoff EA, Moore DJ. "Conversion reactions" in adolescents: a biofeedback-based operant approach. J Behav Ther Exp Psychiatry 1986;17:179–84.
91. Mizes JS. The use of contingent reinforcement in the treatment of a conversion disorder: a multiple baseline study. J Behav Ther Exp Psychiatry 1985;16:341–5.
92. Caldwell TA, Stewart RS. Hysterical seizures and hypnotherapy. Am J Clin Hypn 1981;23:294–8.
93. Elkins GR, Carter BD. Hypnotherapy in the treatment of childhood psychogenic coughing: a case report. Am J Clin Hypn 1986;29:59–63.
94. Williams DT, Singh M. Hypnosis as a facilitating therapeutic adjunct in child psychiatry. J Am Acad Child Psychiatry 1976;15:326–42.
95. Linton SJ. A case study of the behavioural treatment of chronic stomach pain in a child. Behav Change 1986;3:70–3.
96. Masek B, Russo DC, Varni JW. Behavioral approaches to the management of chronic pain in children. Pediatr Clin North Am 1984;31:1113–31.
97. Moene FC, Hoodguin KA, Van Dyck R. The inpatient treatment of patients suffering from (motor) conversion symptoms: a description of eight cases. Int J Clin Exp Hypn 1998;46:171–90.
98. Anbar RD. Subconscious guided therapy with hypnosis. Am J Clin Hypn 2008;50: 323–34.

99. Bloom PB. Treating adolescent conversion disorders: are hypnotic techniques reusable? Int J Clin Exp Hypn 2001;49:243–56.

100. Looper KJ, Kirmayer LJ. Behavioral medicine approaches to somatoform disorders. J Consult Clin Psychol 2002;70:810–27.

101. Mutter CB, Coates ML. Hypnosis in family medicine. Am Fam Physician 1990;42(5 Suppl):70S–3S.

102. Goodyer IM. Hysterical conversion reactions in childhood. J Child Psychol Psychiatry 1981;22:179–88.

103. Liebman R, Honig P, Berger H. An integrated treatment program for psychogenic pain. Fam Process 1976;15:397–405.

104. Walker LS, Zeman JL. Parental response to child illness behavior. J Pediatr Psychol 1992;17:49–71.

105. Palermo TM. Impact of recurrent and chronic pain on child and family daily functioning: a critical review of the literature. J Dev Behav Pediatrics 2000;21:58–69.

106. Wood BL. Physically manifested illness in children and adolescents: a biobehavioral family approach. Child Adolesc Psychiatric Clin N Am 2001;10:543–62.

107. Campo JV, Shafer S, Lucas A, et al. Managing pediatric mental disorders in primary care: a stepped collaborative care model. J Am Psychiatr Nurse Assoc 2005;11:1–7.

108. Fritz GK, Bergman AS. Child psychiatrists seen through pediatricians' eyes: results of a national survey. J Am Acad Child Psychiatry 1985;24:81–6.

109. Smith GR Jr, Monson RA, Ray DC. Psychiatric consultation in somatization disorder. New Engl J Med 1986;314:1407–13.

110. Fallon BA. Pharmacotherapy of somatoform disorders. J Psychosom Res 2004;56:455–60.

111. Stahl SM. Antidepressants and somatic symptoms: therapeutic actions are expanding beyond affective spectrum disorders to functional somatic syndromes. J Clin Psychiatry 2003;64:745–6.

112. Fishbain DA, Cutler RB, Rosomoff HL, et al. Do antidepressants have an analgesic effect in psychogenic pain and somatoform pain disorder? A meta-analysis. Psychosom Med 1998;60:503–9.

113. O'Malley PG, Jackson JL, Santoro J, et al. Antidepressant therapy for unexplained symptoms and symptom syndromes. J Fam Pract 1999;48:980–90.

114. Drossman DA, Toner BB, Whitehead WE, et al. Cognitive-behavioral therapy versus education and desipramine versus placebo for moderate to severe functional bowel disorders. Gastroenterology 2003;125:19–31.

115. Jailwala J, Imperiale TF, Kroenke K. Pharmacologic treatment of the irritable bowel syndrome: a systematic review of randomized, controlled trials. Ann Intern Med 2000;133:136–47.

116. Egger HL, Costello EJ, Erkanli A, et al. Somatic complaints and psychopathology in children and adolescents: stomach aches, musculoskeletal pains, and headaches. J Am Acad Child Adolesc Psychiatry 1999;38:852–60.

117. Campo JV. Coping with ignorance: exploring pharmacologic management for pediatric functional abdominal pain. J Pediatr Gastroenterol Nutr 2005;41:569–74.

118. Hyams JS, Hyman PE. Recurrent abdominal pain and the biopsychosocial model of medical practice. J Pediatr 1998;133:473–8.

119. Phillips KA, Albertini RS, Rasmussen SA. A randomized placebo-controlled trial of fluoxetine in body dysmorphic disorder. Arch Gen Psychiatry 2002;59:381–8.

120. Hollander E, Allen A, Kwon J, et al. Clomipramine vs desipramine crossover trial in body dysmorphic disorder: selective efficacy of a serotonin reuptake inhibitor in imagined ugliness. Arch Gen Psychiatry 1999;56:1033–9.

121. el-Khatib HE, Dickey TO 3rd. Sertraline for body dysmorphic disorder. J Am Acad Child Adolesc Psychiatry 1995;27:1404–5.

122. Sondheimer A. Clomipramine treatment of delusional disorder- somatic type. J Am Acad Child Adolesc Psychiatry 1988;27:188–92.

123. Lewis D, Ashwal S, Hershey A, et al; American Academy of Neurology Quality Standards Subcommittee; Practice Committee of the Child Neurology Society. Practice parameter: pharmacological treatment of migraine headache in children and adolescents: report of the American Academy of Neurology Quality Standards Subcommittee and the Practice Committee of the Child Neurology Society. Neurology 2004;63:2215–24.

124. Siow H, Young W, Silberstein S. Neuroleptics in headache. Headache 2005;45: 358–71.

125. Battistella PA, Ruffilli R, Cernetti R, et al. A placebo-controlled crossover trial using trazodone in pediatric migraine. Headache 1993;33:36–9.

126. Kroenke K, Messina N 3rd, Benattia I, et al. Venlafaxine extended release in the short-term treatment of depressed and anxious primary care patients with multisomatoform disorder. J Clin Psychiatry 2006;67:72–80.

127. Brannan SK, Mallimckrodt CH, Brown EB, et al. Duloxetine 60 mg once-daily in the treatment of painful physical symptoms in patients with major depressive disorder. J Psychiatr Res 2005;39:43–53.

128. Campo JV. Disorders primarily seen in general medical settings. In: Findling RL, editor. Clinical manual of child and adolescent psychopharmacology. Arlington (VA): American Psychiatric Publishing, Inc., 2008. p. 375–423.

129. First MB. Paradigm shifts and the development of the diagnostic and statistical manual of mental disorders: past experiences and future aspirations. Can J Psychiatry 2010;55:692–700.

Somatization in Older People

Chanaka Wijeratne, MD, FRANZCP[a,b,*]

KEYWORDS
• Somatization • Geriatric • Somatoform disorders
• Somatic symptoms

NEGLECT BY GERIATRIC PSYCHIATRY

The popular contention that preoccupation with bodily functions is characteristic of older age has been accepted by the lay and medical community on the basis of received wisdom.[1] The reality is that somatic presentations of distress have been largely ignored by geriatric (or old age) psychiatry for a number of reasons.[2] The resultant paucity of age-specific literature necessarily limits any review of this nature.

The general conceptual failings in the nosology enshrined in the Diagnostic and Statistical Manual (DSM) remain a major impediment to their study in old age.[3] The definition of the somatoform disorders has been described as "among the tallest and most complex conceptual edifices ever erected in medicine."[4] Their essence—the presentation with a physical (ie, somatic) symptom(s) for which there is no, or an inadequate, patho-physiological explanation—is particularly troublesome in older people. The definition also assumes a psychogenic explanation for symptoms, although the category was intended to be etiologically neutral.[5]

Primary care studies have shown that recognition of psychological distress was lower in patients who were older or had a predominantly somatic presentation.[6] Possible reasons for this include the masking effect of physical illness, or the incorrect belief that emotional or somatic distress is apposite to old age. Standardized assessment scales used in research that require raters to determine whether each somatic symptom is "medically explained" may also encourage a conservative approach to diagnosis in the presence of physical disease.

Even if a physical cause is deemed inappropriate, the use of traditional psychiatric hierarchies in which mood and psychotic disorders are favored over "minor" disorders such as somatoform disorders means that depressive disorders may be seen as the next most likely explanation for a somatic presentation.[7]

[a] Academic Department for Old Age Psychiatry, Prince of Wales Hospital, Randwick 2031, NSW, Australia
[b] School of Psychiatry, University of New South Wales, Kensington 2052, NSW, Australia
* Corresponding author: 20 English Street, Kogarah 2217, NSW, Australia.
E-mail address: Chanaka.Wijeratne@sesiahs.health.nsw.gov.au

Psychiatr Clin N Am 34 (2011) 661–671
doi:10.1016/j.psc.2011.05.010
0193-953X/11/$ – see front matter Crown Copyright © 2011 Published by Elsevier Inc. All rights reserved.

Moreover, the somatoform disorders do not fit neatly into the structure of geriatric psychiatry services. The provision of specialist psychiatric services for this age group is dominated by the epidemiological imperative of dementia, which has burdened and, thereby, required a degree of prioritization of services.[8] This pattern of service delivery and focus, although not an explicit one, may well influence referral patterns.

It will also be seen that the general limitations of diagnostic criteria for the somatoform disorders are accentuated in older people.[5]

Given the multiple conceptual and practical concerns about the term "somatoform," an alternate term that will be used in this article is "somatization," a process in which the experience of a somatic symptom is followed by the development of a pathological attribution and the eventual presentation of that symptom to a medical practitioner.[9] Among older people, somatization has been reported to be common, associated with an increased frequency of primary care consultation, and independently predictive of a poorer quality of life.[10,11]

MEASURING AND VALIDATING SOMATIC SYMPTOMS IN OLDER PEOPLE

There are 2 preliminary but seminal issues that must be examined in any consideration of somatic symptoms in older people, namely measurement and clinical validity.

First, somatic symptoms appropriate for use in older people, and rating scales specifically designed for older people, should be employed. The varying somatic symptoms endorsed by older people and reported by the literature are the result of the particular rating scale or questionnaire used and cannot necessarily be extrapolated to suggest specific salience to old age.[12–14] For instance, community-dwelling older adults reported difficulty sleeping, fatigue, nervousness, sadness, unsteadiness on feet, and forgetfulness as the most common symptoms experienced.[12] The problem with this particular list, however, is that the last 2 symptoms overlap with neurological disease.

Similarly, certain items on the PRIME-MD about menstrual pain, pain during intercourse, and fainting spells may be confusing or annoying to older people.[14,15] Neurological symptoms listed within criteria for DSM-IV somatization disorder, such as impaired coordination or balance, deafness, and diplopia, seem inappropriate, as sensory loss and gait difficulties increase with age. Sexual symptoms pose similar difficulties, as erectile dysfunction also tends to increase with age. This raises the psychometric issue of "item bias," in that an instrument may not perform similarly across age or, indeed, across gender or culture.[16,17]

So, how does symptom endorsement vary across age? A US primary care study of older patients who responded to a modified PRIME-MD questionnaire reported musculoskeletal pain, fatigue, back pain, shortness of breath, and difficulty sleeping as the most common symptoms.[14] In fact, this list is similar to the common non-menstrual symptoms (joint pains, back pain, headaches, chest pain, limb pain, abdominal pain, fatigue, and dizziness) reported by 13,538 adults across the entire age spectrum in the multi-community Epidemiological Catchment Area (ECA) study.[18] On the other hand, an Australian community survey of around 2000 respondents across the age spectrum reported that symptoms such as colds, sore throat, flu, headache, palpitations, breathlessness, depression, tiredness, and irritability all *declined* from mid-life and into older age.[13] Thus, it is incorrect to assume that older people report more somatic symptoms.

Secondly, it must be established that somatic symptoms can be adequately distinguished from psychological symptoms. Early primary care research questioned whether somatic symptoms were an independent or valid form of distress, as 2 highly correlated dimensions of anxiety and depression symptoms were shown to underlie the presentation of non-psychotic disorders.[19,20] When similar statistical methods were applied to samples of older people, other researchers again concluded that somatic symptom reporting could be subsumed within depression and anxiety dimensions.[21] A significant reservation about these earlier studies is their use of rating scales that did not adequately record somatic symptoms, potentially creating biased results.

Exploratory factor analysis may be used to reduce a large data set into a smaller number of summary variables, and to explore the theoretical structure underlying symptom endorsement. This method was used in a study of nearly 12,000 older Australians presenting to primary care practices who completed a 34-item questionnaire that assessed a wide range of psychological and somatic symptoms.[22] If the traditional argument that somatic symptoms are secondary to psychological distress is true, then both somatic and psychological symptoms would correlate significantly with one another, with a single underlying dimension or a series of mixed symptom dimensions produced. Instead, a final four factor solution—consisting of specific mood, musculoskeletal, cognitive and fatigue symptom dimensions—was derived, suggesting that somatic symptoms could be distinguished from psychological symptoms and, indeed, from each other.

Another study which examined validity measured the prevalence, co-morbidity, and longitudinal outcome of 3 disorders: chronic fatigue, anxiety, and depressive disorder.[23] Although the majority of cases of chronic fatigue were co-morbid with a psychological disorder, some cases occurred separately. Also, rather than evolving into a psychological disorder or vice-versa, cases of chronic fatigue were longitudinally stable. This study concluded that while chronic fatigue does overlap with psychological disorders, there may also be distinct forms of fatigue, supporting the notion that somatic syndromes may be independent.

In summary, neurological and genitourinary/gynecological symptoms are unsuitable for the study of somatic symptom endorsement by older people because they are more commonly encountered in the elderly. When more appropriate somatic symptoms are used and adequately measured, fatigue and musculoskeletal symptom dimensions may be distinguished from psychological and cognitive symptom dimensions, suggesting somatic symptoms are a form of distress with clinical validity in older people.

THE PREVALENCE OF SOMATIZATION IN OLDER PEOPLE

Reported rates of somatoform disorders in older people have been low, due mainly to the method of diagnosis by exclusion, and high symptom and disability thresholds required by DSM (**Table 1**).[24–30] Indeed, the low overall rates obtained by the ECA studies may have resulted in the failure of subsequent major epidemiological studies, such as the National Comorbidity Survey, to examine somatoform disorders.[31]

Surveys in other countries have found similar results. A 2-phase population survey of elderly Brazilian subjects (aged 75 years and older) reported a one-month, 1.8% prevalence rate of somatoform disorders.[32] This rate may also have been confounded by the use of the semi-structured clinician interview—the Schedules for Clinical Assessment in Neuropsychiatry (SCAN)—which requires the interviewer to determine if somatic symptoms are unexplained or not.[33] Given that two-thirds of the sample reported 3 or more chronic diseases, it is likely interviewers were cautious in their ratings of symptoms as medically explained.

It would be expected that rates increase successively from community samples, to primary care, to specialist psychiatric clinics as patients pass through each layer of medical care.

Table 1
Rates of somatoform and related disorders reported in studies that included older people (60 years and over)

Authors	Cohort	Specific Disorder	Association with Age	Prevalence Rate
Regier et al, 1988[24] (ECA)	Multi-site US community – 30% aged 65yrs+	DSM III somatization disorder	Nil	0.1% overall; 0.1% elderly
Bland et al, 1988[25]	Canadian community – 11% aged 65yrs+	DSM III somatization disorder	Nil	No cases at any age
Australian Bureau of Statistics, 1998[26]	Multi-site Australian community - 17% aged 65yrs+	ICD-10 neurasthenia (a disorder of chronic fatigue)	Decline	1.3% overall; 0.6% elderly
Barsky et al, 1991[27]	Boston primary care	DSM-III-R hypochondriasis	Decline	4.3% overall; 1.6% elderly
Kroenke et al, 1997[28] (PRIME-MD)	Multi-site US primary care	Hypochondriasis Pain disorder Multisomatoform disorder	Decline (for subjects with at least one somatoform disorder)	No age specific data reported
Kirmayer & Robbins, 1991[29]	Montreal primary care - 23% aged 61–75	Hypochondriasis	Not reported	
de Waal et al, 2004[30]	Dutch primary care	Somatoform disorders	Decline across three age groups: 25-44, 45-64 & 65-79 years	16.1% overall; 5.4% in elderly

Table 2
Somatic symptoms reported by older primary care attenders - symptom frequency by chronic physical disease

	Total Sample	Hypertension	Arthritis	Diabetes Mellitus	Coronary Artery Disease	Chronic Heart Failure	Obstructive Lung Disease
Musculoskeletal pain	65%	65%	78%	67%	65%	65%	63%
Tiredness	55%	54%	57%	59%	61%	63%	64%
Back pain	45%	45%	53%	46%	47%	46%	50%
Shortness of breath	41%	40%	41%	40%	53%	57%	70%
Trouble sleeping	37%	36%	40%	39%	43%	40%	40%
Nausea, gas, indigestion	36%	35%	38%	40%	38%	38%	39%
Constipation or diarrhea	34%	34%	36%	39%	34%	39%	35%

The first column indicates the overall frequency of symptom reporting by the total sample; the other columns indicate the proportion of patients diagnosed with that disorder who reported the symptom indicated in each row (*Data from* Sha M, Callahan C, Counsell S, Westmoreland G, Stump T, Kroenke K. Physical symptoms as a predictor of health care use and mortality among older adults. Am J Med 2005;118:301–6.).

A Dutch study of 404 primary care patients, which also used the SCAN, reported the rate of somatoform disorders in patients 65 to 79 years of age was 5.4% when moderate-to-severe clinical impairment was present.[30] The rate of somatoform disorders was even higher (7.2%) when cases with little or no impairment were included, although the equivalent rates of anxiety and depressive disorders were unchanged. What is also noteworthy is that the rate of somatoform disorders was higher than the rate of anxiety disorders (1.8%) and depressive disorders (0.9%), both of which also declined with age.

The rate of somatoform disorders is highest in specialist or multidisciplinary clinics. A UK study reported a rate of 75%, and a Dutch study a rate of 86%; in both samples, pain (joint, back, abdominal) and diagnoses of undifferentiated somatoform disorder were most common.[34,35]

IS SOMATIZATION UNDERDIAGNOSED IN OLDER PEOPLE?

There are several lines of evidence which suggest that somatization may be underestimated in older research and clinical samples.

A large primary care sample of nearly 3500 adults aged 60 years and older (69% being female, 56% African-American with a mean age of 69 years), reported an average of 4.3 symptoms.[14] Data from this study is shown in **Table 2**, which lists the six most common chronic conditions diagnosed by a physician, and patient endorsement of disabling symptoms over the preceding month for each of those diagnoses. Seven symptoms—musculoskeletal pain (65%), fatigue (55%), back pain (45%), shortness of breath (41%), difficulty sleeping (38%), nausea/indigestion (36%), and constipation/diarrhea (34%)—that were endorsed by more than one-third of the sample are shown.

While cardinal symptoms (for example, musculoskeletal pain or back pain) that would logically be due to a specific condition (in this case, arthritis) were more common in that particular condition, it can be observed that many patients without the diagnosis still endorsed the cardinal symptoms. The authors provided another example of this phenomenon, not contained in **Table 2**, in which a combined group of patients with diagnoses of coronary heart disease, cardiac failure, or respiratory disease were shown to report more shortness of breath (57% vs 31%), chest pain (27% vs 14%), and heart racing (31% vs 20%) than patients without one of these 3 diagnoses; these figures emphasize the point that somewhere between 10% and 30% of somatic complaints cannot be attributed to a specific physical disease.[14]

These figures are very similar to English primary care practitioners' ratings of the etiology of their older patients' somatic symptoms. Approximately one-third of attendees were rated as having some psychological component to their somatic presentations, including 13% rated as mainly or entirely of psychological origin.[36] The implication of these studies is that there is an additional large reservoir of background symptoms presenting to primary care practitioners that cannot be attributed to a specific disease, and which are potentially somatoform.[14,18]

Any inclination for clinicians and raters to attribute somatic symptoms to physical disease in older people is understandable due to the DSM principle of diagnosis by exclusion. ECA data showed that older people tended to report a disproportionately high number of raw lifetime symptoms, although the number of medically unexplained somatic symptoms showed no increase with age.[18,37]

Clinicians may feel uneasy about making a diagnosis of a somatoform disorder because of the fear of potentially missing a physical disease. One particular study published nearly 50 years ago, which claimed that one-third of patients with hysteria had been misdiagnosed, may have been influential in instilling this fear, which has been compounded by the medico-legal climate of modern day clinical practice.[38] However, a systematic review reported a rate of misdiagnosis of only 4% in patients with motor and sensory symptoms such as paralysis, seizures, and blindness since the 1970's.[39] Of a small sample (median age 75 years) with chronic medically unexplained somatic presentations referred to a multidisciplinary specialist clinic, only 3 out of 35 patients received a new physical disease diagnosis.[35]

Poor recall is another confounding factor, especially when lifetime rates of disorder are measured in older people. Somatization disorder requires the presence of symptoms beginning before the age of 30, so its diagnosis is especially vulnerable to poor recall. This was demonstrated by the ECA study, in which lifetime rates of somatization disorder showed a successive decline in all age bands in the St. Louis site, and declined from the second youngest age band in the New Haven and Baltimore sites.[40] This is counterintuitive; since onset is before the age of 30, the lifetime rate should have risen from the first (18 to 24 years) to the second (25 to 44 years) age band and plateaued thereafter, as all subjects would have passed through the age of risk. In fact, somatoform presentations to a tertiary referral clinic tended to begin in middle age and persist into old age.[34]

DOES SOMATIZATION PRESENT DIFFERENTLY IN OLDER PEOPLE?

The evidence suggests that the predisposing factors to somatic distress in older people are similar to those in younger adults.[10,23,30] These include female gender, perceived poor social support (which may limit access to a social network from which to seek advice), and physical disease (which may sensitize an individual to somatic distress). High rates of co-morbidity with anxiety, depressive, and substance use disorders have also been reported.[30,35]

The strong overlap between physical disease and psychological disorders was illustrated by a study of over 1000 predominantly older patients with established coronary artery disease, in which angina symptoms were associated with depressive symptoms, but not left ventricular ejection fraction or the degree of cardiac ischemia.[41] In an Australian primary care study of older people suffering from chronic fatigue, greater physical disease morbidity certainly predicted chronic fatigue, but the strength of the association was much stronger for psychological disorder than for physical morbidity.[23]

One potential point of difference across age—cognitive impairment—has been insufficiently explored in the study of somatization in older people. A non-clinical sample of community-dwelling Italians (aged 75 years and over) found that, as Mini Mental State Examination (MMSE) scores declined, reports of somatic symptoms increased.[42]

With regard to prevalence across age, there are only a handful of studies that have reported rates across the adult age span, and as all of these are cross-sectional, cohort effects cannot be excluded (**Table 1**). This limited data suggests that there is a tendency for somatoform disorder rates to decline with age. This parallels similar age-related declines in the rates of depressive and anxiety disorders summarized by previous reviewers.[43] Leaving aside the methodological issues that may have confounded rates per se, it is possible that these findings represent a real decline in prevalence with age.

If we assume that somatoform disorders do become less common with age, then an examination of each part of the process by which patients eventually receive such a diagnosis may highlight possible reasons for this decline.

While the experience of somatic symptoms is universal and constant, it is symptom perception that shapes medical consultation. It has been estimated that community-dwelling older adults report as little as 45% of perceived symptoms to health professionals, with symptom reporting to a relative or friend being just as likely.[12] Cognitions associated with non-disclosure included the symptom being benign, perceived lack of interest from others, not wanting to bother others, and pessimism about treatment.

The attributional style of older patients in response to common somatic symptoms was assessed in a UK study of Oxford primary care practices.[10] The authors used the Symptom Interpretation Questionnaire, in which respondents were asked to choose between a normalizing, psychological, or somatic explanation for 13 symptoms.[44] For instance, possible responses to the scenario, "If I got dizzy all of a sudden, I would probably think it was because . . ." are, "I must be under a lot of stress" (psychological), "I am not eating enough, or I got up too quickly" (normalizing), or "there is something wrong with my heart or blood pressure" (somatic).

A predominantly normalizing attributional style was seen in 73% of older patients, while a somatic style was observed in only 14%.[10] These findings are similar to studies of college students whose mean scores were lowest on the somatic symptom attribution subscale, and highest on the normalizing subscale, but a little counterintuitive given the greater physical disease burden which accompanies age.[44] Two studies of older people from the same authors have found that a somatic attributional style also tended to be a stable phenomenon.[10,45] Non-specific symptoms, such as weakness and aches, were more likely to be attributed to age by older people who may have difficulty distinguishing specific symptoms against background somatic noise.[46]

A tendency to form normalizing attributions and adaptation to chronic disease may help explain the findings of a multi-center primary care study of 3000 adults across the age span. The Patient Health Questionnaire was used to derive a Somatic Symptom Severity score, based on the frequency and severity of 13 commonly presented symptoms.[47] This score was significantly lower in older patients, despite significantly more physical disease diagnoses.[48]

Even after medical presentation, functional impairment and disability determine the need for ongoing management of somatic symptoms. Two studies of chronic pain clinic samples have suggested that older people adapt better psychologically to their symptoms. In comparison to younger sufferers of non-malignant chronic pain, patients aged 65 years and over scored significantly lower on the scale "disease conviction," which measures affirmation of physical disease, symptom preoccupation, and rejection of reassurance by a physician, and also reported less physical and social disability despite greater objective physical disease.[49] The study also noted that the younger group was more likely to report a history of injury prior to the onset of pain and to seek financial compensation for it, which suggests a more conflictual environment in which pain arises, causing persistent stressors such as the inability to work.

Similarly, in a study of oncology patients, despite reporting comparable pain intensity and interference, older patients tended to accept pain as an inevitable part of cancer, and they continued to pursue life goals, and modified their activities to maximize engagement.[50] In contrast, younger patients reported feeling out of control, angry, and unable to accept their pain. Two mental processes, psychological immunization, in which repeated exposure to stress has been hypothesized to increase individual resilience to life events, and increased emotional control, in which coping skills may improve with age, may be protective and attenuate the response to pain in older people.[43,51]

In summary, older people may have difficulty distinguishing somatic symptoms among the background noise of multiple physical co-morbidities and tend to respond to somatic symptoms with a normalizing attribution. Physical illness per se does not seem sufficient to lead to medical presentation; in particular, psychological distress, including anxiety and depression, tend to increase somatic symptom distress. Older people's adaptation to symptoms may be better than younger cohorts so that disability is minimized.

It may be that the current literature reflects, at least partially, a cohort effect whereby people exposed to the deprivations of the Great Depression and a World War have lower expectations of their health and well-being. One wonders if baby boomer and subsequent generations may be more likely to present somatic symptoms to medical care.

MANAGEMENT

It should come as no surprise to learn that there are no formal studies of the management of somatization in older people. The main challenge for geriatric psychiatry is to integrate the care of older patients with complex somatic presentations. The current paradigm, whereby internal medicine labels patients with poorly defined pathology as "psychiatric," is stigmatizing, and psychiatry viewing such symptoms as "psychogenic" is equally unhelpful.[5] Any solution would require psychological assessment to be embedded as a part of routine medical care, and the institution of multi-disciplinary "one-stop" clinics with physicians, psychiatrists, and clinical psychologists working collaboratively.

Prevention consists of using a holistic, biopsychosocial etiological model for all presentations, judicious use of physical investigations and specialist referrals, and avoiding the use of spurious diagnoses and treatments. Formal treatment can only be extrapolated from studies of younger adults. Selective serotonin reuptake inhibitors and tricyclic antidepressants are beneficial in a number of somatic syndromes.[52] Their efficacy in pain syndromes is independent of effects on mood. Cognitive behavior therapy and graded exercise therapy may also be effective.[53]

REFERENCES

1. Pitt B. Psychogeriatrics. An Introduction to the Psychiatry of Old Age. Edinburgh: Churchill Livingstone; 1982.
2. Wijeratne C, Brodaty H, Hickie I. The neglect of somatoform disorders by old age psychiatry: some explanations and suggestions for future research. Int J Geriatr Psychiatry 2003;18:812–9.
3. Mayou R, Sharpe M, Kirmayer L, et al. Somatoform disorders: time for a new approach in DSM-V. Am J Psychiatry 2005;162:847–55.
4. Jablensky A. The concept of somatoform disorders: a comment on the mind-body problem in psychiatry. In: Ono Y, Janca A, Asai M, et al, editors. Somatoform disorders, vol 3. A worldwide perspective. Tokyo: Springer Verlag; 1999. p. 3–10.
5. Sharpe M, Mayou R. Somatoform disorders: a help or hindrance to good patient care? Br J Psychiatry 2004;184:465–67.
6. Hickie I, Davenport T, Scott E, et al. Unmet need for recognition of common mental disorders in Australian general practice. Med J Aust 2001;175(Suppl):S18–24.
7. Wittchen H-U. Comorbidity of mood disorders - diagnosis and treatment. Depression 1995;3:131–3.
8. Jeste D, Alexopoulos G, Bartels S, et al. Consensus statement on the upcoming crisis in geriatric mental health: research agenda for the next 2 decades. Arch Gen Psychiatry 1999;56:848–53.
9. Lipowski Z. Somatization: the concept and its clinical application. Am J Psychiatry 1988;145:1358–68.
10. Sheehan B, Bass C, Briggs R, et al. Somatization among older primary care attenders. Psychol Med 2003;33:867–77.
11. Sheehan B, Lair R, Bass C. Does somatization influence quality of life among older primary care patients? Int J Geriatr Psychiatry 2005;20:967–72.
12. Brody E, Kleban M, Moles E. What older people do about their day-to-day mental and physical health symptoms. J Am Geriatr Soc 1983;31:489–98.
13. Henderson A. Somatization in the elderly. In: Ono Y, Janca A, Asai M, et al, editors. Somatoform disorders. A worldwide perspective. Tokyo: Springer-Verlag; 1999. p. 57–64.
14. Sha M, Callahan C, Counsell S, et al. Physical symptoms as a predictor of health care use and mortality among older adults. Am J Med 2005;118:301–6.
15. Spitzer R, Williams J, Kroenke K, et al. Utility of a new procedure for diagnosing mental disorders in primary care. The PRIME-MD 1000 Study. JAMA 1994;272:1749–56.
16. Kroenke K, Spitzer R. Gender differences in the reporting of physical and somatoform symptoms. Psychosom Med 1998;60:150–5.
17. Escobar J, Burnam M, Karno M, et al. Somatization in the community. Arch Gen Psychiatry 1987;44:713–8.
18. Kroenke K, Price R. Symptoms in the community. Prevalence, classification, and psychiatric comorbidity. Arch Intern Med 1993;153:2474–80.
19. Goldberg D. A dimensional model for common mental disorders. B J Psychiatry 1996;168(Suppl 30):44–9.
20. Goldberg D, Bridges K. Somatic presentations of psychiatric illness in primary care settings. J Psychosom Res 1988;32:137–44.
21. Christensen H, Jorm A, Mackinnon A, et al. Age differences in depression and anxiety symptoms: a structural equation modelling analysis of data from a general population sample. Psychol Med 1999;29:325–39.

22. Wijeratne C, Hickie I, Davenport T. Is there an independent somatic symptom dimension in older people? J Psychosom Res 2006;61:197–204.
23. Wijeratne C, Hickie I, Brodaty H. The characteristics of fatigue in an older primary care sample. Psychosom Res 2007;62:153–8.
24. Regier D, Boyd J, Burke J, et al. One-month prevalence of mental disorders in the United States. Based on five epidemiologic catchment area sites. Arch Gen Psychiatry 1988;45:977–86.
25. Bland R, Newman S, Orn H. Prevalence of psychiatric disorders in the elderly in Edmonton. Acta Psychiatr Scand Suppl 1988;338:57–63.
26. Australian Bureau of Statistics. Mental health and wellbeing. Profile of adults, Australia, 1997. Canberra: Australian Bureau of Statistics; 1998.
27. Barsky A, Frank C, Cleary P, et al. The relation between hypochondriasis and age. Am J Psychiatry 1991;148:923–8.
28. Kroenke K, Spitzer R, deGruy F, et al. Multisomatoform disorder. An alternative to undifferentiated somatoform disorder for the somatizing patient in primary care. Arch Gen Psychiatry 1997;54:352–8.
29. Kirmayer L, Robbins J. Three forms of somatization in primary care: prevalence, co-occurrence and sociodemographic characteristics. J Nerv Ment Dis 1991;179: 647–55.
30. de Waal M, Arnold I, Eekhof J, et al. Somatoform disorders in general practice. Prevalence, functional impairment and comorbidity with anxiety and depressive disorders. Br J Psychiatry 2004;184:470–6.
31. Kessler R, Merikangas K. The National Comorbidity Survey Replication (NCS-R): background and aims. Int J Methods Psychiatr Res 2004;13:60–8.
32. Costa E, Barreto S, Uchoa E, et al. Prevalence of International Classification of Diseases, 10th Revision common mental disorders in the elderly in a Brazilian community: The Bambui Health Ageing Study. Am J Geriatr Psychiatry 2007;15: 17–27.
33. Division of Mental Health WHO. Schedules for Clinical Assessment in Neuropsychiatry. Geneva: World Health Organization; 1992.
34. Wilkinson P, Bolton J, Bass C. Older patients referred to a consultation-liaison psychiatry clinic. Int J Geriatr Psychiatry 2001;16:100–5.
35. Hilderink P, Benraad C, van Driel D, et al. Medically unexplained physical symptoms in elderly people: a pilot study of psychiatric geriatric characteristics. Am J Geriatr Psychiatry 2009;17:1085–8.
36. Sheehan B, Bass C, Briggs R, et al. Do general practitioners believe that their older patients physical symptoms are somatized? J Psychosom Res 2004;56:313–6.
37. Simon G, vonKorff M. Somatization and psychiatric disorder in the NIMH Epidemiologic Catchment Area study. Am J Psychiatry 1991;148:1494–1500.
38. Slater E, Glithero E. A follow-up of patients diagnosed as suffering from "hysteria". J Psychosom Res 1965;9:9–13.
39. Stone J, Smyth R, Carson ASystematic review of misdiagnosis of conversion symptoms and "hysteria". BMJ 2005;331(7523):989.
40. Robins L, Helzer J, Weissman M, et al. Lifetime prevalence of specific psychiatric disorders in three sites. Arch Gen Psychiatry 1984;41:949–58.
41. Ruo B, Rumsfeld J, Hlatky M, et al. Depressive symptoms and health-related quality of life: the heart and soul study. JAMA 2003;290:215–21.
42. Frisoni G, Fedi V, Geroldi C, et al. Cognition and the perception of physical symptoms in the community-dwelling elderly. Behav Med 1999;25:5–12.
43. Jorm A. Does old age reduce the risk of anxiety and depression? A review of epidemiological studies across the life span. Psychol Med 2000;30:11–22.

44. Robbins J, Kirmayer L. Attributions of common somatic symptoms. Psychol Med 1991;21:1029–45.
45. Sheehan B, Philpott M, Banerjee S. Attributions of physical symptoms in patients of an old age psychiatry service. Int J Geriatr Psych 2002;17:61–4.
46. Leventhal E, Prohaska T. Age, symptom interpretation, and health behavior. J Am Geriatr Soc 1986;34:185–91.
47. Spitzer R, Kroenke K, Williams J. Patient Health Questionnaire Primary Care Study Group. Validity and utility of a self-report version of PRIME-MD: the PHQ Primary Care Study. Primary care evaluation of mental disorders. Patient health questionnaire. JAMA 1999;282:1737–44.
48. Klapow J, Kroenke K, Horton T, et al. Psychological disorders and distress in older primary care patients: a comparison of older and younger samples. Psychosom Med 2002;64:635–43.
49. Wijeratne C, Shome S, Hickie I, et al. An age-based comparison of chronic pain clinic patients. Int J Geriatr Psychiatry 2001;16:477–83.
50. Gagliese L, Jovellanos M, Zimmermann C, et al. Age-related patterns in adaptation to cancer pain: a mixed-method study. Pain Med 2009;10:1050–61.
51. Henderson A. Does ageing protect against depression? Soc Psychiatry Psychiatr Epidemiol 1994;29:107–9.
52. O'Malley P, Jackson J, Santoro J, et al. Review: Antidepressant therapy for unexplained symptoms and symptom syndromes. J Fam Pract 1999;48:980–90.
53. Allen L, Woolfolk R. Cognitive behavioral therapy for somatoform disorders. Psychiatr Clin N Am 2010;33:579–93.

Functional Somatic Syndromes and Somatoform Disorders in Special Psychosomatic Units: Organizational Aspects and Evidence-Based Treatment

Andreas Schröder, MD, PhD*, Per Fink, prof., MD, PhD, DMSc

KEYWORDS

- Bodily distress • Functional somatic syndromes
- Somatoform disorders • Treatment • Organization of care
- STreSS intervention

A substantial number of patients encountered in different medical settings complain of physical symptoms not attributable to any known conventionally defined disease, that is, "medically unexplained" or functional somatic symptoms.[1–3] In this paper, we name this phenomenon "bodily distress."[4] In most cases, such symptoms are mild and self-limiting; however, some patients are severely disabled. These patients are frequently given functional somatic syndrome diagnoses such as fibromyalgia, chronic fatigue syndrome, or irritable bowel syndrome; others may receive a somatoform disorder diagnosis. Research into the pathophysiology of these syndromes has suggested some unifying mechanisms, including aberrant functions of efferent neural pathways, such as the autonomic nervous system and the hypothalamic–pituitary axis, and alterations in central processing of sensory input.[5–8] The syndromes may thus be viewed as different expressions of bodily distress, namely, (patho)physiologic responses to prolonged or severe mental or physical stress in genetically susceptible individuals.[9] Bodily distress is hence not conceptualized as a maladaptive psychological response to somatic sensations, symptoms, or diseases.[1] Nevertheless, psychological and behavioral factors may be involved in the initiation and perpetuation of bodily distress.[10,11]

The Research Clinic for Functional Disorders and Psychosomatics, Aarhus University Hospital, Noerrebrogade 44, DK-8000 Aarhus C, Denmark
* Corresponding author.
E-mail address: andreas.schroeder@aarhus.rm.dk

Psychiatr Clin N Am 34 (2011) 673–687
doi:10.1016/j.psc.2011.05.008
0193-953X/11/$ – see front matter © 2011 Elsevier Inc. All rights reserved.

Beside causing a substantial decrease in quality of life,[12] such illnesses are costly for society because of high health care use and missed working years.[1–3,13] The prevalence of somatoform disorders in the general population is about 6%, the same as for depressive disorders.[14] Despite a high need for care, however, bodily distress constitutes a low-priority area in most health care systems across the world and is grossly ignored in general psychiatry, even by many psychosomatic services.[15,16] Most countries offer no or very limited specialized care for these patients, because most treatment options are reserved for patients with a particular symptom profile, namely, patients with specialty-specific functional somatic syndrome diagnoses. Consequently, the majority of patients with bodily distress are not offered evidence-based treatment.[10]

In this paper, we examine the status of treatment and organizational models for specialized care for these patients.

CLASSIFICATION

A major obstacle in the organization of treatment of bodily distress is the inconsistent use of terminology for classification. Although psychiatrists may use somatoform disorder diagnoses according to the DSM-IV classifications, most patients are seen by general practitioners and specialists and receive specialty-specific syndrome diagnoses such as fibromyalgia, irritable bowel syndrome, chronic fatigue syndrome, or non-cardiac chest pain.[3,17] There is disagreement as to whether these diagnoses and syndromes that include patients presenting with functional somatic symptoms represent a single disorder or multiple disorders. From the "lumping" point of view, functional somatic syndrome diagnoses are believed to be an artifact of medical specialization—caused by the diagnostic heterogeneity that exists across the different medical specialties.[3,4,17]

Increasingly, scientific evidence suggests that these conditions belong to the same family of disorders. Studies have indicated a huge overlap in symptoms and illness pictures between patients who have received different diagnostic labels.[18–25] Moreover, functional somatic syndromes share similarities in etiology,[26] pathophysiology,[5] neurobiology,[7] psychological mechanisms,[27] patient characteristics,[3,24,28] and treatment response,[29] which speaks in favor of a common family of disorders. Some studies, however, support the "splitting" point of view, especially with regard to triggering factors and risk profiles for specific syndromes.[30–33] Moreover, some studies indicate that symptoms of bodily distress cluster in groups of gastrointestinal, cardiopulmonary, and musculoskeletal symptoms,[34] supporting the existence of different subtypes of bodily distress.[1,35,36] Nevertheless, because there seem to be more similarities than differences between the functional somatic syndromes, it seems rational to treat them within the same service. To do this, a common language and a theoretical framework for understanding of bodily distress across medical specialties are highly needed.[2] Although the new suggested somatic symptom disorder category of the DSM-V lumps most of the current subcategories of the DSM-IV somatoform diagnoses,[37] it only captures patients with evident psychological or behavioral disturbances, thereby splitting patients with bodily distress into a group whose conditions are regarded as medical and a group whose conditions are conceptualized as psychiatric.[34]

A new, empirically established approach is based on the identification of bodily distress syndrome (BDS) as a diagnosis in its own right that encompasses both the "non-psychiatric" functional somatic syndromes and "psychiatric" somatoform disorders.[1] The diagnosis includes a multiorgan subtype and 4 single-organ subtypes (**Fig. 1**),[24] and is hence not a pure lumping or splitting approach, but both a lumping

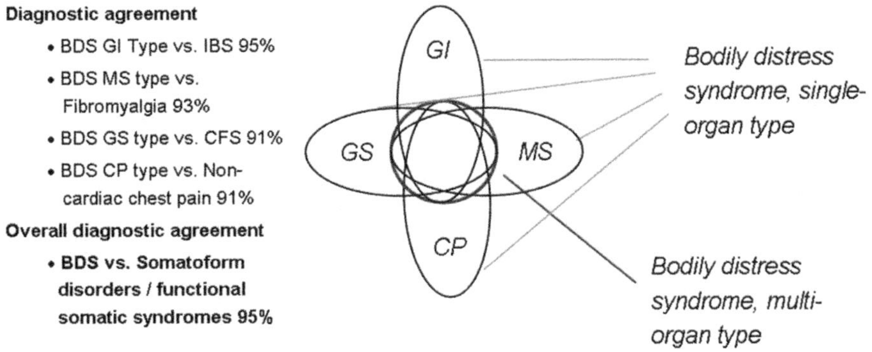

Diagnostic agreement

- BDS GI Type vs. IBS 95%
- BDS MS type vs. Fibromyalgia 93%
- BDS GS type vs. CFS 91%
- BDS CP type vs. Non-cardiac chest pain 91%

Overall diagnostic agreement

- **BDS vs. Somatoform disorders / functional somatic syndromes 95%**

Bodily distress syndrome, single-organ type

Bodily distress syndrome, multi-organ type

Fig. 1. Theoretical model of BDS and empirical diagnostic agreement of its subtypes with existing diagnostic categories. CFS, chronic fatigue syndrome; CP, cardiopulmonary; GI, gastrointestinal; GS, general symptoms (fatigue, headache, dizziness, memory and concentration difficulties); IBS, irritable bowel syndrome; MS, musculoskeletal. (*Data from* Fink P, Toft T, Hansen MS, et al. Symptoms and syndromes of bodily distress: an exploratory study of 978 internal medical, neurological, and primary care patients. Psychosom Med 2007;69:30–9; and Fink P, Schröder A. One single diagnosis, Bodily distress syndrome, succeeded to capture ten diagnostic categories of functional somatic syndromes and somatoform disorders. J Psychosom Res 2010;68:415–26.).

and a splitting concept. In contrast with the DSM-V's somatic symptom disorder category, the BDS diagnosis does not require specific psychopathology or behavioral features. Nevertheless, first evidence suggests that the BDS diagnosis captures patients with somatoform disorders according to DSM-IV as well as the functional somatic syndromes.[24] In this paper, we focus on the diagnoses covered by the BDS concept, that is, the most important functional somatic syndromes and the somatoform disorders that are primarily characterized by physical symptoms. We do not discuss hypochondriasis/health anxiety or body dysmorphic disorder, which are primarily characterized by anxiety and cognitive symptoms rather than bodily distress.[38]

TREATMENT

Most systematic reviews and meta-analyses in the field of bodily distress are focused on single-syndrome diagnoses. Only few studies have reviewed the whole area systematically.[29,39,40] Both these comprehensive reviews and reviews focused on specific syndromes[41–43] conclude that pharmacologic agents working on the central nervous system are preferable to organ-oriented treatments and that interventions based on active patient involvement such as exercise and cognitive–behavioral therapy are currently the most promising treatments. There seems to be no clear differences between various functional somatic syndromes in terms of which treatment type works, namely, the specific symptom profiles seem to be nonessential for the choice of treatment strategy (**Table 1**).

Some evidence suggests that a combination of pharmacotherapy, exercise, and psychological interventions in multicomponent management programs is effective.[29,62] These programs may also further include some types of organ-oriented treatments. For instance, various organ-oriented and symptomatic treatments have shown effect in the management of irritable bowel syndrome (eg, probiotics).[63] The same is true for other functional somatic syndromes.[29] Organ-oriented treatment

Table 1
Evidence for antidepressants, aerobic exercise and psychological interventions in different subtypes of bodily distress

Symptom Profile (BDS subtype) and Corresponding Functional Somatic Syndrome or Diagnostic Label	GS-Type/Chronic Fatigue Syndrome	MS-Type/Fibromyalgia	GI-Type/Irritable Bowel Syndrome	CP-Type/Non-Cardiac Chest Pain	Multiorgan Type/Multiple Medically Unexplained Symptoms and Somatization Disorder
Type of treatment					
Antidepressants	+[29,41]	+++[44]	+++[45,46]	?	++[39,40,47]
Exercise	+++[41,48,49]	+++[50,51]	?	?	+[52]
Psychological treatment (mainly CBT)	+++[41,49,53]	+++[54,55]	++[45,56,57]	++[58]	+++[39,40,47,52,59-61]

Symptom profiles are ordered according to the BDS concept (see **Fig. 1**), whereas references refer to the corresponding diagnostic categories. Evidence ratings are based on Henningsen and colleagues[29] and recent meta-analyses or high-quality, randomized, controlled trials. Only the most important references are listed.

Symbols: +++, strong evidence; ++, moderate evidence; +, weak evidence; ?, no evidence, or lack of studies.

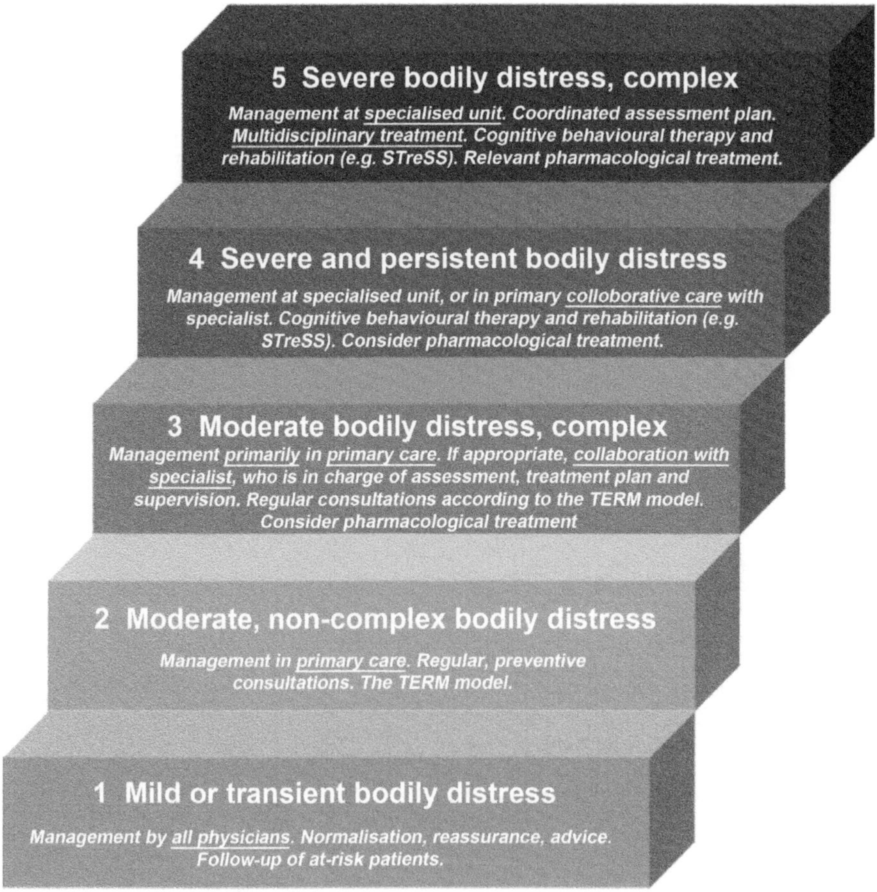

5 Severe bodily distress, complex
Management at specialised unit. Coordinated assessment plan. Multidisciplinary treatment. Cognitive behavioural therapy and rehabilitation (e.g. STreSS). Relevant pharmacological treatment.

4 Severe and persistent bodily distress
Management at specialised unit, or in primary colloborative care with specialist. Cognitive behavioural therapy and rehabilitation (e.g. STreSS). Consider pharmacological treatment.

3 Moderate bodily distress, complex
Management primarily in primary care. If appropriate, collaboration with specialist, who is in charge of assessment, treatment plan and supervision. Regular consultations according to the TERM model. Consider pharmacological treatment

2 Moderate, non-complex bodily distress
Management in primary care. Regular, preventive consultations. The TERM model.

1 Mild or transient bodily distress
Management by all physicians. Normalisation, reassurance, advice. Follow-up of at-risk patients.

Fig. 2. Stepped care model for treatment of bodily distress (*Data from* Refs.[17,29,69]).

may therefore play an additional role in the management of different subtypes of bodily distress. However, we do not know whether multicomponent treatment is more effective than single treatment elements, nor can we currently estimate the relative effects of the interventions that form part of multicomponent treatment approaches.

Despite a clear body of evidence for the efficacy of behavioral and cognitive treatments (**Table 1**), there seems to be some reluctance to recommend such treatments in non-psychiatric specialties. Thus, in the European rheumatologists' guidelines for treatment of fibromyalgia, cognitive–behavioral therapy is only recommended as an optional treatment element for a limited number of patients, whereas such treatment according to the American Pain Society and meta-analyses plays an essential part in the management.[62,64] Cognitive-behavioral interventions may even be the treatment of choice,[54] since they are effective also in the absence of evident psychopathology.[65] The mechanisms how these interventions reduce bodily distress are not fully understood, but evidence suggests that they have the potential to modify symptom experience and pain perception[65,66] and to restore central nervous system abnormalities that are linked with functional impairment.[67]

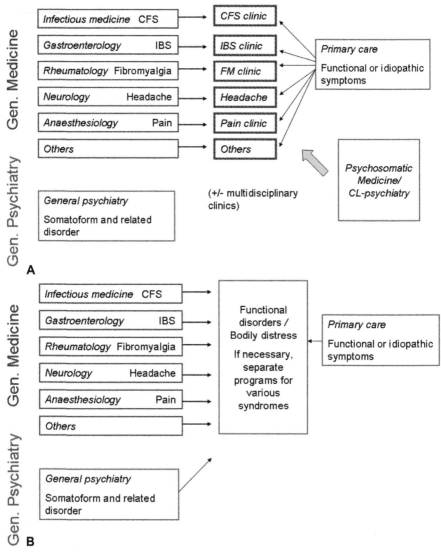

Fig. 3. (*A*) Fractionated specialized clinics model. (*B*) Specialized clinic for bodily distress, including functional somatic syndromes and somatoform disorders (*From* Fink P, Burton C, de Bie J, et al. Current state of management and organisation of care. In: Creed F, Henningsen P, Fink P, editors. Medically unexplained symptoms, somatisation and bodily distress: developing better clinical services. Cambridge: Cambridge University Press; 2011; with permission.).

ORGANIZATION OF CARE: MODELS AND RECOMMENDATIONS

Although no studies on the topic exist, there seems to be a general agreement among experts that management of patients with bodily distress should be organized according to a stepped care model (**Fig. 2**) in which milder distress is treated in primary care[68] and the more severe or complex cases are treated in secondary care.[10,17,29] Specialist care for severe bodily distress (steps 4 and 5) can be organized in 2 ways (**Fig. 3**): Specialist services for single syndromes and diagnoses (eg, chronic fatigue syndrome, fibromyalgia, somatization disorder), and specialist services for all types combined, that is, BDS including both functional somatic syndromes and somatoform disorders.

Syndrome-Specific Specialized Clinics

Medical specialists have developed facilities for treating "their own" functional somatic syndrome within their own service such as rheumatologists treating fibromyalgia or infectious medicine treating chronic fatigue syndrome. This is a natural consequence of the large number of patients with these disorders they receive at their services (see **Fig. 3**A). Health care in these clinics is often mono-disciplinary, and dominated by pharmacologic treatment methods.[64]

The mainly mono-disciplinary nature of such fractionated specialized clinics is a drawback. The multidisciplinary model seems the most suitable for patients with severe and complicated BDS,[29] but even if various specialty-specific clinics for single functional somatic syndromes were organized according to a multidisciplinary model, this may not be a rational strategy. First, establishing multiple different clinics, one for each functional somatic syndrome, is costly and inappropriate given that these clinics deliver very similar treatments. Second, the existence of various syndrome-specific clinics confirms the separate, specialty-dominated view on bodily distress and hence perpetuate fragmented care instead of moving toward a more generic model. Finally, and most important, fractionated specialized clinics may not be prepared to deal with patients who have symptoms from multiple organ systems. These patients often fulfill the diagnostic criteria for multiorgan BDS, and it may therefore be random which type of clinic they attend, or even worse, they may attend several clinics simultaneously and receive several, parallel, uncoordinated treatments.

Specialized Integrated Clinics for Bodily Distress

Integrated specialized clinics for bodily distress treat patients with different diagnostic labels under one hat (see **Fig. 3**B). The integrated approach has some clear advantages. First, it is obvious that patients with multiorgan BDS belong in such a clinic to prevent simultaneous treatment by different services or sequential treatment in different clinics. Second, it would make referrals much easier for family physicians and other doctors as they do not need to decide which service is the best for the patients—there is only one entrance to care. This also provides better possibilities for shared care models as the family physicians only need to relate to one multidisciplinary service rather than several, which is the case in the fractionated model. Presumably, most patients are happy to be treated for their multiple symptoms at a single clinic instead of several clinics, but this requires that specialists and primary care physicians are able to explain to the patients that their symptoms are expressions of bodily distress not caused by a medical disease and thus not requiring medical specialist treatment.

A third advantage of the integrated model is that it is cost-effective and ensures synergy between therapists and different medical specialists. A drawback, however, may be that it is difficult to warrant the presence of the necessary medical expertise in an integrated model because it involves nearly all medical specialties. Moreover, it can be necessary to tailor subtypes of treatment programs to special types of problems or to patients with single-organ BDS, which requires several similar treatment programs at the same clinic.

In conclusion, although there are arguments to support both integrated and fractionated approaches (**Box 1**), the integrated approach seems to provide more advantages, and it has achieved broad international support.[10,29]

> **Box 1**
> **Integrated versus fractionated treatment**[69,70]
>
> **Arguments supporting integrated treatment**
>
> Increasing evidence suggests that fibromyalgia, irritable bowel syndrome and other functional somatic syndromes belong to the same family of disorders.[71]
>
> The same treatment strategies have proven effective for these disorders (see **Table 1**).[29]
>
> Close cooperation including several medical specialties facilitates effective assessment of patients with multiple symptoms or substantial comorbidity.
>
> It seems unrealistic and inefficient to establish specific treatment offers for every individual functional somatic syndrome.
>
> **Arguments supporting fractionated treatment:**
>
> It may be beneficial to target treatments according to subtypes of bodily distress, for example, patients who suffer primarily from muscle pain, fatigue or abdominal discomfort.
>
> Patients with bodily distress are encountered in all medical specialties and it may be advantageous not to refer them to another department.
>
> Organ-focused symptomatic treatment may be needed and require the expertise of a specific medical specialty.[29]

RECOMMENDATIONS FOR A SPECIALIZED SERVICE

The basic structure of services for BDS should be the same as that for other disorders or diseases in the health care system, that is, that appropriate treatment is provided in primary care with referral of more severely affected patients to specialized services for BDS at general hospitals or specialist clinics. There should be highly specialized services at university hospitals, which should also carry responsibility for training and research. The specialized service for BDS could also be part of a comprehensive psychosomatic or consultation–liaison (C-L) psychiatry service outside of university hospitals, but the necessary specific assessment and treatment skills should be available to those patients who require them.

The recommended form of service for BDS requires a multidisciplinary team, which includes both psychological/psychiatric and medical–surgical expertise. Because patients with severe BDS may be chronically ill with a high risk of being excluded from the labor market, occupational medicine and rehabilitation expertise are also needed, together with expertise in physical training. The number of experts needed from various specialties could be quite large, so a realistic way of organizing this would be that the specialists/counselors have a partial attachment to a clinic, but are employed elsewhere.

Each discipline relies on input from other specialists. For instance, a psychologist seeing a patient with bodily distress should collaborate with an general physician because medical knowledge is often required. However, psychologists are important when it comes to psychological treatment provided they have the backup from psychiatrists and physicians.

Because of the multidisciplinary approach, specialist clinics for BDS are best located at general hospitals to promote collaboration with other medical specialties and promote patient acceptance, although it is unclear whether such clinics should be organized under psychiatry or general medicine. However, most patients with bodily distress find it odd to attend a psychiatric hospital or clinic for their mainly physical ailment. Consequently, patients with BDS are rarely seen in general psychiatric services, and only patients displaying prominent emotional symptoms or who have a concurrent mental disorder are referred to psychiatric services.

Psychosomatic medicine is the only medical or psychiatric subspecialty having BDS as one of their target groups, and patients with BDS are frequently referred to such services. An early survey of a C-L psychiatry service in the United States found that 38% of referrals were for somatization.[72] A more recent, large survey of patients referred to an American C-L psychiatry service found that approximately 10% of referrals from the medical inpatient units had a somatoform disorder,[73] and studies from the UK reported that medically unexplained symptoms or somatoform disorders accounted for up to 30% of referrals to C-L psychiatry services.[74,75] In a large European study of general hospital patients referred to 56 C-L psychiatry services in 11 countries, 19% of the patients were referred because of "medically unexplained symptoms," but only 8 of these 56 C-L psychiatry services had a marked preponderance of such patients; these were mainly psychosomatic services in Germany.[76] In the United States, a well-organized subspecialty of psychosomatic medicine has been established, but there are no clinics in the United States that specifically treat patients with bodily distress.[77] This means that although patients with bodily distress are frequently referred to C-L psychiatry and psychosomatic services, they are mostly not the services' main target group and may therefore not receive appropriate assessment and treatment even in those services.[15,16]

The best way of developing a good clinical service for patients with BDS may, therefore, be to establish the area as a specialty of its own as is the case for psychosomatic medicine in Germany. In most parts of the world, however, this may not be a realistic first goal. A certain amount of pragmatism is necessary for local adaptations. For instance, in countries with specialized clinics for chronic fatigue syndrome, a strategy could also be to establish programs for a broader range of BDS.[10]

One may wonder why such specialized clinics are not implemented more widely; this seems to be an evident way of obviating many of the drawbacks of the current, unsuitable, fractionated treatment of bodily distress. We speculate that a range of strong academic, political, economic, and social interests may be invested in the status quo concerning some of the functional somatic syndrome diagnoses.[78] Pharmaceutical companies, lawyers, clinics, insurance companies, patient organizations, and research milieus may have economic or interests in presenting certain functional somatic syndromes as valid and generally accepted diagnoses, even if their validity may be dubious. Less speculative is our assumption that the status quo is maintained by the increasing subspecialization of health care and by the fact that psychiatric and non-psychiatric services are often organized in separate organizations which makes it difficult to get funding for services for disorders in the "no-man's land" between psychiatry and general medicine.

One of the very few university hospital departments specialized in patients with BDS is located in Denmark. Herein, the treatment for BDS is described.

SPECIALIZED TREATMENT FOR SEVERE BODILY DISTRESS: A PRACTICAL EXAMPLE

The Specialized Treatment for Severe Bodily Distress Syndromes (STreSS) program was developed to treat patients with persistent multiorgan BDS.[70] STreSS was based on a cognitive–behavioral approach and, to maximize its potential cost effectiveness, designed to be delivered as group treatment. The department that offers the STreSS program is not part of the mental health service, but is located at a university general hospital as part of the Neurocenter, which enhances acceptability for both patients

Table 2
Elements of the STreSS intervention
1 Letter with management recommendation for functional somatic symptoms sent to primary care physician.
2 Treatment manual, including schedule, symptom diary, education material, worksheets, and homework assignment for the 9 treatment modules. Patients are handed relevant chapters at the beginning of each module. Nonattending patients receive the chapters by mail. The treatment manual is available at www.functinaldisorders.dk.
3 Consultancy service on the phone for primary care physicians and specialists.
4 The 9 treatment modules, 3.5 hours each, are based on a cognitive–behavioral approach, delivered in groups of 9 patients by 2 physicians, at weeks 1, 2, 3, 4, 6, 8, 10, 12, and 16 (see Table 2) Each patient is allowed to receive 2 supplemental individual consultations in case of new, important symptoms or major psychiatric problems.
5 Close cooperation with social authorities or the patient's employer, when needed.

and doctors. The treatment program is open to patients referred by physicians, and the department receives patients from all over Denmark. The Danish national health insurance covers the expenses for the treatment amounting to US$6500 for the STreSS program and US$2200 for the preceding clinical assessment.

Before patients are offered the STreSS program, they undergo a thorough clinical assessment at the department, which includes a review of clinical records, a semistructured psychiatric interview,[79] physical and neurologic examinations, and a laboratory screening battery. This assessment not only aims to ensure that a patient's symptoms are not due to an undiagnosed medical or psychiatric condition, but also to provide the patient with a positive and evidence-based understanding of his or her illness and to enhance the patient's motivation to engage in a cognitive–behavioral group treatment. If an undiagnosed medical condition is suspected, the patient is referred to the relevant department. If comorbid anxiety and depression are present, written individualized advice on treatment is given to the patient's family physician in the expectation that he or she will treat this psychiatric disorder.[70,80]

The STreSS program consists of several elements (**Table 2**), some of which (elements 1 and 3) do not aim to influence the patients directly, but to change the "usual care" they receive from their family physicians, both during and after treatment at the department. Furthermore, the STreSS program includes close cooperation with social authorities and the patients' employers, when needed (element 5). The core of the treatment is 9 modules of manualized psychotherapy (element 4) based on a cognitive–behavioral approach, each of 3.5 hours duration and delivered to groups of 9 patients by 2 psychiatrists (consultants or senior residents in psychiatry with at least 2 years of training in cognitive–behavioral therapy and expertise in the field of bodily distress). **Table 3** gives a brief overview of the 9 modules. The patients are given the relevant chapter of the treatment manual (element 2)[70] at the beginning of each module, including educational material, a symptom diary, worksheets, and homework assignments.

Recently, the department has treated patients with multiorgan BDS[24] of at least 2 years' duration. This threshold has been used to ensure that the department is concerned primarily with patients with severe and disabling bodily distress. The efficacy of STreSS has been tested in a randomized, controlled trial, and the results showed an immediate, clinically relevant effect on the patients' self-reported physical health and their perceived bodily distress.[70] This effect was sustained at the 1-year follow-up. These results suggest that it is feasible to treat patients diagnosed with the

Table 3
Overview of treatment modules in the STreSS program

Module	Week	Content
1	1	Introduction to STreSS
2	2	Bodily symptoms and their interpretation
3	3	Illness perceptions, stress response, and treatment goals
4	4	Negative automatic thoughts and dysfunctional behaviors
5	6	Cognitive distortions and emotional awareness
6	8	From illness behavior to health behavior I
7	10	From illness behavior to health behavior II
8	12	Becoming your own therapist; relapse prevention
9	16	How to maintain learned skills and coping strategies

unifying BDS diagnosis together, regardless of the diagnostic label they may have received previously. Therefore, we regard the STreSS program as a promising example of a unified treatment approach that overcomes current shortcomings in the organization of care for patients with severe bodily distress.

SUMMARY

Based on our current knowledge and clinical experience, this article outlines evidence for the implementation of unified treatment programs for functional somatic syndromes and somatoform disorders at specialized multidisciplinary psychosomatic services. An essential rationale is our knowledge that both psychological–behavioral and psychopharmacologic interventions are effective, regardless of the diagnostic label and the patient's symptom profile, although organ-specific treatments may play an additional role in the management of bodily distress. Different organizational models are evaluated asking the question whether they have the potential to improve the quality of care for patients with bodily distress. An integrated approach seems to be preferable compared with fractionated specialized clinics for various functional somatic syndromes. Specific recommendations for the implementation of such integrated services for bodily distress are given. Finally, the authors have provided an example of a unified treatment approach for patients with severe bodily distress from their own clinic, the STreSS intervention.

REFERENCES

1. Fink P, Toft T, Hansen MS, et al. Symptoms and syndromes of bodily distress: an exploratory study of 978 internal medical, neurological, and primary care patients. Psychosom Med 2007;69:30–9.
2. Fink P, Rosendal M, Olesen F. Classification of somatization and functional somatic symptoms in primary care. Aust N Z J Psychiatry 2005;39:772–81.
3. Wessely S, Nimnuan C, Sharpe M. Functional somatic syndromes: one or many? Lancet 1999;354:936–9.
4. Creed F, Guthrie E, Fink P, et al. Is there a better term than "Medically unexplained symptoms"? J Psychosom Res 2010;68:5–8.
5. Bradley LA. Pathophysiologic mechanisms of fibromyalgia and its related disorders. J Clin Psychiatry 2008;69(Suppl 2):6-13.6-13.
6. Clauw DJ. Potential mechanisms in chemical intolerance and related conditions. Ann N Y Acad Sci 2001;933235–53.

7. Wood PB. Neuroimaging in functional somatic syndromes. Int Rev Neurobiol 2005; 67119–63.
8. Yunus MB. Central sensitivity syndromes: a new paradigm and group nosology for fibromyalgia and overlapping conditions, and the related issue of disease versus illness. Semin Arthritis Rheum 2008;37:339–52.
9. Schweinhardt P, Sauro KM, Bushnell MC. Fibromyalgia: a disorder of the brain? Neuroscientist 2008;14:415–21.
10. Fink P, Burton C, de Bie J, et al. Current state of management and organisation of care. In: Creed F, Henningsen P, Fink P, editors. Medically unexplained symptoms, somatisation and bodily distress: developing better clinical services. Cambridge: Cambridge University Press; 2011.
11. Deary V, Chalder T, Sharpe M. The cognitive behavioural model of medically unexplained symptoms: a theoretical and empirical review. Clin Psychol Rev 2007;27:781–97.
12. Harris AM, Orav EJ, Bates DW, et al. Somatization increases disability independent of comorbidity. J Gen Intern Med 2009;24:155–61.
13. Barsky AJ, Orav EJ, Bates DW. Somatization increases medical utilization and costs independent of psychiatric and medical comorbidity. Arch Gen Psychiatry 2005;62: 903–10.
14. Wittchen HU, Jacobi F. Size and burden of mental disorders in Europe—a critical review and appraisal of 27 studies. Eur Neuropsychopharmacol 2005;15:357–76.
15. Bass C, Peveler R, House A. Somatoform disorders: severe psychiatric illnesses neglected by psychiatrists. Br J Psychiatry 2001;17911–4.
16. Creed F. Should general psychiatry ignore somatization and hypochondriasis? World Psychiatry 2006;5:146–50.
17. Fink P, Rosendal M. Recent developments in the understanding and management of functional somatic symptoms in primary care. Curr Opin Psychiatry 2008;21:182–8.
18. Aaron LA, Buchwald D. A review of the evidence for overlap among unexplained clinical conditions. Ann Intern Med 2001;134:868–81.
19. Aaron LA, Burke MM, Buchwald D. Overlapping conditions among patients with chronic fatigue syndrome, fibromyalgia, and temporomandibular disorder. Arch Intern Med 2000;160:221–7.
20. Kato K, Sullivan PF, Evengard B, et al. Chronic widespread pain and its comorbidities: a population-based study. Arch Intern Med 2006;166:1649–54.
21. Cole JA, Rothman KJ, Cabral HJ, et al. Migraine, fibromyalgia, and depression among people with IBS: a prevalence study. BMC Gastroenterol 2006;626.
22. Weir PT, Harlan GA, Nkoy FL, et al. The incidence of fibromyalgia and its associated comorbidities: a population-based retrospective cohort study based on International Classification of Diseases, 9th Revision codes. J Clin Rheumatol 2006;12:124–8.
23. Nimnuan C, Rabe-Hesketh S, Wessely S, et al. How many functional somatic syndromes? J Psychosom Res 2001;51:549–57.
24. Fink P, Schröder A. One single diagnosis, Bodily distress syndrome, succeeded to capture ten diagnostic categories of functional somatic syndromes and somatoform disorders. J Psychosom Res 2010;68415–26.
25. Nimnuan C, Hotopf M, Wessely S. Medically unexplained symptoms. An epidemiological study in seven specialities. J Psychosom Res 2001;51:361–7.
26. Kato K, Sullivan PF, Evengard B, et al. A population-based twin study of functional somatic syndromes. Psychological Med 2009;39:497–505.
27. Rief W, Broadbent E. Explaining medically unexplained symptoms-models and mechanisms. Clin Psychol Rev 2007;27:821–41.
28. Barsky AJ, Borus JF. Functional somatic syndromes. Ann Intern Med 1999;130:910–21.

29. Henningsen P, Zipfel S, Herzog W. Management of functional somatic syndromes. Lancet 2007;369:946–55.
30. Moss-Morris R, Spence M. To "lump" or to "split" the functional somatic syndromes: can infectious and emotional risk factors differentiate between the onset of chronic fatigue syndrome and irritable bowel syndrome? Psychosom Med 2006;68:463–9.
31. Kato K, Sullivan PF, Pedersen NL. Latent class analysis of functional somatic symptoms in a population-based sample of twins. J Psychosom Res 2010;68:447–53.
32. Kanaan RA, Lepine JP, Wessely SC. The association or otherwise of the functional somatic syndromes. Psychosom Med 2007;69:855–9.
33. Hamilton WT, Gallagher AM, Thomas JM, et al. Risk markers for both chronic fatigue and irritable bowel syndromes: a prospective case-control study in primary care. Psychological Med 2009;1–9.
34. Schröder A, Fink P. The proposed diagnosis of somatic symptom disorders in DSM-V: Two steps forward and one step backward? J Psychosom Res 2010;68: 95–6.
35. Gara MA, Silver RC, Escobar JI, et al. A hierarchical classes analysis (HICLAS) of primary care patients with medically unexplained somatic symptoms. Psychiatry Res 1998;81:77–86.
36. Simon G, Gater R, Kisely S, et al. Somatic symptoms of distress: an international primary care study. Psychosom Med 1996;58:481–8.
37. Dimsdale J, Creed F. The proposed diagnosis of somatic symptom disorders in DSM-IV to replace somatoform disorders in DSM-IV—a preliminary report. J Psychosom Res 2009;66:473–6.
38. Fink P, Ørnbøl E, Toft T, et al. A new, empirically established hypochondriasis diagnosis. Am J Psychiatry 2004;161:1680–91.
39. Kroenke K. Efficacy of treatment for somatoform disorders: a review of randomized controlled trials. Psychosom Med 2007;69:881–8.
40. Sumathipala A. What is the evidence for the efficacy of treatments for somatoform disorders? A critical review of previous intervention studies. Psychosom Med 2007; 69:889–900.
41. Whiting P, Bagnall AM, Sowden AJ, et al. Interventions for the treatment and management of chronic fatigue syndrome: a systematic review. JAMA 2001;286: 1360–8.
42. Prins JB, van der Meer JW, Bleijenberg G. Chronic fatigue syndrome. Lancet 2006;367: 346–55.
43. Goldenberg DL, Burckhardt C, Crofford L. Management of fibromyalgia syndrome. JAMA 2004;292:2388–95.
44. Hauser W, Bernardy K, Uceyler N, et al. Treatment of fibromyalgia syndrome with antidepressants: a meta-analysis. JAMA 2009;301:198–209.
45. Ford AC, Talley NJ, Schoenfeld PS, et al. Efficacy of antidepressants and psychological therapies in irritable bowel syndrome: systematic review and meta-analysis. Gut 2009;58:367–78.
46. Rahimi R, Nikfar S, Rezaie A, et al. Efficacy of tricyclic antidepressants in irritable bowel syndrome: a meta-analysis. World J Gastroenterol 2009;15:1548–53.
47. Jackson JL, O'Malley PG, Kroenke K. Antidepressants and cognitive-behavioral therapy for symptom syndromes. CNS Spectr 2006;11:212–22.
48. Edmonds M, McGuire H, Price J. Exercise therapy for chronic fatigue syndrome. Cochrane Database Syst Rev 2004;3:CD003200.
49. White PD, Goldsmith KA, Johnson AL, et al. Comparison of adaptive pacing therapy, cognitive behaviour therapy, graded exercise therapy, and specialist medical care for chronic fatigue syndrome (PACE): a randomised trial. Lancet 2011;377:823–36.

50. Busch AJ, Barber KA, Overend TJ, et al. Exercise for treating fibromyalgia syndrome. Cochrane Database Syst Rev 2007;4:CD003786.
51. Hauser W, Klose P, Langhorst J, et al. Efficacy of different types of aerobic exercise in fibromyalgia syndrome: a systematic review and meta-analysis of randomised controlled trials. Arthritis Res Ther 2010;12:R79.
52. Donta ST, Clauw DJ, Engel CC Jr, et al. Cognitive behavioral therapy and aerobic exercise for Gulf War veterans' illnesses: a randomized controlled trial. JAMA 2003; 289:1396–404.
53. Price JR, Mitchell E, Tidy E, et al. Cognitive behaviour therapy for chronic fatigue syndrome in adults. Cochrane Database Syst Rev 2008;3:CD001027.
54. Glombiewski JA, Sawyer AT, Gutermann J, et al. Psychological treatments for fibromyalgia: A meta-analysis. Pain 2010;151:280–95.
55. Bernardy K, Fuber N, Kollner V, et al. Efficacy of cognitive-behavioral therapies in fibromyalgia syndrome: a systematic review and metaanalysis of randomized controlled trials. J Rheumatol 2010;37:1991–2005.
56. Zijdenbos IL, de Wit NJ, van der Heijden GJ, et al. Psychological treatments for the management of irritable bowel syndrome. Cochrane Database Syst Rev 2009;1: CD006442.
57. Lackner JM, Mesmer C, Morley S, et al. Psychological treatments for irritable bowel syndrome: a systematic review and meta-analysis. J Consult Clin Psychol 2004;72: 1100–13.
58. Kisely SR, Campbell LA, Skerritt P, et al. Psychological interventions for symptomatic management of non-specific chest pain in patients with normal coronary anatomy. Cochrane Database Syst Rev 2010;1:CD004101.
59. Allen LA, Woolfolk RL, Escobar JI, et al. Cognitive-behavioral therapy for somatization disorder: a randomized controlled trial. Arch Intern Med 2006;166:1512–18.
60. Kroenke K, Swindle R. Cognitive-behavioural therapy for somatization and symptom syndromes: a critical review of controlled clinical trials. Psychother Psychosom 2000;69:205–15.
61. Kleinstauber M, Witthoft M, Hiller W. Efficacy of short-term psychotherapy for multiple medically unexplained physical symptoms: a meta-analysis. Clin Psychol Rev 2011; 31:146–60.
62. Hauser W, Bernardy K, Arnold B, et al. Efficacy of multicomponent treatment in fibromyalgia syndrome: a meta-analysis of randomized controlled clinical trials. Arthritis Rheum 2009;61:216–24.
63. Moayyedi P, Ford AC, Talley NJ, et al. The efficacy of probiotics in the treatment of irritable bowel syndrome: a systematic review. Gut 2010;59:325–32.
64. Hauser W, Thieme K, Turk DC. Guidelines on the management of fibromyalgia syndrome: a systematic review. Eur J Pain 2010;14:5–10.
65. Creed F, Guthrie E, Ratcliffe J, et al. Does psychological treatment help only those patients with severe irritable bowel syndrome who also have a concurrent psychiatric disorder? Aust N Z J Psychiatry 2005;39:807–15.
66. Lackner JM, Jaccard J, Krasner SS, et al. How does cognitive behavior therapy for irritable bowel syndrome work? A mediational analysis of a randomized clinical trial. Gastroenterology 2007;133:433–44.
67. de Lange FP, Koers A, Kalkman JS, et al. Increase in prefrontal cortical volume following cognitive behavioural therapy in patients with chronic fatigue syndrome. Brain 2008;131:2172–80.
68. Fink P, Rosendal M, Toft T. Assessment and treatment of functional disorders in general practice: the extended reattribution and management model—an advanced educational program for nonpsychiatric doctors. Psychosomatics 2002;43:93–131.

69. Schröder A, Fink P, Fjorback L, et al. Towards a unified treatment approach for functional somatic syndromes and somatization (Behandlingsstrategi for funktionelle syndromer og somatisering). Ugeskr Laeger 2010;172:1839–42.

70. Schröder A. Syndromes of bodily distress. Assessment and treatment [PhD dissertation]. Denmark: Faculty of Health Sciences, Aarhus University; 2010.

71. Fink P, Rosendal M, Lyngså Dam M, et al. New unifying diagnosis of functional diseases (Ny fælles diagnose for de funktionelle sygdomme). Ugeskr Laeger 2010; 172:1835–8.

72. Katon W, Ries RK, Kleinman A. A prospective DSM-III study of 100 consecutive somatization patients. Compr Psychiatry 1984;25305–14.

73. Rundell JR, Amundsen K, Rummans TL, et al. Toward defining the scope of psychosomatic medicine practice: psychosomatic medicine in an outpatient, tertiary-care practice setting. Psychosomatics 2008;49:487–93.

74. Creed F, Guthrie E, Black D, et al. Psychiatric referrals within the general hospital: comparison with referrals to general practitioners. Br J Psychiatry 1993;162204–11.

75. The psychological care of medical patients. Recognition of need and service provision (vol. CR35) London: Royal College of Physicians & Royal College of Psychiatrists; 1995. p. 97.

76. Huyse FJ, Herzog T, Lobo A, et al. Consultation-Liaison psychiatric service delivery: results from a European study. Gen Hosp Psychiatry 2001;23:124–32.

77. Fink P, Fritzsche K, Söllner W, et al. Training. In: Creed F, Henningsen P, Fink P, editors. Medically unexplained symptoms, somatisation and bodily distress: developing better clinical services. Cambridge University Press; 2011.

78. Wolfe F. Fibromyalgia wars. J Rheumatol 2009;36:671–8.

79. WHO.SCAN. Schedules for Clinical Assessment in Neuropsychiatry, version 2.1. Geneva (Switzerland): World Health Organization, Division of Mental Health; 1998.

80. Creed F, van der Feltz-Cornelis C, Guthrie E, et al. Identification, assessment and treatment of individual patients. In: Creed F, Henningsen P, Fink P, editors. Medically unexplained symptoms, somatisation and bodily distress. Cambridge: Cambridge University Press; 2011.

Teaching Trainees about the Practice of Consultation-Liaison Psychiatry in the General Hospital

Marlynn H. Wei, MD, JD, John Querques, MD, Theodore A. Stern, MD*

KEYWORDS
- Consultation-Liaison Psychiatry • Psychosomatic Medicine
- Teaching Psychiatry • Education • Teaching Rounds

Learning about the scope of psychiatric practice in the general hospital is essential for trainees and their patients. Consultation-liaison (C-L) psychiatry (officially named psychosomatic medicine), the subspecialty of psychiatry that deals with the care of patients with comorbid psychiatric and medical/surgical illness, is taught through formal didactics, teaching and bedside rounds, and demonstration of specific skills (eg, critical thinking, autognosis [self-knowledge]).[1] Both the process and the content of these educational forums are equally important. In this article, we discuss the theory, place, techniques, and challenges of teaching the craft of consultation psychiatry.

ADULT LEARNING THEORY

Adult learning theory, as developed by Knowles (who coined the term "andragogy" to describe his theory of adult education), has provided an approach to teaching in several areas of medicine that can enhance self-directed and independent learning of trainees in C-L psychiatry.[2–5] Several assumptions of adult learning models are useful in crafting an effective approach to, and an optimal learning environment for, teaching about psychosomatic medicine:

- Adult learners need to understand why learning something is important before they learn it
- Adults prefer being responsible for their decisions and they want their education to be self-directed

Department of Psychiatry, Massachusetts General Hospital, 55 Fruit Street, Warren Building, Room 605, Boston, MA 02114, USA
* Corresponding author.
E-mail address: TStern@Partners.org

Psychiatr Clin N Am 34 (2011) 689–707
doi:10.1016/j.psc.2011.05.009
0193-953X/11/$ – see front matter © 2011 Published by Elsevier Inc.

Table 1
Adult learning theory: Principles and examples

Learning Principle	Examples
Establish an effective learning climate where trainees feel safe while expressing their opinions	Participate in an open discussion of difficult patients or complex decision-making, accepting complex situations
Involve trainees in the development and planning of the curriculum	Organize conferences with broad topics that are related to psychosomatic medicine
Involve trainees in the categorization of their educational needs to increase internal motivation	Have trainees identify an area of desired growth (such as academic writing, the teaching of medical students, or the delivery of lectures)
Encourage trainees to develop their own learning objectives	Encourage a trainee to learn about a specific area (such as a neuropsychiatric problem or capacity assessment)
Support trainees in the identification of resources (and how to use their resources) to achieve their learning objectives	Encourage trainees to conduct a literature search and perform research on specific topics to address case-based questions that arise during C-L rounds
Encourage trainees to carry out their learning plans	Have trainees monitor their own development and progress
Encourage trainees to reflect critically on, and to evaluate, their progress and learning	Conduct formal feedback sessions (mid-term and at the end of the rotation) and provide informal feedback after bedside interviews with patients

- Adults have more experience to draw on and, therefore, want individualized approaches and learning strategies
- Adults learn when they realize how specific knowledge can be integrated into real-life situations
- Adults are more interested in problem-oriented and task-centered approaches than in subject-centered ones
- Adults are more responsive to internal rather than external motivation.[2]

These principles encourage teachers to foster a learning environment that promotes self-initiation, self-direction, and pragmatic learning solutions, and can be applied to clinical education in general, and psychosomatic medicine specifically. The learning climate should allow trainees to feel safe while expressing themselves and formulating their own needs and learning objectives; this enhances internal motivation.[3] For example, during teaching rounds, the trainee can be given more control over his or her learning by being asked, "What is your specific question regarding this case?", rather than being told what is important about the case. Learning theory also posits that trainees should identify resources and self-directed strategies to achieve their learning objectives. For example, trainees can be encouraged to find relevant articles about their cases, and to contribute to the literature by writing case reports and reviews. Finally, trainees should be afforded the opportunity to evaluate their own learning and to develop critical reflective skills through formal and informal bidirectional feedback about their learning experience. Overall, principles derived from adult learning theory furnish a framework for teachers of psychosomatic medicine that can support trainees and maximize education and development (**Table 1**).

EDUCATIONAL VENUES

The learning objectives for psychosomatic medicine encompass the core competencies set forth by the Accreditation Council for Graduate Medical Education (ACGME), as well as the didactic content and the practical skills required for psychiatric consultation and patient care in the medical/surgical setting (as set forth in the recommended training and practice guidelines of the Academy of Psychosomatic Medicine (APM) and the general practice guidelines of the American Psychiatric Association).[6–16] This content and skill set include the following: (1) ensuring the safety and stability of the patient within the medical environment, (2) collecting sufficient history and medical data from appropriate sources, (3) conducting a mental status examination and neurological and physical examinations as necessary, (4) interpreting laboratory tests, (5) synthesizing all of this data in a comprehensive, differential diagnosis and a coherent formulation of the patient's problem(s) (which may include an appreciation of the interaction among the patient, his or her family, the consultant, and the medical/surgical team), and (6) initiating (and/or implementing) a treatment plan and/or making recommendations for diagnostic procedures and treatment.[8] We advocate a multi-layered approach to imparting this knowledge that occurs in several forums: teaching rounds, bedside teaching and individual supervision, formal didactics, and conferences. Each of these is suited for teaching in different ways.

Teaching Rounds

Teaching rounds are a core clinical and educational activity in teaching hospitals.[17,18] Setting the agenda and purpose for rounds before they begin maximizes their educational impact. The goals of C-L rounds are: to teach trainees how to present cases concisely and effectively; to hone a resident's interviewing skills; to learn how to conduct a thorough evaluation, create a complete differential diagnosis, and plan and implement effective and timely treatment; to apply a comprehensive biopsychosocial approach (that also includes existential and cultural aspects); to develop a formulation; to hone autognostic skills; and to learn the subtle art of being a consultant while collaborating and communicating with other clinicians in the general hospital. Broader aims of C-L rounds are: to encourage trainees to participate and engage in the process of discussion and analysis of cases and related concepts; to instill curiosity about unfamiliar diseases and the motivation to acquire new knowledge about them; and to maintain a positive and affectively engaged attitude toward each case, regardless of how banal or seemingly benign the case initially appears.

Psychosomatic medicine emphasizes an integrated biopsychosocial model for case discussions and formulations.[19] The biopsychosocial model integrates the anatomical, structural, and molecular aspects of disease, psychological and developmental factors (including patients' reactions to illness), and sociocultural and environmental influences on patients' experience of illness.[20] Existential approaches to, and aspects of, psychosomatic cases are also part of this model, particularly among patients who are facing death and are having difficulty coping with end-of-life issues.[21]

Unfortunately, some residents develop role confusion and conflate the style and content of presentations at C-L rounds with the more detailed narrative and sequence-driven style of process notes used in psychotherapy supervision. Creating a map of C-L case presentations that tracks in real time the sequence of the information presented can help demonstrate the importance of a clear and organized

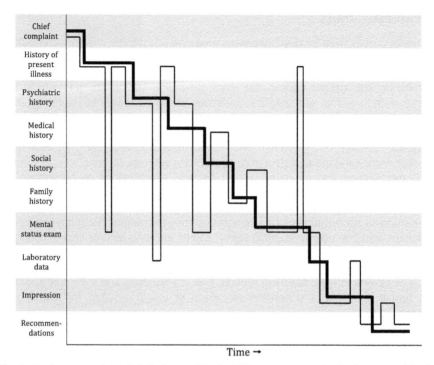

Fig. 1. Oral presentation of clinical cases. The bold line represents the "staircase model," the correct way to present a case, proceeding over time (x axis) through the different elements of the presentation (y axis) in an orderly fashion. The thin line represents the "skyline model," an inefficient way to present a case, "jumping" from one element to another.

case presentation (**Fig. 1**). Cogent case presentations in rounds can facilitate clear and effective note-writing.

C-L rounds provide an opportunity for residents to examine the boundaries of their knowledge in a non-judgmental and non-shaming way that underscores the philosophy of lifelong learning and training. The willingness to acknowledge that one may not have all the data or information available about a case presents the opportunity to search resources (eg, PubMed, articles, textbooks, Web sites) and to access information (eg, medication lists, imaging results, laboratory data, previous clinical notes) in real time during the course of C-L rounds.

Maintaining an atmosphere that promotes the notion that every clinical case can stimulate interest and be the fountain from which teaching flows helps trainees appreciate the diversity and complexity of C-L psychiatry. Focal points for analysis of cases can include etiology, peculiar manifestations or complications, associated laboratory abnormalities, emotional reactions of trainees (eg, fascination, reactions to the grotesque or the provocative), difficult or even tragic elements, and psychodynamically-informed understanding of interactions with the patient and other clinical personnel. Using a list of C-L rounds topics for each rounds helps to track and ensure that all subjects are covered in each of the domains (**Table 2**). The list can be used routinely in C-L rounds to keep track of what topics have been discussed, to document training, and to indicate which areas should be addressed in the future so that each trainee will have covered all areas.

The Socratic style of teaching during C-L rounds facilitates critical thinking and the development of analytical skills rather than rote memorization of characteristics or complications of an illness or process.[22] The strategy uses individual cases as starting points to examine and question general concepts and topics; it facilitates a non-directive style that requires participants to make explicit their analytical approach. Questions asked during C-L rounds should foster creation of a broad differential diagnosis (that includes medical/surgical diagnoses) and encourage a safe, comprehensive, and thoughtful approach that eschews premature conclusions. We favor questions that cultivate a sense of mastery and responsibility, stimulate trainees to articulate their own questions about a case, and heighten internal motivation for learning. For example, questions that place the decision-making in the hands of the trainee enhance a sense of ownership: "What questions do you have about the case?" and "What options did you consider and why?" Other questions such as "What did you decide to do to help the patient?" or "How did you help the team to resolve the issue at hand?" can help guide trainees in their role as a consultant and frame the relationship with the consultee.

Specific methods (eg, creation of Venn diagrams [for clustering of symptoms]) to determine more probable diagnoses can be useful; this approach, in concert with the principle of Occam's razor (or diagnostic parsimony [where alternative hypotheses exist, the one involving the fewest assumptions is preferable]) can assist in pattern recognition necessary for making a diagnosis. This principle can be balanced by Hickam's dictum, a counter-argument to Occam's razor, which asserts that patients may have several diagnoses.[23] Hickam's dictum acknowledges that patients can have several common diseases rather than one rare disease.

Bedside Teaching and Individual Supervision

Bedside teaching provides numerous opportunities for trainees. Attending physicians can observe trainees' interviews, examinations, and bedside manner, enabling direct and timely feedback. In turn, trainees can observe attending physicians demonstrate the wide range of interviewing styles and psychotherapeutic techniques in the inpatient setting. The style or strategy can be discussed beforehand to create a coordinated patient encounter and worthwhile learning experience. We advise that, by the end of the C-L rotation, almost equal time has been spent by each party observing the other.

Trainees can be taught to observe the patient prior to entering the room and to notice what materials (eg, magazines, food, cards) are in the patient's proximity (or notably absent) and to use this information in formulation of a differential diagnosis. Interviewing strategies (eg, motivational interviewing, following the flow of the patient's associations), bedside neuropsychiatric examinations, and use of rating scales can be demonstrated. Teaching note-writing skills to achieve succinct and efficient documentation of the case and its formulation can be discussed in these venues.

Formal Didactics

Formal didactics occur before and during the rotation. A typical orientation C-L psychiatry seminar series might cover common and problematic clinical domains (**Box 1**). Trainees should be encouraged to supplement this didactic instruction with reading and researching primary sources (ie, journal articles) that are relevant to their cases, not just secondary synopses (eg, textbooks, various medical Web sites).

Table 2
C-L psychiatry rounds topic list

Dx	W/u	Tx	Topic	Models				
				Biological	Psychological	Sociocultural	Existential
			Aggressive patients				
			Alcohol-related problems (chronic/acute)				
			Anxious patients and families				
			Autognosis				
			Burn patients				
			Capacity assessments				
			Catatonia/NMS/serotonin syndrome				
			Coping with illness/inpatient psychotherapy				
			Delirium				
			Dementia				
			Depression of the inpatient				
			Difficult patients				
			Drug abuse (management and pain control)				
			Eating disorders				
			ECT - when and how to recommend				
			End-of-life issues				
			Ethical issues				
			Factitious illness				
			Geriatric patients				
			HIV-infected patients				

(continued on next page)

Table 2
(continued)

Hypnosis
ICU patients
Legal aspects of psychiatric consultation
Neurologic conditions:
*Seizures
*CVD
*Traumatic brain injury
*Movement disorders
*Multiple sclerosis
*Others
Neuropsychological testing
Pain
Paper-writing
Paraplegia
Peri-partum patients
Psychooncology
Psychopharmacology of medical patients
Psychosis

Abbreviations: CVD, cerebrovascular disease; Dx, diagnosis; ECT, electroconvulsive therapy; HIV, human immunodeficiency virus; ICU, intensive care unit; NMS, neuroleptic malignant syndrome; Tx, treatment; W/u, work-up.

Box 1
Typical C-L psychiatry orientation lecture series

- The psychiatric consultation
- Differential diagnosis of mental status change
- Delirium recognition and management
- Approaches to neuropsychiatric dysfunction
- Neuropsychiatric testing
- Patients with memory problems
- Capacity evaluations
- Trauma and stress syndromes
- Depression in the medically ill
- Normal and maladaptive responses to illness
- Patients with multiple physical complaints
- Assessment and management of the substance-abusing patient
- Coping with medical illness
- Approach to the patient with seizures
- Mental disorders due to a general medical condition
- Assessment and management of the suicidal patient
- Alcohol abuse and withdrawal
- Psychopharmacology in the medically ill
- The use of seclusion and restraints
- Factitious disorders and malingering
- Difficult patients

Conferences

Weekly conferences focused on specific aspects of C-L psychiatry afford trainees the opportunity for self-motivated learning, public speaking, and academic participation. Trainees are encouraged to review the literature, present the review orally, prepare a written version of the talk, and submit the review for publication. Invited discussants from various fields contribute to the education of trainees and enhance interdisciplinary communication and learning that is critical to being an effective consultant.

THE ART OF BEING A CONSULTANT: TEACHING TOLERANCE AND RESPONSIBILITY

"The fundamental act of medical care is assumption of responsibility."

—F.D. Moore, *Metabolic Care of the Surgical Patient*, 1959, vii

A major aspect of teaching psychosomatic medicine is to educate the fledgling consultant about how to manage interactions with medical/surgical teams with regard to consultation requests, diagnostic and treatment recommendations (and their acceptance or refusal), and communication and management of differences in opinion.

Medical and surgical teams often lack the expertise, knowledge, or specific language (or all of these) to convey a clearly delineated request for a psychiatric consultation. In fact, clinicians' uncertainty about their question belies their need for the consultation in the first place. Therefore, a core skill of the consultant is aiding the consultee in framing the question of interest. While the consultant may consider the consultee to be more ignorant about psychiatry than he or she is about medicine or surgery, and may see a residue of stigma in that discrepancy, taking a practical stance and helping craft the consultee's question is often more productive than waging a philosophical battle.[24,25]

Table 3
Specific techniques in psychosomatic medicine

Teaching Technique Use of:	Examples
Humor	Observation of shifting moods and laughter during a case presentation of a recidivistic, depressed, diabetic, homeless man with angry and bizarre interactions with staff leads to a discussion of his coping strategies and defenses.
Autognosis	The trainee is asked: "What did you like about the patient?", "How did you feel when you saw the patient?", "Why did you use this gesture (eg, hands as if praying, pointing to the speaker) when speaking about this patient or that point?"
Role-playing	Trainees engage in role-playing in situations of patient, family, or staff conflicts (eg, an attending physician interrupts a consultant trainee during an interview of a patient without addressing the consultant). Discussion focuses on what the trainee should say or do and how the trainee should approach this issue.
Psychotherapeutic techniques	Examination of the stress responses, personality types (eg, hysterical, obsessive, narcissistic, oral, masochistic, schizoid, paranoid), and defenses commonly seen and their management[35]
Motivational interviewing	Discussion of the different ways to respond to resistance, including reflective responses and shifting the focus[37]
Limbic probes	Testing limbic function of patients with the Frank Jones story by examining a patient's emotional and cognitive responses to an absurd proposition[49]
Metaphor	Using a metaphor involving professional athletes and coaches may show a patient how to prevent anxiety from interfering with optimal performance and to allow for the process of constructive feedback.
Modeling	Demonstration of a bedside neuropsychiatric exam

Even though the consultee asks for the consultant's help, he or she is not obligated to heed the consultant's suggestions for diagnostic and therapeutic interventions. At a certain level, this does not make sense because, if the consultee knew what to do, he or she would not have requested the consultation. While neophyte psychiatric consultants (and even seasoned practitioners) find this grating, it is wise to remember that, as a consultant, one cannot ultimately control how a patient is treated. Furthermore, one cannot pin his or her self-esteem on whether or not his or her recommendations are followed.

Parallel to the consultee's not being beholden to the consultant, the consultant is not obligated to continue seeing a patient if his or her suggestions are persistently not implemented or are outrightly ignored, especially if no rationale is documented or forthcoming when sought. Discerning how often to see a patient and how and when to follow peripherally, or to sign off, is productive grist for the mill of teaching and bedside rounds.

SPECIFIC TECHNIQUES

Several techniques can be helpful in evaluating and treating patients, and are particularly useful to the psychiatric consultant. Over time, these techniques become part of one's repertoire when working with patients and consultees (**Table 3**).

Humor

Part of feeling safe while openly expressing oneself rests upon encouraging an environment that accepts the use of humor; teaching about and understanding why and when humor is being used can further illuminate a case.[26] Humor can be used as a method both in and outside the patient's presence, and can help one to understand a case's subtleties. Subsequent analyses of the reactions of the patient, trainees, or both can furnish insight into the complexities of a patient.

Humor can have several motives (eg, aggressive, self-deprecating, playful).[27] Various theories (eg, psychoanalytic, relief, incongruity, and superiority theories) examine how humor may mitigate stress, may occur after rules have been violated, and may enhance bonding and camaraderie with others in a group setting.[28] Depending on the situation and place, humor can be used as a leavening agent to facilitate an interpretation or comment that would otherwise be too difficult to absorb. Humor can also "even the playing field" of the asymmetric relationship of patient and doctor (as well as trainee and teacher).

For example, during discussion on rounds of an angry patient who had been difficult to manage during his frequent hospitalizations, which had led to a consultation request for behavioral management, the trainee reported that the patient's T-shirt read: "I have an attitude and know how to use it." This description elicited laughter from those at C-L rounds. The question "Why might the mood in the room be brighter?" and the comic exaggerations of the patient's actions and expressions led to an analysis of what the patient might be experiencing, his level and sources of depression, his ability to interact with friends, and his ability to cope with his medical illness.

When humor is used, this technique should be made transparent to trainees at all levels, particularly those with less experience. The challenge of using humor includes recognizing that humor can be perceived as derogatory or derisive to patients and staff—an issue that should be made explicit with trainees (along with how humor can provide insight into a clinical case).[29–32] The perception of humor and its motivation are related to the level of training and to the clinical experience of the trainee, particularly medical students who may not understand that, in psychiatry, humor is used as a probe of a patient's limbic reactions.[33]

Autognosis

An analysis of a consultant's reactions both outside of and during rounds (in real time) helps to guide the understanding of patients presented at C-L teaching rounds.[34] During the case presentation and discussion, psychiatric residents often unintentionally and unknowingly channel different, relevant aspects of the patient, whether imitating patients' speech patterns or using seemingly innocuous hand gestures to demonstrate the affect surrounding a case and the behavior of a patient. For example, a female resident speaking about an angry, frustrated male patient shook her index finger when describing the patient in rounds; a male resident held his hands in a praying position when reflecting on a patient who turned out to have strong religious beliefs that were relevant to the resident's clinical decision-making. Residents also unintentionally alter their speech patterns (eg, to one slower than normal) when describing elderly patients with dementia, or they make more grammatical errors when discussing patients who speak English as a second language. Pointing out these gestures and patterns of responses to residents helps them to understand the subtle characteristics of the patient and the significance of their own reactions as the consultant.

Role-Playing

Role-playing can be useful for helping trainees consider in real time possible interventions and relevant questions to ask patients. For example, in dealing with an agitated patient attempting to leave the hospital against medical advice, role-playing can entail the attending's standing up and leaving the room, thereby allowing the trainee to choose a suitable reaction (including verbal discussion, confrontation, or summoning security). Questions that emerge during the role play (eg, "How do you decide which strategy to use?", "What tone might you use with the patient?", "What body language or gestures would you use and what would they convey to patients?", "What relevant information would help you determine which strategy will be the most effective?") can help generate several hypotheses.

Role-playing can also be used when illustrating various options for resolving potential challenges between the consultant and the consultee in complex cases. For example, take the situation of a consultee who requested that the consultant (who has been asked to assess the capacity of a patient) not document the capacity assessment in the chart because it differed from the opinion of the consultee. Or, consider an attending physician in another discipline who interrupted a consultant's interview without acknowledging the consultant. Role-playing in these situations can help to illuminate the most effective approach (eg, different tones of voice) to speaking and working with the consultee, without creating or exacerbating conflict. Role-playing can unearth which factors (such as the power differential between the consultant and consultee, the shared or disparate goals for patient care, differences in understanding the nature of the patient's clinical issues, or other nuances) are important in the art of consultation.

Psychotherapeutic Techniques

Specialized psychotherapeutic techniques are crucial to the management of psychiatric illness in the medically ill as well as crucial in helping patients cope effectively with medical/surgical illness.[35] Isolating the individual, hospital, and broader environmental factors that both enhance and hinder a patient's ability to cope and adapt to illness, as well as helping trainees elucidate these attributes, are key. Ascertaining patients' assets (eg, faith, family, friends) and liabilities (eg, homelessness, unemployment, lack of social supports) helps craft a collaborative and therapeutic treatment plan. While not performing psychotherapy in a formal or usual way, one can still use certain techniques more frequently employed in the consulting room at the medical bedside. For example, one might invite patients to say whatever is on their mind, even if they think it is irrelevant; follow the flow of a patient's associations and discern potential meaning in apparently random thoughts; permit both oneself and the patient to remain silent at certain junctures; say what one thinks the patient would say if he or she were less inhibited or anxiety-ridden, and inquire if that captures what the patient is thinking or feeling.

Psychodynamic formulation allows the consultant to propose a practical program of management that is informed by an understanding of a patient's level of psychological development and defenses, especially those that are common in hospitalized, medically ill individuals.[36] An appreciation that all patients in the hospital are under stress and, thus, prone to regression to earlier developmental levels (characterized by less mature defenses) is key to avoiding over-diagnosis of personality disorders in this setting as well as to most fully appreciating the wide panorama of different reactions to adversity.

Motivational Interviewing

Motivational interviewing is a therapeutic approach that combines relationship-building principles with cognitive-behavioral methods that target the patient's stage of change.[37] Principles of motivational interviewing can frame a patient-centered approach that explores and helps to resolve ambivalence about altering problematic behavior.[38] Although the methods are directive, the consultant-therapist does not explicitly persuade the patient to change. The patient discusses his or her resistance to change; the therapist listens reflectively to help the patient begin to see the importance of change. The trainee learns to assess the patient's own readiness for change as a product of the importance of change for the patient, and the confidence that the patient has about being able to make that change successfully.[38]

Motivational interviewing as an intervention for alcohol and other substance abuse has shown mixed results and is less effective individually than in groups.[39–45] Motivational interviewing has also been suggested to help in childhood chronic disease (eg, diabetes, obesity), smoking cessation, and medication adherence.[46–49] Brief motivational interviewing techniques in C-L psychiatry may be useful in patients who smoke, do not adhere to prescribed medications, or refuse recommended medical tests or treatment.

For example, consider a patient with a history of alcohol dependence—with daily use and multiple recent admissions for alcohol withdrawal—whom the consultant is asked to see for substance abuse counseling. The patient is willing to speak about addiction treatment options because his drinking is causing marital strife, but he is worried that becoming sober means he will not be able to socialize with his friends. He is skeptical that treatment will help him because he has relapsed so often.

The consultant can apply several different techniques of motivational interviewing to help the patient begin to address his concerns about change. Open-ended questions are useful to begin the conversation:

- "What has happened since your last hospitalization?"
- "What is different for you this time?"
- "How can I help you with some of the difficulties you are experiencing?"
- "What is most important to you right now?"

In order to help the patient start to talk about change, the consultant can ask "What would you like to see different about your current situation?" or "What makes you feel that it might be time for change?" Reflective listening is another technique that can validate how a patient is feeling (eg, "It sounds like your drinking is causing difficulties with your relationship with your wife." or "The sense that you want to change, but you have concerns about becoming sober."). Normalizing the difficulties of changing also helps patients understand that change is commonly difficult ("A lot of people find it very difficult to become sober."). Affirmative statements convey recognition of strengths and efforts to change ("It's clear that you are trying very hard to become sober." or "By the way you have continued to try to be sober, you have shown a lot of determination and strength.").

Finally, summaries can be useful to end and frame the conversation, and can reflect any ambivalence that the patient has expressed. For example, the consultant can let the patient know that he or she has heard the patient's dilemmas (ie, "It sounds like you are concerned about your drinking because of how much it costs in terms of both money and your relationship with your wife, but you're also worried that you won't be able to be as social without drinking. That doesn't sound like an easy decision."). Motivational interviewing techniques provide multiple approaches to empathize with patients, to meet them where they are, and to elicit talk of change from patients themselves rather than forcing them to change by persuasion.

Limbic Probes

C-L psychiatry involves patients who may have neuropsychiatric impairment that is not obvious in everyday hospital interactions or detected with screening tools. The limbic system mediates motivation, attention, emotion, and memory; limbic "probing" helps to screen patients for neuropsychiatric impairment.[50] One example of the clinical application of limbic probing is George Murray's Frank Jones story.[50] By ascertaining a patient's cognitive and affective responses to the statement, "I have a friend, Frank Jones, whose feet are so big he has to put his pants on over his head," the trainee can assess higher cortical function in a patient who might otherwise appear unimpaired. Through education about limbic probes, the trainee can learn to observe how the patient processes and interacts with the world around him or her. Other methods of limbic probing include using humor with patients and observing whether and how the patient participates, responds, or interprets the humor, and (in some patients) using salty or even vulgar language (to do this decorously, it is advisable to ask the patient if he or she minds if the examiner uses "bad language").

Metaphor

Metaphor can serve as a framework for, and a memorable description of, complex concepts and approaches in C-L psychiatry. For example, the metaphor of athlete and coach can be useful to trainees in helping to encourage self-motivation, continued learning, and improvement in a non-judgmental setting. During presentations in teaching rounds, when trainees use metaphor, even if they are not aware of it, they tap into a rich vein of material which they and the audience can use to understand the patient both diagnostically and therapeutically. For example, a trainee may describe a patient as speaking to the staff as a stand-up comedian would—a metaphor that affords insight into how the patient may seek to perform for others, make light of difficult situations, or use humor as a defense in coping with serious medical problems.

Modeling

Modeling can be useful as a strategy both at the bedside and in rounds. For example, components of the neuropsychiatric examination (eg, frontal release signs, calculations, limb and facial praxis, figure and clock drawing, cortical sensory testing, Luria maneuvers, alternating sequences) can be demonstrated for the trainee at rounds and at the bedside.[51] Specific nuances of these examinations can be clarified with the modeling technique. Modeling can also be used to demonstrate interviewing skills, clear and organized case presentations, and therapeutic interactions with patients (eg, use of body language, posture, and tone).

CHALLENGES AND LIMITATIONS

Several challenges exist in teaching C-L psychiatry. Some of these challenges can be identified and addressed, while others cannot necessarily be as easily altered. However, recognition of these limitations can help optimize the C-L training experience.

Different Levels of Knowledge and Skills

Medical students, visiting medical students, international trainees, and postgraduate trainees at several levels of training and from various fields (eg, internal medicine, neurology) possess a different fund of knowledge that necessitates tailoring the level of discussion and teaching. Even among similar levels of training, knowledge and skills can differ widely. The time of year (ie, earlier in the academic calendar, earlier in training generally) and the corresponding level of training will affect how one should address and approach teaching the trainee.

Trainees should learn specific techniques and treatment-planning skills for certain populations. For example, psychiatric consultation for patients with somatoform disorder (characterized by the presence of physical symptoms in the absence of known pathophysiology) requires specific knowledge and understanding of how to work with these patients. Patients with multiple, unexplained physical complaints benefit most from a long-term empathic relationship with a primary care physician.[52] Trainees should be taught that the goals of treatment for a somatizing patient include focus on care, rather than cure. Trainees should learn that treatment goals also include treating any physical or comorbid psychiatric disorder (eg, obsessive-compulsive or delusional disorder), decreasing any conversion symptoms, and maintaining and improving overall function of a patient.[52]

Trainees also need to develop a clinical approach for a pattern of medically unexplained complaints that provides support and reassurance rather than confrontation. For example, consider a young woman who was admitted for worsening paralysis of her right arm and shoulder. The work-up reveals no medical explanation and suggests a diagnosis of conversion paralysis. The trainee consultant is faced with the challenge of how to speak with the patient about her condition, as well as how to direct the medical team to work with the patient. It is often unhelpful to tell the patient "There is nothing wrong with your arm." Rather, reassurance, combined with suggestions, can be helpful for both the consultant and the medical team: "We will set you up with a physical therapist who will help you increase the strength and mobility of your arm over the next week."

The trainee consultant is also challenged by how to guide the medical team in working effectively with a patient with a somatoform disorder. The trainee can learn to work with medical teams on how to make a clear treatment plan (which depends on the specific somatoform diagnosis). For example, psychiatrists can help primary care physicians with patients with somatization disorder. Psychiatric consultation includes helping the consultant understand how and when to deliver the diagnosis, that the patient's main contact with the health care system should be the primary care physician, that regularly scheduled appointments should be planned every 2 to 6 weeks, and that patients should have a list of prioritized problems.[52]

Trainees should be encouraged to work with the patient to identify precipitants or stressors that may be connected with the disability. In this case, further discussion with the woman with arm paralysis revealed that her husband, who is in the US Army, recently sustained a gunshot wound to the right arm in combat and had multiple surgeries of his right arm over the past month. Subsequent discussion with the patient about her concerns about her husband's health improved both her anxiety and her paralysis. The trainee thus begins to build knowledge and skills in understanding how to work effectively with populations commonly seen as a consultant.

Different Learning Styles

Another difference among trainees is learning styles that can vary significantly. An effective teacher should assess the learning styles of the trainees and respond by using layers of learning and methods to communicate knowledge and build skills among the trainees.

Lack of Camaraderie

Camaraderie is important within every group learning C-L psychiatry; the amount of solidarity and teamwork that exists within each group of trainees varies. C-L rounds and other learning environments are most effective when trainees are comfortable with asking questions of each other and with interacting in a team-building and interdisciplinary manner. *Esprit de corps* among the attending staff of the C-L service helps model for trainees the collegial relations that can and should exist among professionals at all levels of training. It also provides a pleasant environment in which trainees can most profitably learn and work, and buffers the stresses of C-L practice. The sense of camaraderie and openness in the learning environment depends highly on the successful development of trust amongst trainees, as well as between the trainees and their supervisors.

Lack of Trust

Trust is necessary for trainees to feel comfortable when discussing perceived mistakes or problems, and when asking questions without fear of shame, retribution, or a poor evaluation. Maintaining an open, trust-enhancing atmosphere for learning can be compromised by many factors that may not be readily changed or controlled. An awareness of the group dynamic of the trainees, particularly on C-L rounds, and an ability to foster trust and respond to group dynamics in real time are challenging but useful.

Insufficient Funding or Manpower

Other factors that influence the teaching environment for C-L psychiatry include the realities of available funding and manpower (eg, staffing, number of trainees, level of training of trainees). Balancing service with education can create conflicts if the number of cases that need to be staffed daily butts up against duty-hour restrictions. One teaching strategy is to spend time discussing and teaching at the bedside commensurate with the severity or complicated nature of a case. In an alternative style, the available time is distributed evenly among all cases.

Fear of Evaluation, Retaliation, or Feedback Assessment and Delivery

Evaluation of and feedback given to trainees are essential parts of clinical teaching; however, some avoid giving feedback due to fears that it may be interpreted as an insult or that it will provoke defensiveness.[53] Recommended feedback techniques include being respectful, open-minded, non-judgmental, and specific, with a focus on behaviors and observations rather than personality.[54] Feedback should be based on a set of well-defined and shared goals that are openly discussed with the trainee.[54] Implementing prescribed techniques is just as important as avoiding proscribed ones.[54] One model describes 6 important points to heed during feedback (**Box 2**).[54]

The feedback session should be done in-person and in private; it should invite the trainee's participation and provide an opportunity to discuss the observations and suggestions. Feedback can occur formally during a feedback session, and should

---

Box 2
Feedback techniques

- Create an appropriate orientation and climate for the feedback session.
- Elicit self-assessment from the trainee regarding his or her knowledge, skills, and attitudes.
- Provide an assessment of areas of improvement and offer corrective feedback, including a discussion of how this area is related to well-defined and shared goals.
- Develop a specific plan for improving these areas (eg, invite the trainee's suggestions as well as provide one's own such as relevant articles or reading).
- Apply these planned steps to future cases or issues.
- Review and check with the trainee to make sure he or she agrees with the proposed shared plan.

---

also occur consistently throughout the rotation in individual supervision with attending physicians and during bedside teaching (outside of the patient's presence). Even the best athletes in the world need coaching; this sports analogy can serve as an example to trainees that evaluative feedback is intended to be encouraging, supportive, and stimulating to enhance successful clinical performance.

Feedback from the trainee to the service director as well as to each individual attending faculty member is also equally important. Eliciting feedback from trainees during and after the C-L rotation about, for example, the service-to-education balance and effective teaching styles can help the service develop and can enhance the learning experience for future trainees.

SUMMARY

Teaching C-L psychiatry is most effective with a multi-layered approach in accord with the principles of adult learning theory; it should integrate many different techniques that are tailored to the specific teaching forum and the learning styles of the trainees.

REFERENCES

1. Academy of Psychosomatic Medicine. Proposal for the designation of Consultation-Liaison Psychiatry as a subspecialty: internal report. Chicago, IL, Academy of Psychosomatic Medicine, June 1992.
2. Knowles M. The adult learner. A neglected species. 4th edition. Houston (TX): Gulf Publishing; 1990.
3. Kaufman DM. ABC of learning and teaching in medicine: applying educational theory in practice. Br Med J 2003;326:213–6.
4. Green ML, Ellis PJ. Impact of an evidence-based medicine curriculum based on adult learning theory. J Gen Int Med 1997;12:742–50.
5. David TJ, Patel L. Adult learning theory, problem based learning, and paediatrics. Arch Dis Childhood 1995;73:357–63.
6. Accreditation Council for Graduate Medical Education. Common Program Requirements Language: General Competencies, Feb. 13, 2007. Available at: http://www.acgme.org/outcome/comp/GeneralCompetenciesStandards21307.pdf. Accessed June 19, 2011.
7. Bronheim HE, Fulop G, Kunkel EJ, et al. The Academy of Psychosomatic Medicine practice guidelines for psychiatric consultation in the general medical setting. Psychosomatics 1998;39:S8–30.
8. Cohen-Cole SA, Haggerty J, Raft D. Objectives for residents in consultation psychiatry: recommendations of a task force. Psychosomatics 1981;23:699–703.

9. Hayes JR. Consultation-liaison psychiatry residency training guidelines: another milestone. Psychosomatics 1996;37:1–2.
10. Gitlin DF, Schindler BA, Stern TA, et al. Recommended guidelines for consultation-liaison psychiatric training in psychiatry residency programs. Psychosomatics 1996; 37:3–11.
11. American Psychiatric Association. Practice guideline for psychiatric evaluation of adults. Am J Psychiatry 1995;152(Suppl):65–80.
12. American Psychiatric Association: Guidelines on confidentiality. Am J Psychiatry 1987;144:1522–6.
13. American Psychiatric Association. Practice guideline for the treatment of patients with substance use disorders: alcohol, cocaine, opioids. Am J Psychiatry 1995; 152(Suppl):1–59.
14. American Psychiatric Association. Practice guideline for the treatment of patients with bipolar disorder. Am J Psychiatry 1994;151(Suppl):1–36.
15. American Psychiatric Association. Practice guideline for major depressive disorders in adults. Am J Psychiatry 1993;150(Suppl):207–28.
16. American Psychiatric Association. Practice guideline for eating disorders. Am J Psychiatry 1993;150(Suppl):207–28.
17. Elliot DL, Hickam DH. Attending rounds on in-patient units: differences between medical and non-medical services. Med Educ 1993;27:503–8.
18. Walton JM, Steinert Y. Patterns of interaction during rounds: implications for work-based learning. Med Educ 2010;44:550–8.
19. Engel GL. The need for a new medical model: a challenge for biomedicine. Science 1977;196:129–36.
20. Campbell WH, Rohrbaugh RM. The Biopsychosocial Formulation Manual: A Guide for Mental Health Professionals. New York: Routledge; 2006.
21. Havens LL. The development of existential psychiatry. J Nerv Ment Dis 1972;154: 309–31.
22. Birnbacher D. The Socratic method in teaching medical ethics: potentials and limitations. Med Health Care Philos 1999;2:219–24.
23. Miller WT. Occam versus Hickam. Semin Roentgenol 1998;33:213.
24. Caplan JP, Epstein LA, Stern TA. Consultants' conflicts: a case discussion of differences and their resolution. Psychosomatics 2008;49:8–13.
25. Caplan JP, Querques J, Epstein LA, et al. Consultation, communication, and conflict management by out-of-operating room anesthesiologists: strangers in a strange land. Anesthesiology Clin 2009;28:111–20.
26. Chiarello MA, Shinrigaku K. Humor as a teaching tool. J Psychosoc Nurs Ment Health Serv 2009;80:397–404.
27. Tsukawaki R, Koshi R, Higuchi M, Fukada H. Investigation into the motives for different expressions of humor. Shinrigaku Kenkyu 2009;80:397–404.
28. Wilkins J, Eisenbraun AJ. Humor theories and the physiological benefits of laughter. Holist Nurs Pract 2009;23:349–54.
29. Aultman JM. Against humor: when humor in the hospital is no laughing matter. J Clin Ethics 2009; 20:227–34.
30. Berk R. Derogatory and cynical humour in clinical teaching and the workplace: the need for professionalism. Med Educ 2009;43:7–9.
31. Wear D, Aultman JM, Varley JD, Zarconi J. Making fun of patients: medical students' perceptions and use of derogatory and cynical humor in clinical settings. Acad Med 2006;81:454–62.

32. Wear D, Aultman JM, Zarconi J, Varley JD. Derogatory and cynical humour directed towards patients: views of residents and attending doctors. Med Educ 2009;43:34–41.
33. Parsons GN, Kinsman SB, Bosk CL, Sankar P, Ubel PA. Between two worlds medical student perceptions of humor and slang in the hospital setting. J Gen Intern Med 2001;1:544–9.
34. Stern TA, Prager LM, Cremens MC. Autognosis rounds for medical house staff. Psychosomatics 1993;34:1–7.
35. Scholzman S, Groves JE, Gross AF. Coping with illness and psychotherapy of the medically ill. In: Stern TA, Fricchione GL, Cassem NH, et al, editors. MGH handbook of general hospital psychiatry. 6th edition. Philadelphia: Saunders; 2010. p. 425–32.
36. Groves JE. Introduction: four "essences" of short-term therapy: brevity, focus, activity, selectivity. In: Groves JE, editor. Essential papers on short-term dynamic therapy. New York: New York University; 1996. p. 1–26.
37. Burke BL, Arkowiz H, Menchola M. The efficacy of motivational interviewing: a meta-analysis of controlled clinical trials. J Consult Clin Psychology 2003;71:843–61.
38. Miller WR, Rollnick S. Responding to resistance. In: Motivational interviewing: preparing people for change. New York: Guilford Press; 2002. p. 98-110.
39. Lundahl B, Burke BL. The effectiveness and applicability of motivational interviewing: a practice-friendly review of four meta-analyses. J Clin Psychol 2009;651232–45.
40. Dunn C, Deroo L, Rivara FP. The use of brief interventions adapted from motivational interviewing across behavioral domains: a systematic review. Addiction 2001;96: 1725–42.
41. McQueen J, Howe TE, Allan L, et al. Brief Intervention for heavy alcohol users admitted to general hospital. Cochrane Database Syst Rev 2009;3:CD005191.
42. Vasilaki EI, Hosier SG, Cox WM. The efficacy of motivational interviewing as a brief intervention for excessive drinking: a meta-analytic review. Alcohol 2006;41:328–35.
43. Miller WR, Yahne CE, Tonigan JS. Motivational interviewing in drug abuse services: a randomized trial. J Consult Clin Psychology 2003;71:754–63.
44. Barrowclough C, Haddock G, Wykes T, et al. Integrated motivational interviewing and cognitive behavioural therapy for people with psychosis and comorbid substance misuse: randomised controlled trial. BMJ 2010;341:c6325.
45. McCambridge J, Strang J. The efficacy of single-session motivational interviewing in reducing drug consumption and perceptions of drug-related risk and harm among young people. Addiction 2004;99:39–52.
46. Gregory JW, Channon S. Motivational interviewing to improve blood-glucose control in childhood diabetes. J Paediatr Child Health 2009;19:331–4.
47. Resnicow K, Davis R, Rollnick S. Motivational interviewing for pediatric obesity: conceptual issues and evidence review. J Am Diet Assoc 2006;106:2024–33.
48. Lai DT, Cahill K, Qin Y, et al. Motivational interviewing for smoking cessation. Cochrane database Syst Rev 2010;1:CD006936.
49. Borrelli B, Riekert KA, Weinstein A, et al. Brief motivational interviewing as a clinical strategy to promote asthma medication adherence. J Allergy Clin Immunol 2007;120: 1023–30.
50. Murray GB, Kontos N. Limbic music. In: Stern TA, Fricchione GL, Cassem NH, et al, editors. MGH handbook of general hospital psychiatry. 6th edition. Philadelphia: Saunders; 2010. p. 45–51.
51. Shulman K, Shedletsky R, Silver I. The challenge of time: clock drawing and cognitive function in the elderly. Intl J Geriatr Psychiatry 1986;1:135–40.

52. Calabrese L, Stern, TA. The patient with multiple physical complaints. In: Stern TA, Herman JB, Slavin PL, editors. MGH guide to primary care psychiatry. 2nd edition. New York: McGraw-Hill; 2004. p. 269–78.

53. Ende J. Feedback in clinical medical education. JAMA 1983;250:777–81.

54. Hewson MG, Little ML. Giving feedback in medical education. J Gen Intern Med 1998;13:111–6.

Index

Note: Page numbers of article titles are in **boldface** type.

Psychiatr Clin N Am 34 (2011) 709–716
doi:10.1016/S0193-953X(11)00069-4
0193-953X/11/$ – see front matter © 2011 Elsevier Inc. All rights reserved.

psych.theclinics.com

Printed and bound by CPI Group (UK) Ltd, Croydon, CR0 4YY

03/10/2024

01040455-0001